36.95

DATE DUE

MAY 28 '93		
DEC 1 1993		
DEC 14 1993		
	DEC 21 2004	
MAY 3 0 1995	MAY 2 3 2005	
DEC 0 4 1995		
OCT 2 9 1997	Aug 2, 2005	
NOV 1 8 2000		
MAY 1 4 2002		
JUL 1 1 2002		
DEC 1 6 2002		
NOV 2 5 2003		
MAY 1 3 2004		
GAYLORD		

SURROGATE
MOTHERHOOD

MEDICAL ETHICS SERIES

David H. Smith and
Robert M. Veatch, Editors

SURROGATE
MOTHERHOOD

Politics and Privacy

Edited by
Larry Gostin

Indiana University Press
Bloomington and Indianapolis

This book is based on a special issue of *Law, Medicine & Health Care* (16:1–2, spring/summer, 1988), a journal of the American Society of Law & Medicine. Many of the essays have been revised, updated, or corrected, and five appendices have been added. ASLM coordinator of book production was Merrill Kaitz.

Manufactured in the United States of America

⊗ ™

The paper used in this publication meets the minimum requirements of American National Standard for Information Sciences—Permanence of Paper for Printed Library Materials, ANSI Z39.48-1984.

Library of Congress Cataloging-in-Publication Data

Surrogate motherhood : politics and privacy / edited by Larry Gostin.

p.   cm. — (Medical ethics series)

Includes bibliographical references.

ISBN 0-253-32604-4 (alk. paper)

1. Surrogate mothers—Legal status, laws, etc.—United States.

2. Surrogate mothers—Civil rights—United States.

3. Surrogate mothers—United States.   I. Gostin, Larry O. (Larry Ogalthorpe) II. Series.

KF540.A75S87   1990

346.7301'7—dc20

[347.30617]   89-45474

                                    CIP

1 2 3 4 5   94 93 92 91 90

CONTENTS

ETHICS

WOMEN'S AUTONOMY

PUBLIC HEALTH

CASE REVIEW ESSAYS
The New Jersey Supreme Court Baby M Decision

APPENDIXES

INTRODUCTION

Larry Gostin

When the American Civil Liberties Union appointed me as chair of the ACLU Special Committee on Surrogate Parenting, the task seemed relatively straightforward. It quickly became apparent that each side in the surrogacy debate claimed that civil liberties principles supported its own preconceived view. Proponents of surrogacy argued that the right to reproductive freedom required the judicial enforcement of contracts. Opponents of surrogacy countered that the same civil liberty (this time focused exclusively on women's autonomy) militated against surrogacy agreements. The ACLU Committee had the task of unraveling the competing claims and of proposing a policy-neutral civil liberties framework for surrogacy. My chapter is built upon the ACLU's deliberations and conclusions on surrogacy.

The validity of these opposing arguments depends upon whether there is a constitutional right to privacy in making a surrogacy agreement. John Robertson argues forcefully that there is a right to contract with consenting collaborators for the purposes of reproduction. He sees this right as virtually equivalent to the constitutional protection afforded to coital reproduction. If there is a constitutionally protected privacy interest in surrogacy, then the state must show a compelling interest in order to ban or regulate it. Robertson's argument is that the state could never show a compelling interest in banning surrogacy (a conclusion shared by the ACLU), but that it might have a compelling interest in regulating surrogacy, primarily to protect the interests of the child.

There is little doubt that Robertson's argument would prevail if non-coital reproduction received the same level of constitutional protection as traditional reproduction. The Supreme Court has enunciated a fundamental right "whether to bear or beget a child." But Supreme Court reproduction cases have been concerned with sterilization, contraception, and abortion. These cases involved questions of sexual intimacy, personal and family relationships, and deep expectations of privacy. The Court has never decided a case involving non-coital reproduction. One could argue that the right to form a contract with a stranger for sterile artificial insemination has little to do with the loving and private relationships the Supreme Court has protected.

In effect, the Robertson argument uses the name "reproduction" to assert a constitutional right to privacy. But reliance upon the words used in Supreme Court precedent is not the same as an argument about *why* surrogacy is a truly intimate relationship deserving protection under the privacy doctrine. One reason given is that the private character of reproduction is not the loving relationship between two people, but the mere fact of reproducing an offspring that is biologically related to the couple. To feminists, it is anathema to suggest that a male's right to reproduce from his own gene line is the core value in the ethos of privacy.

In the view of George Annas, the "core reality of surrogate motherhood is that it is both classist and sexist: a method to obtain children genetically related to white males by exploiting poor women." Annas uses symbols entirely different from those of Robertson, so their arguments seldom meet. To Annas, the question is not whether there is a constitutional right to privacy. His argument is that the reasons advanced for surrogate reproduction are abhorrent to commonly accepted social values. The implications are that a man has no "right" to a biologically related child; that women are exploited by fulfilling the man's desire for such a child; and that babies are treated as consumer products, which is immoral. This is a highly judgmental perspective on the free decisions of genetic fathers and gestational mothers, even though the judgments are powerfully stated and "ring true." But judgmental they are, for they say to men and women that they cannot do what they believe would make them happy, because others with a "finer" ethical sense should decide the "right way" to reproduce.

The "commodification" argument is extended and strengthened by Alex Capron and Margaret Radin. They meet Robertson's constitutional argument merely by asserting that there is no "absolute right to paid surrogacy." What is needed to sustain their argument is a careful analysis of *why* the considerable Supreme Court precedent cannot be applied to surrogacy arrangements. The chapter leaves several questions unanswered: How is surrogacy different from coital reproduction and the right to privacy? If there is no absolute right to paid surrogacy, is there a presumptive right? Were the state to ban all surrogacy—whether or not renumeration were offered—would such a ban fall afoul of the Constitution?

The privacy argument is not merely theoretical, because it goes straight to the heart of Capron and Radin's thesis. They assert, with considerable eloquence and force, that commercial surrogacy should be banned on the grounds that it is potentially harmful to children. But they put forward no evidence to suggest that children born in surrogacy arrangements are less well off than other children, or even that their chances of thriving are any lesser. If non-coital reproduction is not constitutionally protected, Capron and Radin give us ample reason for the state to intervene, for the state must show only that its intervention is related to a valid governmental interest—e.g., to provide a clear rule in advance about who will be the lawful custodial parent. But if surrogate parents do have a constitutionally protected privacy interest, it is doubtful that Capron and Radin have demonstrated a sufficiently compelling interest to ban it. Their arguments about harm to children are speculative. They express philosophical concerns that "commodification" would undermine the social fabric, but they provide little data to suggest that children are imperiled.

The argument that the child's interests are the most important in assessing surrogacy arrangements was first enunciated by Angela Holder in a seminal article in *Law, Medicine & Health Care* (12:3, June, 1984). At that time Holder represented a minority, perhaps even an eccentric, view. Today, of course, this view is very well respected and has the persuasive support of the New Jersey Supreme Court in the *Baby M* case. (Excerpts from the *Baby M* decision are reproduced in Appendix I.)

The *Baby M* case has influenced state legislatures across the country. Legislators are now having to make decisions about surrogacy: Should states regulate the enterprise? Should states permit surrogacy arrangements and even require the enforcement of contracts under certain circumstances? Do special rules for parental rights and custody apply? The choices for state legislators are wide and the policy questions complex. R. Alta Charo was instrumental in drafting the report on reproductive technology for the Office of Technology of the U.S. Congress. Her chapter in this volume provides a wealth of practical information on states' activities in this area. It provides clear options for state legislators developing public policy on surrogacy.

Alta Charo's chapter is complemented by Appendix II, written by Marilyn Adams of the National Council of State Legislatures. Five states have enacted substantive legislation: Florida, Indiana, Kentucky, Michigan, and Nebraska. The legislation is remarkably uniform in content, very much in keeping with the *Baby M* decision. The definition of a surrogate parenting contract is similar in each statute: a contract by which a woman is to be compensated for bearing the child of a man who is not her husband. The approach taken in all five states is to declare such contracts void and unenforceable as contrary to public policy.

The only slightly different approaches are found in the Michigan and Kentucky statutes. The Kentucky statute makes the implicit assumption that surrogacy arrangements are tantamount to the selling or purchasing of a child for the purpose of adoption. It bans this "commodification" of children, as well as any advertising for these purposes.

The Michigan statute is the first in the country to make it a felony to arrange a surrogate-mother contract for money. It provides for a maximum $50,000 fine and five years in prison for a surrogate broker.

Those interested in legislation and public policy will find Appendixes III and IV to be invaluable. Appendix III contains model surrogacy acts from the section of family law of the American Bar Association and from the National Conference on Uniform State Laws. In addition, Appendix IV contains policy statements representing the diverse viewpoints of leading groups across the country: the American Civil Liberties Union, the American College of Obstetricians and Gynecologists, the American Medical Association, the American Fertility Association, the New York State Task Force on Life and the Law, and the Institute on Women and Technology.

The division of opinion over constitutional and legislative principles can just as easily be recast as a series of ethical dilemmas. From one perspective any decision to ban commercial surrogacy could deny infertile couples the opportunity to have a child. On the other hand, if all parties consent to the agreement and perceive it to be in their own interest, there appear to be strong ethical grounds for allowing the practice. Just as in constitutional theory, some weight of ethical value must be assigned to protecting this private surrogacy arrangement. Does allowing surrogacy further some important social or personal value such as autonomy, happiness, or privacy among those entering the arrangement? Balanced against the value of surrogacy in helping infertile couples are the detriments to the gestational mother, the child, and society. Some ethical discourse finds that surrogacy demeans women by asking them to be fetal containers. To other ethicists, it is the potential harm to the child that takes precedence. To others, paying a surrogate is abhorrent because it places a price tag on a child. Treating the child as "chattel," the argument suggests, undermines well-established social values. Bonnie Steinbock, Ruth Macklin, and Lisa Cahill take us through the ethics of surrogacy. But each takes her own tightly argued ethical position, based upon social utility, or upon personal or religious values.

One of the most challenging questions regarding surrogacy is that of its impact on women's autonomy. Surrogacy presents a classic example of the equal/special treatment debate. Should the gestational mother be treated like others who are bound by contract? Or do the special circumstances involved in bearing a child mean that the gestational mother cannot or should not be bound by her word? The concept that contract principles— "a deal is a deal"—should govern the birth of a human being is, to some, inconceivable.

Lori Andrews brings to her essay a well-respected and carefully thought out analysis about a woman's right to do what she wants with her body. The gestational mother not only possesses this right as a theoretical matter, but she can also profit financially.

Joan Mahoney also believes in the woman's right to autonomy. But she would draw a bright line where the woman's freedoms end and the child's interests begin. Professor Mahoney believes strongly in the right of the child not to be purchased. She would ban payment of money in exchange for a binding promise to terminate parental rights.

The objective of this series of essays is to bring together the leading authorities with diverse perspectives on reproductive freedoms. We did not forget that surrogacy has important public health aspects. The public health impact is felt by both the health care professional (HCP) and the infertile couple. Karen Rothenberg has produced the first comprehensive examination of the impact of surrogacy on the health care professions. She posits a number of unanswered questions about the role of the HCP in the surrogacy process: How will HCPs effectively evaluate, counsel, and obtain informed consent from the gestational mother? What obligations do HCPs have to screen potential sperm donors and gestational mothers for such things as sexually transmitted diseases (and HIV), drugs, or genetic problems? Should HCPs in any way respect contract provisions which limit the autonomy of gestational mothers in such matters as amniocentesis, abortion, smoking, or lifestyle decisions? Should HCPs be able to intervene after the birth to affect such fundamental decisions as custody and parental rights? In sum, Karen Rothenberg has alerted us to the fact that the rights, duties, and practices of HCPs can have a major impact at every stage of surrogacy arrangements.

Nadine Taub explains how surrogacy and other forms of assisted reproduction have become so important throughout the developed world because of the increasing human, social, and technological problems of human infertility. Professor Taub suggests a number of preventive public health approaches to infertility. Surrogacy, she reminds us, can assist only a small number of infertile couples. Government and employers should devise more broadly based public health strategies to help prevent infertility.

Many deep societal issues are involved in the surrogate motherhood controversy. Although surrogacy is more a social and ethical problem than a legal one, it is being resolved in our courts and legislatures. We should be relieved that the first major surrogacy decision was handed down by the New Jersey Supreme Court, widely respected as one of the foremost judicial bodies in the country. *Baby M* may have been one of the most publicized cases in the history of American jurisprudence. The case is majestically written, whether or not one agrees with all of its conclusions. Professor Walter Wadlington of the University of Virginia School of Law drew together two informative and provocative views on *Baby M*, those of George Smith II and Randall Bezanson. Professor Wadlington's objective was to present essays that were not merely descriptive but richly evaluative and oriented to the future.

This series of essays, then, is for all of us who are concerned with civil liberties, ethics, women's autonomy, or the law, and who may once have felt that the issue of surrogacy was, after all, quite straightforward.

SURROGATE MOTHERHOOD

CIVIL LIBERTIES

A Civil Liberties Analysis of Surrogacy Arrangements

Larry Gostin

Proponents of surrogacy arrangements[1] assert that a married couple's right to "procreative autonomy" includes the right to contract with consenting collaborators for the purposes of bearing a child. The right to "genetic continuity" and to rear offspring are all part of the right of reproductive choice for the contracting father and his partner.[2]

Critics of surrogacy arrangements similarly cite "reproductive autonomy" as the basis for their claim that women cannot be compelled by contract to use their bodies in particular ways—either to forgo the right to abortion or to be "fetal containers." The right to autonomy over her own body and to rear the offspring she has borne are all part of the mother's reproductive freedom.[3]

Both proponents and critics of surrogacy arrangements, therefore, claim that their positions maximize freedom and liberty. Each position, of course, focuses on the autonomy of the party the commentator favors; the analysis is invariably outcome-determinative, without enunciating a neutral civil liberties framework. Neither proponents nor critics define clearly what the "right to procreate" entails, or what resolution is warranted when there is a conflict. What is absent from the debate, and what I wish to offer, is a civil liberties analysis of surrogacy arrangements.

In this essay I come to the following conclusions based upon a civil liberties analysis. First, surrogacy arrangements cannot be prohibited or criminalized. Second, the state cannot ban the exchange of money for surrogacy services, provided the money is paid for conception, gestation, and birth. Money, however, cannot be paid on condition that the gestational mother waive her parental rights over the child. Third, contractual provisions that require the gestational mother to waive her parental rights or her rights to privacy and autonomy are void and unenforceable. Fourth, when the child is born, both the gestational mother and the genetic father are the legal parents. If the gestational mother declines to relinquish her parental rights and a custody battle ensues, custody of the child should be determined under a "best interests" standard.

Non-specific performance of the surrogacy agreement is not an elegant result from the perspective of contract law. It also creates risks for those who enter into surrogacy arrangements. It does not foreclose the practice of surrogacy, but would encourage those considering this path to think carefully before planning to bring a child into the world using this method of reproduction. There would be no guarantee that the gestational mother would, after birth, waive her parental rights. If she refused to do so, however, the genetic father and she would find themselves in no worse position than that of any two parents involved in a custody dispute.

I want to enunciate the positions taken in this essay very clearly because they are, to some extent, contrary to the elegant decision of the New Jersey Supreme Court in the Baby M case.[4] The New Jersey Supreme Court treated that surrogacy arrangement as a simple custody matter, as I do. However, the court went further by banning, if not criminalizing, commercial surrogacy.

WHERE REPRODUCTIVE FREEDOMS COINCIDE

The parties in a surrogacy arrangement have substantial civil liberties interests: the rights to privacy in making an intimate personal decision about reproduction; the right to autonomy in decisions affecting the health and welfare of the mother and the offspring; and the right to association with future offspring. In this section I will demonstrate the human and constitutional interests at stake in surrogacy arrangements. I will argue that if a private consensual arrangement promotes happiness and contentment for both parties, and involves the exercise of constitutional rights to privacy and autonomy, then the state should not interfere with these arrangements in the absence of a clearly demonstrated harm to the child. This civil liberties analysis balances the strong reproductive rights that the gestational mother and genetic father have individually and collectively, on the one hand, with the government's speculative interests in protecting the unborn child, on the other. I conclude that the state has no sufficient ground for banning or criminalizing surrogacy arrangements.

What interests do constitutional rights to privacy place beyond the reach of government? The Constitution's promise of privacy and autonomy enfolds a constellation of intimate sexual, social, and family relationships, including bodily integrity, personal choice, and future association with offspring. Privacy is a "sensitive, key relationship of human existence, central to family life, community welfare and the development of human personality."[5]

The U.S. Supreme Court has enunciated a fundamental right "whether to bear or beget a child."[6] Citizens have a privacy right to decide whether, how, and when to bear a child. *Griswold*,[7] *Loving*,[8] and *Zablocki*[9] defined that right within the marital relationship. The Court in *Griswold* regarded marriage as "an association . . . a harmony of living . . . a bilateral loyalty, not a commercial or social project." In *Eisenstadt*[10] and *Carey*[11] the Court extended *Griswold* to non-married couples, using unequivocal language in its defense of interpersonal relationships. Contraception, it stated, concerns "the most intimate of human activities and relationships"[12]; a couple is "an association of two individuals each with a separate intellectual and emotional makeup."[13]

The Constitution's promise of privacy protects not only human relationships but also the right to decide whether to conceive and to carry a fetus to term. *Roe v. Wade*[14] concerned the potential detriments to pregnant women of being made to carry an unwanted fetus to term—the medical and psychological harm of having to bear and, possibly, to raise the child, and the distress of having their own choices about their bodies overriden by the state. Later, in *Akron*[15] and *Thornburgh*,[16] the Supreme Court refocused its thinking on abortion, describing it as the woman's private informed choice, which is for her and her physician alone to make.

The contraception cases decided by the Supreme Court also concern the right to make choices about future offspring. In *Griswold v. Connecticut*,[17] the first privacy case decided by the Court, the state had imposed a criminal penalty upon a physician for advising and prescribing contraception to a married couple, despite the fact that pregnancy would have jeopardized the woman's health. The Court overturned the statute, noting that there was a "zone of privacy created by several constitutional guarantees."[18] By criminalizing the *use* of contraception the government had exerted a "maximum destructive impact" upon privacy.[19]

Finally, the Supreme Court has held that natural parents have a constitutionally protected interest to rear their child.[20] The "fundamental liberty interest" in the care, custody, and management of the child extends even to the unwed father.[21] A father's interest is constitutionally protected when he "act[s] as a father toward his children."[22] It is difficult for any unwed father to demonstrate his parental attachment to a newborn. But a father's desire to reproduce and his financial and emotional attention to the welfare of the fetus help create a meaningful paternal involvement.

Surrogacy arrangements, then, deserve constitutional protection because of the private relationships and procreative intention of the parties, the woman's control over her own body, and the rights of genetic parents to association with their child.

The gestational mother has a particularly strong right of privacy and autonomy, founded upon several factors: her experience of artificial insemination, the changes in her body, her emotional commitment, her nurturing of the fetus for nine months, and the labor and pain of giving birth. The fact that she did not originally intend to keep the child does not dispose of this complex constitutional and social issue. Her bonding and identification with a baby born of her own body is an understandable and real human experience.

Supporters of surrogacy contracts ask the gestational mother to alienate herself from the child she is carrying, to become a dispassionate incubator for the growing fetus. The gestational mother's claims to control her own body and to be involved in the parenting of her child cannot be so easily trivialized. Her physical and psychological burdens deserve respect beyond the artificial confines of a sterile contract.

The genetic father and his partner use the surrogacy arrangement for the purpose of having a child, implementing their personal decision to procreate and to obtain the right to intimate association with the future offspring. The genetic father has a deep desire to reproduce and to care (usually tenderly) for a child. It is the father's intention to procreate that begins the process of reproduction; without his desire to reproduce, there would be no conception and birth. He has demonstrated by his personal decision to enter into the arrangement that he has paternal feelings and desires similar to those of a father in a conventional relationship. His psychological commitment and human desire to raise and care for a child entitles him to be treated as a parent and to assert a privacy right consistent with that status.

It is true that the donation of sperm does not involve the intensely private sexual and social relationship of conventional reproduction. Nor does a man have an unqualified right to use his power in the marketplace to inseminate a stranger for a fee. The principle enunciated in *Griswold*, that privacy protects an intimate sexual and social relationship but not a commercial project, is apt to demonstrate that the genetic father's privacy rights are not without limit.

Critics would either ban or criminalize surrogacy because of the greater stake the gestational mother brings to the arrangement.[23] This weighing of human interests in favor of the gestational mother may have meaning where there is a discernible conflict of interests. But the logic of those who would ban surrogacy falters considerably when the interests of both contracting parties coincide—as they usually do. In such cases the gestational mother's constitutional interests militate against state restrictions on surrogacy, not in favor of them.

Balanced against the powerful individual and collective interests in surrogacy arrangements are the undocumented and speculative interests of the state. Some persuasively argue that the state has a compelling interest in protecting the child.[24] But surrogacy arrangements do not pose any clear harm to children. There is the academic argument that no matter how maltreated or unwanted a child may be, she is better off than never having been born.[25] This is not a powerful argument because the state may well have a legitimate interest in preventing the birth of babies whom no one will want or care for. There are, however, no data to demonstrate that children born as the result of surrogacy contracts are worse off by any measure—that they suffer more neglect, abandonment, and physical abuse, or that they receive less nurturing and love.

The *Baby M* court acknowledged that the long-term effects of surrogacy contracts are not known, only "feared."[26] The court noted that the child might suffer from the knowledge that she was born as a result of a commercial transaction, and that the natural father and gestational mother might suffer when they "realize the consequences of their conduct."[27] The fact is that children are often born in adverse circumstances. Children can thrive when there is only one parent to love them. The infant born of a surrogacy arrangement is not necessarily disadvantaged, for she has a genetic father, an adoptive mother, and a gestational mother who may each come to treasure her. The *Baby M* court, moreover, is wrong to suppose that the parents will invariably, or even frequently, regret their decision. In the majority of cases the parties see the arrangement as in their own best interests. The hurt and human sadness evident in the Baby M case should not be used as a benchmark to judge all surrogacy arrangements.

Others point to the irreconcilable problems posed when the surrogate's baby turns out to have a physical deformity or a genetically inherited disease, or to be mentally retarded.[28] Men who sign surrogacy agreements, it is suggested, want perfect babies in their own images, and would be more likely to reject an imperfect child. It is true that surrogacy arrangements appear to stack the deck against an imperfect child, since neither party has any clear stake in the child. The gestational mother is invited not to think of the baby as her own. The contracting father has a certain image of how the child should be. He will be less likely to bond with the infant if he has not seen it growing in a woman he loves, seen it being born, or had a relationship with it in the early days and weeks of its life. While the possibility of both parents disclaiming responsibility for an imperfect child is an understandable concern, no data, again, are available to support it. Many handicapped infants are abandoned, and it is not at all certain that surrogacy arrangements would have any significant impact on the rate of abandonment.

Those who would ban or criminalize surrogacy have a heavy burden to explain why they would allow the state to stifle an activity that fulfills a human need without imposing any tangible harm on others.

Families in our society take many different forms, and a great deal of latitude in "private ordering" should be encouraged. Tolerance of diversity among families, and in the way they are formed, is part of a rich civil liberties tradition. Society should not be too quick to judge those who, for whatever reason, use surrogacy as a method of reproduction.

The New Jersey Supreme Court in the Baby M case found "no offense to our current laws where a woman voluntarily and without payment agrees to act as a 'surrogate' mother, provided that she is not subject to a binding agreement to surrender her child."[29] However, it found that the constitutional right to procreate does not extend as far as claimed by the parties to a surrogacy arrangement. "The right to procreate very simply is the right to have natural children, whether through sexual intercourse or artificial insemination. It is no more than that."[30] The court suggested that Mr. Stern and Ms. Whitehead had not been deprived of the right to procreate as defined, because Baby M is their child.[31] It may be true that these two people were not denied their constitutional right to procreate. However, the decision of the court to ban, or even criminalize, commercial surrogacy will obstruct, or certainly chill, the procreative rights of persons using this method of reproduction in the future. Had the New Jersey Supreme Court come to this decision previously, it is clear, Baby M would not have been born.

The New Jersey court held that the payment of money as part of a surrogacy agreement is contrary to state law and policy. Commercial surrogacy is "illegal, perhaps criminal, and potentially degrading to women."[32] In the following section I examine the question of whether the payment of money should change a legal, possibly constitutionally protected, activity into an unlawful, possibly criminal, enterprise.

THE STATE SHOULD NOT PERMIT THE PAYMENT OF MONEY IN RETURN FOR A BINDING WAIVER OF PARENTAL RIGHTS

If parties have a privacy right to enter into surrogacy arrangements, should there be any bar to the exchange of money? I will argue that payments that are made expressly on condition that the gestational mother agree to a binding termination of her parental rights are tantamount to the purchase of a baby and should be prohibited. However, the state should not ban payments to the woman for the conception, gestation, and birth of the child.

Legal and ethical objections to surrogacy often turn on the payment of money to the gestational mother and to a third-party broker. The British, as their media vividly expressed, were revolted by the idea of paying a price for a human being. The Surrogacy Arrangements Act 1985, which was hastily enacted before the Warnock Committee[33] presented its report to the government, prevents third parties (i.e., brokers) from deriving financial benefits.[34] The act does not expressly ban payments to the gestational mother.

The most articulate voice in the United States for banning commercial surrogacy has been the New Jersey Supreme Court. In the *Baby M* decision it stated:

> This is the sale of a child, or, at the very least, the sale of a mother's right
> to her child, the only mitigating factor being that one of the purchasers
> is the father. Almost every evil that prompted the prohibition of payment
> of money in connection with adoptions exists here.[35]

Treating a child as a commodity is unconstitutional and contrary to public policy. The Thirteenth Amendment to the Constitution prohibits involuntary servitude, or the buying and selling of human beings. The Pennsylvania Supreme Court, for example, held that certain payments by adoptive parents that appeared to be for the child were unconstitutional. The state constitution declared that all people are born with inalienable rights, including the right not to be bought or sold.[36]

State statutes make it a criminal offense to pay to adopt a child. Surrogacy contracts are markedly similar to paid adoption. In both cases the payment is for delivery of a baby: there is no substantive difference between paying a woman to gestate a child and then to deliver it, and paying a woman to deliver an already "produced" child. Both use a brokerage mechanism— an adoption agency or a surrogacy broker.[37] It was on the basis of the state adoption statute that the Supreme Court of New Jersey found the Baby M contract to be unlawful. The court saw the same conflict with public policy as exists in private adoptions for money. There is the "inducement of money," the "coercion of contract," and the "total disregard of the best interests of the child."[38]

A Gestational Mother Has the Right to Be Paid for Her Services

If paying for the termination of parental rights is wrong, is it also wrong to compensate the gestational mother for her services in being artificially inseminated and carrying the fetus to term? I argue, firstly, that banning payment for gestational services would deprive the woman of the right to be paid for valued labor. Secondly, it is important to get beyond the term "baby-selling." Rather, we should ask what harms would accrue from paying a woman for gestational services, and how those harms can be minimized. Finally, a flat prohibition on the payment of money would chill the practice of surrogacy so thoroughly as to be a *de facto* ban. This would deprive the parties of their reproductive rights as surely as a prohibition on payment for other reproductive services such as contraception or abortion.

A human being has a right to contract with another to be paid for the performance of services, even highly personal services. The "women's work" of conception, gestation, and birth is arduous, and has a high social worth. For the state to prohibit payment for such work would deprive women of compensation for valued labor. They are entitled to economic gain for the physical changes in their bodies, the changes in lifestyle, the work of carrying a fetus, and the pain and medical risk of labor and parturition. Critics of surrogacy assert that it enslaves the woman. But performing personal services and labor in exchange for money is not equivalent to slavery. There is no slave-master relationship, no involuntary peonage, and no entitlement to control any human being.

Some advocates claim that paying women to provide reproductive services exploits poor or uneducated women, who are "coerced" by the marketplace into selling their intimate personal services.[39] As the *Baby M* court put it: the "essential evil is . . . taking advantage of a woman's circumstances."[40] This is analogous to prostitution, which is a criminal offense.

A woman's decision to sell her intimate services may well constitute an indignity for all women and may well mean that she is allowing herself to be exploited. Nonetheless, that choice is not for the state or the body politic but for the woman alone to make. As the American Civil Liberties Union policy on prostitution states, "whether a person chooses to engage in sexual activity for purposes of recreation, or in exchange for something of value, is a matter of individual choice, not for governmental interference."[41] A woman has a privacy right to determine how she will use her own body, and whether or not she will seek compensation. The state may not approve of the decision she makes, but it has no right to override it. It is particularly paternalistic to assume that the state can dictate a woman's choice because it knows better than she what is in her interests as a human being.

The *Baby M* court states that the "evils inherent in baby bartering are loathsome for a myriad of reasons."[42] However, examination of those reasons shows they are neither loathsome nor uncorrectable—and that they are not caused by money changing hands. It is important to get beyond the charged term "baby-selling" to examine what harm would accrue to the child, the parties, or society.

I have already referred to the lack of any demonstrable evidence that the baby in a surrogacy arrangement is harmed by any objective measure. There is no indication that the potential harm is any greater than the risk we already tolerate in other births. We do not, for example, restrict the reproductive freedoms of unwed mothers or "conventional" families with a history of child neglect, drug or alcohol abuse, or congenital disease such as AIDS.

Most commentators concede that there is not enough evidence of potential harm to the children to justify banning commercial surrogacy. Rather, they argue that the commercialization of reproduction degrades humankind.[43] All personal attributes (e.g., sex, race, height, eye color, intelligence) would be given a dollar value. This is also a speculative argument, since it does not rely on any tangible injury to the parties or to society. The "commodification" argument assumes that it is morally wrong to pay money for reproductive services. It is not for government to judge the morality of payment by a genetic father and his partner, particularly when it is the only way a couple can reproduce. Further, parents in a surrogacy arrangement want children for reasons probably no less humane or understandable than those of parents who reproduce by conventional means. Conventional parents, like surrogate parents, have children for many reasons, some for love, some for money, and some because they have a certain image of the offspring they would like to have. There is no "ideal" reason for choosing a mate and having a baby.

Finally, there is no evidence for the "slippery slope" argument that commercial surrogacy will lead to market values being placed on particular genetic traits. As conceived here, surrogacy would be carefully regulated and non-enforceable by the courts—hardly a strong encouragement to a free marketplace for babies.

The remaining reasons given by the *Baby M* court for banning commercial surrogacy are eminently correctable. The court was concerned that there is "no counseling, independent or otherwise, of the natural mother, no evaluation, no warning"[44] and that the genetic father knows "little about the natural mother, her genetic makeup, and her psychological and medical history."[45] The same can be said of any private adoption. The legislature has ample regulatory power to require counseling, as well as social, medical, and psychological reports. The law, then, can require all that is necessary to ensure full information and the fitness of the parties to enter into the surrogacy arrangement.

The New Jersey Supreme Court's other criticisms of surrogacy can also be rectified by adherence to the civil liberties principles set out in this essay. The court was concerned that the gestational mother is irrevocably committed "before she knows the strength of her bond with her child."[46] The court's ruling that the gestational mother's contractual waiver is void means that she is free to change her mind and to contest custody under a "best interests" standard. The parties to a surrogacy agreement as envisaged here are in much the same position as unwed parents who have a custody dispute. The evils of surrogacy do not arise because of the exchange of money, but because of the contract's irrevocable waiver. Voiding that contractual provision would eradicate much of the social concern over surrogacy.

The final argument against banning the payment of money is that it would thoroughly chill the practice of surrogacy. A ban on payment will virtually ensure that the would-be parents' individual and collective reproductive rights are never expressed. Payment for services in our society has become so essential that prohibiting compensation would virtually ban the practice. "All parties concede that it is unlikely that surrogacy will survive without money."[47] One need only contemplate the prospect of banning payment for other reproductive services, such as contraception or

abortion, to understand the barrier it would pose to continuation of surrogacy arrangements.

THE DIFFERENCE BETWEEN PAYING FOR
GESTATIONAL SERVICES AND FOR THE TERMINATION
OF PARENTAL RIGHTS

I have drawn a civil liberties distinction between payment for a binding
agreement to terminate parental rights and for gestational services. The
distinction is supported by the analysis in the following section, stating
why a woman should not be bound by an agreement to terminate her
parental rights. If the distinction is accepted, it provides guidance on how
surrogacy arrangements can be structured so as not to involve the purchase
of a child.

Surrogacy contracts are equivalent to "baby-selling" if they essentially
offer payment for the delivery of an uncluttered title to the child. The state
could block this approach by proscribing payment of any fee contingent
upon termination of the woman's parental rights, while allowing periodic
payments throughout the pregnancy to compensate the woman for her
services and health care expenses.

It will be argued that structuring a contract as payment for services rather
than for delivery of the child is a "nice" legal distinction, but that this
nonetheless remains merely a pretense for baby-selling. After all, when a
person pays for labor, he or she is really paying for the commodity that
the labor produces. The genetic father is not interested in the gestational
mother's childbearing experiences. He wants, and believes he is paying
for, her baby. The New Jersey Supreme Court had

> no doubt whatsoever that the money is being paid to obtain an adoption
> and not . . . for the personal services of Mary Beth Whitehead. . . . It
> strains credulity to claim that these arrangements, touted by those in the
> surrogacy business as an attractive alternative to the usual route leading
> to an adoption, really amount to something other than a private placement
> adoption for money.[48]

That is true when a gestational mother can be compelled by contract to
give up her baby. It is not true, however, where she is entitled to maintain
her parental rights. The issue is not what a contracting father wants or
what a private broker promises, but what the law will allow. If the law
does not allow payment in exchange for the child, and if the courts will
not enforce any contractual provision in which the woman waives her
parental rights, then the distinction between payment for the baby and

payment for gestational services is real, and not a pretense. The surrogacy contract would provide no entitlement to the child.

The Supreme Court of Kentucky, in *Surrogate Parenting v. Com. Ex Rel. Armstrong*,[49] considered whether a valid constitutional distinction could be drawn between payment for gestational services and payment for the child. The court held that payments to the woman under a surrogacy contract were for her services, not the baby. The woman could not be forced by the contract to forgo her parental rights; therefore, there was no selling of the baby. This decision is consistent with the civil liberties arguments presented here, except for the manner in which payment was actually made:

> [A] portion of the fee is paid in advance for the use of her body as an incubator, but a portion of the payment is withheld and is not paid until her child is delivered unto the purchaser, along with the equivalent of a bill of sale, or quit claim deed, to wit—the judgment terminating her parental rights. How can it be denied that this last payment is in fact payment for the baby?[50]

A civil liberties theory of surrogacy would avoid this inconsistency by prohibiting payments under a contract in exchange for the waiver of the parental rights of the gestational mother.

A GESTATIONAL MOTHER CANNOT WAIVE HER RIGHTS TO DETERMINE HER OWN LIFESTYLE, TO HAVE AN ABORTION, OR TO PARENT HER CHILD

One simple way to determine parental rights over the child born of a surrogacy agreement is to grant them to the father. After all, the gestational mother signed a contract in which she probably made a series of promises about her lifestyle, medical treatment, and, most importantly, parental rights over the child.[51] Many surrogacy contracts provide for specific performance of these promises.[52] Why shouldn't the gestational mother be compelled in a court of law to fulfill her contractual obligations?[53]

The legal question of whether a person can waive[54] privacy and parental rights is unsettled. There is a strong presumption against waiver of constitutional or fundamental rights.[55] A person cannot waive constitutional rights unless she does so knowingly, voluntarily, and intelligently, "with sufficient awareness of the relevant circumstances and likely consequences."[56] This "voluntariness and knowledge" standard might be applied in individual cases to show that the gestational mother did or did not make a fully informed choice when she signed the contract.

There are some rights, however, that cannot be *irrevocably* waived—that is, the person can change her mind even after she has agreed to waive her rights.[57] For example, criminal defendants cannot irrevocably waive the right to be present at trial in a capital case,[58] to raise a plea of incompetence to stand trial,[59] or to assert a privilege against self-incrimination.[60]

Advance waiver of a constitutional right is particularly troublesome, because the person cannot foresee all the circumstances that will affect a future decision. Therefore, some rights can be waived only at the time they could be invoked. A federal Court of Appeal refused for this reason to recognize a woman's waiver of her due-process rights when signing a foster-care contract, because the relationship the foster parent sought to protect did not exist at the time she signed the contract.[61]

The courts, therefore, have been highly suspicious of advance waivers of fundamental rights. However, there has been no specific judicial guidance on whether the courts would refuse, on constitutional grounds, to enforce the various promises that are often made in surrogacy contracts.[62] I will argue that to hold a woman to a promise to waive her human rights sometime in the future diminishes her constitutional entitlements. I am not suggesting, however, that a gestational mother cannot waive the exercise of her rights at the time they have to be invoked. She can choose not to avail herself of her right to an abortion or to conduct her life the way she pleases. A gestational mother can also decide not to assert her parental rights when the child is born or, preferably, after a period of time following the birth. This is analogous to state adoption statutes that allow a woman who has agreed to relinquish her parental rights over her baby to change her mind any time before the baby is born. In most states the mother has a grace period after birth in which she can still decide to keep the child.

The rights of a gestational mother to make future decisions about her body, lifestyle, and an intimate future relationship with her child are so important to her dignity and human happiness that they should be regarded as inalienable. First, consider the contractual provisions that seek to deprive the gestational mother of her right to make decisions about her medical treatment and lifestyle: restricting or prohibiting smoking, use of alcohol or drugs (prescription as well as recreational), sex or other "strenuous" activity, and abortion; or requiring regular prenatal examination, amniocentesis, and abortion if the baby is likely to be severely handicapped.

The rights to choose one's lifestyle and medical treatment are among the most private aspects of human life. The government itself cannot restrict these activities unless it demonstrates that the person is incompetent or that there is some compelling health purpose.[63] No such health purpose exists in surrogacy, particularly where these activities take place in private and do not affect the public. Since the government cannot reach into this intensely private domain, it is difficult to envisage a private party having the power to do so based upon a contractual obligation.

The genetic father will point to the potential harm to the fetus as the rationale for intervention. This makes the mother and fetus into adversaries, locked in a conflict over whose health and well-being will prevail.[64] While courts recently have been prepared to intervene in cases of immediate and substantial threat to the fetus (e.g., to require a Cesarean delivery),[65] the government does not have a general right to control how a pregnant woman lives her life or the medical treatment she chooses. It would be unconscionable if pregnant women could have private decisions forced on them in ways that would be wholly unimaginable for others. Pregnancy, although it entails another life to consider, should not become a license for denying women their basic right to be left alone to make the health decisions they choose.

Neither government nor a private party has the right to dictate deeply personal choices to the gestational mother, even if they have extracted a promise in exchange for money. Just as important is the deep invasion of privacy involved in monitoring and possibly enforcing the gestational mother's compliance with her promises. There is no lawful and ethical way to determine how a gestational mother is behaving within her own home. Various monitoring and enforcement methods themselves pose threats to individual privacy and autonomy—e.g., testing blood for alcohol or drug use. And to compel submission to a medical procedure such as a gynecological examination, amniocentesis, or abortion is tantamount to a battery—an unconscionable violation of the woman's bodily integrity.[66]

There has not been much caselaw in these areas. However, an analysis of the Supreme Court's abortion decisions indicates that choices affecting privacy and autonomy are for the woman alone to make. In *Planned Parenthood v. Danforth*[67] the Supreme Court held that a husband does not have the right to veto his wife's decision to seek an abortion. "Since the State cannot regulate or proscribe abortion . . . the State cannot delegate authority to any particular person, even the spouse, to prevent abortion."[68] In *Belotti v. Baird*[69] the Supreme Court also invalidated a state statute that required a woman to get her parents' consent to an abortion.[70] As neither husbands nor parents can overrule a woman's decision to get an abortion, the courts would be highly unlikely to give this right to the father in a surrogacy arrangement.[71]

The second major right that surrogacy contracts seek to deny the gestational mother is her choice to assert parental claims over her child. Natural parents have parental rights over their children unless there is a judicial finding that their behavior is seriously detrimental to the child's interests. Decisions about parenthood, like treatment and lifestyle decisions, are essential to dignity and future happiness. These rights may seem abstract and unimportant before they need to be invoked. The gestational mother signs the contract because, at the time, she may have no interest in having a baby herself and she sees the arrangement as offering financial compensation for work performed.[72] Yet once the gestational mother is faced with the actual decision, her rights become of utmost importance. Understandably, the gestational mother's feelings may change once she has nurtured the fetus, given birth to a human being whom she recognizes as part of herself and then holds, cares for, and comes to love. Any parent who has experienced birth and the discovery of the infant's unique human qualities and character cannot help but appreciate the possibility of such changes in feelings, judgment, and outlook.

Irreversible decisions about child-rearing, then, ought not to be forced on any mother nine months before her rights have any real meaning. The decision to give up one's own child for a lifetime is an awesome responsibility to place on any human being.

Proponents of surrogacy repeatedly assert that to hold these personal rights inalienable is indefensibly paternalistic, and disparaging of the decision-making capacity of women.[73] To hold the parental right inalienable, they suggest, is to degrade women by implying they need to be protected from their "irrational" or "whimsical" impulses, and that they cannot understand the import of relinquishing a child.

These arguments show an almost willful blindness to the true meaning of paternalism and to the reasons why fundamental rights should be inalienable. It is paternalistic to make a decision for another person because you believe you know better than she what is in her true interests. To hold the parental right inalienable is not paternalistic at all. Rather, it respects the woman's final decision regarding her bodily integrity and future associations. The principle of inalienability indicates that the woman controls her own destiny and cannot be prevented by contract from making the decision herself when it becomes important.

This argument is not gender-based. There are certain things that we can contract about—property, goods, and services. But there are other things so important to human flourishing and self-respect that they should not be specifically enforceable by contract, whether the subject is male or female. We do not call patients "fickle," for example, if they decide to withdraw their previously given consent to a medical procedure. It is insulting to suggest that because the law allows gestational mothers to withdraw consent to a waiver of parental rights, the women are indecisive or need protection.

DETERMINING CUSTODY WITHIN A CIVIL
LIBERTIES FRAMEWORK

When a child is born of a surrogacy arrangement, the woman who gave birth to the child is the legal mother unless she relinquishes her parental status through adoption. The man who entered into the agreement and who donated his sperm is the legal father. Termination of the parental rights of the gestational mother or the genetic father can be judicially determined only under statutory criteria in each state. Most states will not terminate parental rights unless it is demonstrated that the parent is unfit; a mere showing that it would not be in the child's best interests to live with a parent is insufficient to terminate the parent's wider parental rights, including visitation.[74]

The two genetic parents in a surrogacy arrangement may each want custody of the child. If one of them declines to waive a claim to the child and a dispute ensues, who should have custody? And by what standard should the question be determined?

Custody determinations are potentially so harmful to the child that many believe the law should intervene with a clear rule favoring the genetic father or the gestational mother.[75] Undoubtedly, custody battles should be avoided wherever possible because of the potential trauma to the child. But a judicial determination becomes necessary when each parent seeks custody over the child, and it is not obvious in every case which placement would be in the child's best interests. The adoption of an automatic rule foreclosing the parental rights of the man or the woman would be iniquitous. First, "bright line" rules deter deeper inquiry into the best interests of the child in each case. Using sex as a proxy for a thoroughgoing assessment of the child's interests would not serve those interests well. Second, the parental interests of either the father or the mother would not be respected. Natural parents have substantive and procedural due process rights to assert a claim to custody before a court.[76] A "clear rule" would determine which parent could exercise the fundamental right of association with one's children by presumption, rather than by individual findings of fact. Third, a "clear rule" amounts to a rigid form of discrimination based upon gender. Whether a court uses the contract to favor the father or sees the woman's unique reproductive capabilities as a reason to favor the mother,[77] it is really using the parents' sex, rather than a best-interests standard, to determine custody. This would permit custody to be based on status criteria traditionally used to discriminate against individuals.

These reasons against a clear rule are all based upon strong civil liberties principles, which should not be abridged except for compelling reasons. Both sides in the surrogacy debate argue that there are compelling reasons for a clear rule in their favor. I have already shown why there should not be a paternal presumption based upon the surrogacy contract. Nor should economic status be the sole determining factor for assessing a child's best interests. Economic status usually favors the father—particularly in a surrogacy arrangement, which virtually guarantees a marked disparity in the wealth of the mother and the father. Material advantage is not an important measure for the best interests of the child, and has a discriminatory effect on women. The "best interests" test is designed to help the child become a "well integrated person who might reasonably be expected to be happy with life.''[78] The court should not be concerned with the kind of "idealized life that money can buy."[79]

Advocates of the rights of the gestational mother say she has contributed most to the surrogacy arrangement. Her nine months of gestation not only make her deserving of the child but also put her in a much better position to form a bond and to care for the child.[80] It is argued, moreover, that the present law on parentage already provides a clear preference for the gestational mother. A woman who gives birth to a child is held legally responsible for its welfare, whereas sperm donors cannot assert a parental claim over any child born by use of their sperm.

The comparison between a genetic father who simply donates sperm and one who enters into a surrogacy agreement is inapt, however. Once a donor gives his sperm to a bank in return for a fee he has completed his "transaction"; he has no intention to reproduce and has not committed himself to, or prepared for, the responsibilities of parenthood. Moreover, once the man has donated his sperm he knows nothing further of its use. In short, he has not acted like a father and has no ground for asserting the rights of a father. By contrast, a genetic father in a surrogacy arrangement initiates the whole procreative process. His psychological, emotional, and financial investment in planning the birth, care, and nurturance of the child may be considerable. He acts like a father in the sense that he has an intent to procreate and desires a relationship with the child.

The Supreme Court in *Stanley v. Illinois*[81] held that an unwed father is entitled to notice and a hearing before a court determines that he has no right to custody of his child. Subsequent cases, involving foreclosure of parental rights through adoption rather than denial of custody,[82] do limit the principle enunciated in *Stanley*. Those cases suggest that a father acquires due process rights only when he "act[s] as a father toward his children."[83] Thus, an unwed father who visited and supported his child only irregularly had no constitutional right to a hearing.[84] Conversely, where the father established a relationship by living with, caring for, and supporting the child, he did have due process rights.[85]

Most troubling about the *Stanley* line of cases is that the Court appears to be concerned with the custodial, personal, and financial relationship the father *actually* established. The father's intent and good-faith efforts to establish a relationship with his child are insufficient. In *Lehr v. Robertson*,[86] the putative father had taken every opportunity to establish a relationship with his child. He lived with the mother for two years until the birth and visited the child in the hospital every day; he never ceased in his efforts to locate the child after the mother concealed her; and he offered financial support. The Court, nonetheless, held that he had no right to a hearing before termination of his parental rights.

In a surrogacy arrangement the genetic father ought not to be foreclosed from a hearing on the best interests of the child. He had the paternal intention to procreate, and he may have done all that he could to prepare for the child and to seek a relationship with her. We should not automatically assume that it is always in the best interests of the child to remain with the mother.

Civil liberties principles, therefore, require that such factors as sex and economic status should not become proxies for assessing an individual child's best interests. Neither factor is a good predictor of the ability to parent well—although both should be considered, to the extent strictly relevant to the child's best interests.

Custody should also be determined without regard to the existence of the surrogacy agreement. The fact that the mother entered into a surrogacy agreement should not be held against her in determining custody; she has not neglected, abandoned, or adversely affected her child in any way. A woman is no less able to parent her child because she originally decided to surrender her legitimate claim as its true mother. This conclusion is consistent with the civil liberties approach taken here that contractual provisions requiring an irrevocable waiver of parental rights should be void. To use a surrogacy agreement against the gestational mother in a custody dispute would inhibit the exercise of her constitutional right to associate with her child.

CONCLUSION

The approach to custody taken in this essay is simple and consistent with current law and practice. If the surrogacy arrangement goes as planned, as so many have in the past, then the child will grow up with parents probably as stable and secure as the parents of any conventionally born child. I also treat surrogacy arrangements that break down in the same way as the law treats marriages that break down or births out of wedlock. None of these cases of parents tugging at their child for custody are happy ones. Yet none create insurmountable obstacles to the future well-being of the child. So long as the law treats the child as a person wanted by both parents and sensitively allocates parental rights and responsibilities, including custody, there is every reason to believe that the child can, and will, flourish.

REFERENCES

I want to warmly acknowledge the contribution of the members of the Special Committee on Surrogate Parenting, which I chair for the American Civil Liberties Union. The committee formed the core of analysis on this essay. The members of the ACLU Surrogacy Committee are Leslie Harris, Joan Mahoney, Wendy Williams, and Susan Wolf. Stacey DeBroff is staff liaison to the committee.

1. There are three distinct roles that are potentially involved in a surrogacy arrangement: the woman who gestates the child and who gives birth (whom I will refer to as the gestational mother); the woman who donates an egg without bearing the baby (the egg donor is usually, but not necessarily, the gestational mother); and the man who provides the sperm (whom I will refer to as the genetic father).

2. See, e.g., John Robertson, "Procreative Liberty and the Control of Conception, Pregnancy, and Childbirth," *Virginia Law Review,* 69 (April 1983): 405; John Robertson, "Surrogate Mothers: Not So Novel after All," *Hastings Center Report* (October 1983): 28.

3. See, e.g., George Annas, "Pregnant Women as Fetal Containers," *Hastings Center Report* (Dec. 1986): 13; George Annas, "The Baby Broker Boom," *Hastings Center Report* (June 1986): 30.

4. In re Baby M, 217 N.J. Super. 313 (1987), *rev'd in part,* 525 A.2d 1128, 1988 W L 6251, Slip Op A-39–87, decided Feb 3, 1988.

5. Paris Adult Theatre I v. Slaton, 413 U.S. 49, 63 (1973).

6. Carey v. Population Services International, 431 U.S. 678, 97 S. Ct. 2010, 2016 (1977); Eisenstadt v. Baird, 405 U.S. 438, 453 (1972). See Skinner v. Oklahoma, 316 U.S. 535 (1942).

7. Griswold v. Connecticut, 85 S. Ct. 1678 (1965).

8. Loving v. Virginia, 388 U.S. 1 (1967).

9. Zablocki v. Redhail, 434 U.S. 374 (1978).

10. Eisenstadt v. Baird, 405 U.S. 438 (1972).

11. Carey v. Population Services International, 431 U.S. 678, 97 S. Ct. 2010 (1977).

12. Carey v. Population Services International, 97 S. Ct. at 2016 (1977).

13. Eisenstadt v. Baird, 92 S. Ct. at 1038 (1972).

14. 410 U.S. 113 (1973).

15. City of Akron v. Akron Center for Reproductive Health, 462 U.S. 416 (1983).

16. Thornburgh v. American College of Obstetricians and Gynecologists, 476 U.S. 747 (1986).

17. 85 S. Ct. 1678 (1965).

18. 85 S. Ct. at 1682.

19. Id.

20. Santosky v. Kramer, 455 U.S. 745, 753 (1982). See Myer v. Nebraska, 262 U.S. 390, 399 (1923); Pierce v. Society of Sisters, 268 U.S. 510 (1925); Prince v. Massachusetts, 321 U.S. 158 (1944).

21. Stanley v. Illinois, 405 U.S. 645 (1972).

22. Stanley v. Illinois, 405 U.S. at 650 (unwed father is a parent whose existing relationship with his children must be considered); Caban v. Mohammed, 441 U.S. 380 (1978) (statute that prevented unwed father, but not unwed mother, from vetoing adoption of natural child was unconstitutional when the father had a relationship with the children comparable with the mother's).

23. See George Annas, "Pregnant Women," supra note 3, at 13.

24. In re Baby M, slip op A-39–87 (1988); Angela Holder, "Surrogate Motherhood: Babies for Fun and Profit," *Law, Medicine & Health Care,* 12 (1984): 115.

25. John Robertson, "Procreative Liberty and the Contract of Conception, Pregnancy and Childbirth," *Virginia Law Review,* 69 (1983): 405, 416.

26. In re Baby M, slip op A-39–87, p. 51.

27. Id.

28. H. T. Krimmel, "The Case Against Surrogate Parenting," *Hastings Center Report* (Oct. 1983): 35.

29. In re Baby M, slip op. A-39–87, p. 5.

30. Id.: 62.

31. Id.: 62–68.

32. Id. 4.

33. *Report of the Committee of Inquiry in Fertilisation and Embryology* (London: H. M. Stationery Office, Cmnd 9314, 1984).

34. D. Brahms, "The Hasty British Ban on Commercial Surrogacy," *Hastings Center Report* (Feb. 1987): 16.

35. In re Baby M, slip op. A-39–87, p. 46.

36. In re Baby Girl D, 517 A.2d 925 (1986).

37. Margaret Jane Radin, "Market-Inalienability," *Harvard Law Review*, 100 (1987): 1849 at 1928–29.

38. In re Baby M, slip op. A-39–87, p. 21.

39. Radin, supra note 37, at 1849.

40. In re Baby M, slip op A-39–87, p. 48.

41. ACLU Policy #262.

42. In re Baby M, slip op A-39–87, p. 26.

43. Radin, supra note 37.

44. In re Baby M, slip op A-39–87, p. 44.

45. Id.: 46.

46. Id.: 45.

47. Id.: 47.

48. Id.

49. 704 S.W.2d 209 (Ky. 1986).

50. Dissenting opinion of Vance, J., 704 S. W. at 214. The contract in the Baby M case was structured in much the same way.

51. See Brophy, "A Surrogate Mother Contract to Bear a Child," *Journal of Family Law*, 20 (1982): 263.

52. See Note, "Developing a Concept of the Modern 'Family': A Proposed Uniform Surrogate Parenthood Act," *Georgetown Law Journal*, 73 (1985): 1283.

53. Two very strong articles by members of my committee add weight to the argument. See Susan Wolf, "Enforcing Surrogate Motherhood Agreements: The Trouble with Specific Performance," *New York Law School Human Rights Annual*, vol. 4; Joan Mahoney, "An Essay on Surrogacy and Feminist Thought," *Law, Medicine & Health Care*, 16 (1988): 81.

54. "Waive" means to forgo the exercise of a right. I will distinguish between a current waiver, which takes place at the time the right could have been invoked, and a future waiver (or alienation), which is a promise now to waive a right in the future. See "Rumpelstiltskin Revisited: The Inalienable Rights of Surrogate Mothers," *Harvard Law Review*, 99 (1986): 1936, 1941.

55. See Johnson v. Zerbst, 304 U.S. 458, 464 (1938) (courts must indulge in every reasonable presumption against waiver of fundamental rights); Glasser v. U.S., 315 U.S. 60, 70 (1942) (same presumption applies to rights enumerated in the Bill of Rights).

56. Brady v. U.S., 397 U.S. 742, 748 (1970) (waiver of right to trial). See Boykin v. Alabama, 393 U.S. 238 (1969); Rubin, "Toward a General Theory of Waiver," *UCLA Law Review*, 28 (1981): 478, 487.

57. See Lawrence Tribe, *American Constitutional Law* (1978), 469; Kreimer, "Allocational Sanctions: The Problem of Negative Rights in a Positive State," *University of Pennsylvania Law Review*, 132 (1984): 1293.

58. Diaz v. United States, 223 U.S. 442, 455 (1912); Lewis v. U.S., 146 U.S. 370, 372 (1892).

59. Pate v. Robinson, 383 U.S. 375, 384–85 (1966).

60. Stevens v. Marks, 383 U.S. 234, 244 (1986).

61. Rivera v. Marcus, 696 F.2d 1016, 1206 (1982). But see Reimche v. First National Bank of Nevada, 512 F.2d 187 (9th Cir. 1975); In re Shirk's Estate, 186 Kan. 311, 350 P.2d 1 (1960).

62. The New Jersey Supreme Court refused to enforce the Baby M contract on statutory, not constitutional, grounds.

63. The Supreme Court has on numerous occasions decided that a person has the right to physical autonomy unless there is a strong countervailing state interest, such as public health (Jacobson v. Massachusetts, 197 U.S. 11 [1905]), or the life of a viable fetus (Roe v. Wade, 410 U.S. 113 [1973]). See Larry Gostin, "The Future of Communicable Disease Control: Toward a New Concept in Public Health Law," *Milbank Quarterly*, 64, Supp. 1 (1986): 79–96.

64. See Nancy Rhoden, "Cesareans and Samaritans," *Law, Medicine & Health Care*, 15 (1987): 118–25.

65. Jefferson v. Griffin Spaulding County Hospital Authority, 274 S.E.2d 457 (Ga. 1981). See V. E. B. Kolder, J. Gallagher, and M. T. Parsons, "Court-Ordered Cesarean Deliveries," *New England Journal of Medicine*, 316 (1987): 1192–96.

66. Ruth Macklin, "Is There Anything Wrong with Surrogate Parenting?: An Ethical Analysis," *Law, Medicine & Health Care*, 16 (1988): TK.

67. 428 U.S. 52 (1976).

68. Id.: 69.

69. 443 U.S. 622 (1979).

70. See Jones v. Smith, 278 So.2d 339 (Fla. 1973), *cert. denied*, 415 U.S. 958 (1973) (denying an illegitimate child's potential father the right to prevent the mother from having an abortion); Ponter v. Ponter, 135 N.J. Super. 50, 342 A.2d 574 (Ch. Div. 1975) (denying husband the right to prevent wife from undergoing sterilization).

71. Coleman, "Surrogate Motherhood: Analysis of the Problems and Suggestions for Solutions," *Tennessee Law Review*, 50 (1982): 71, 85; Lawrence Tribe, "The Abortion Funding Conundrum: Inalienable Rights, Affirmative Duties, and the Dilemma of Independence," *Harvard Law Review*, 99 (1985): 330, 336.

72. Phillip Parker, "Motivation of Surrogate Mothers: The Initial Findings," *American Journal of Psychiatry*, 140 (1983): 117–18.

73. McConnell, "The Nature and Basis of Inalienable Rights," *Law and Philosophy*, 3 (1984): 25, 41; Radin, supra note 37, at 1898; Robertson, "Procreative Liberty," supra note 2.

74. Baby M, slip op A-29–87.

75. Statement of Margaret Radin and Alexander Capron at a hearing on surrogate parenting before the Senate Committee on Health and Human Resources of the California Legislature, Dec. 11, 1987.

76. See infra, notes 81–86.

77. For an excellent discussion of the importance of a woman's unique reproductive capabilities in assessing gender discrimination, see Wendy Williams, "Equality's Riddle: Pregnancy and the Equal Treatment/Special Treatment Debate," *Review of Law & Social Change*, 13 (1984): 325–80.

78. In re Baby M, slip op A-39–87, p. 81.

79. Id.

80. The gestational mother's early bonding to and nurturance of the baby is likely to result in her being granted temporary custody. In re Baby M, p. 84. These concerns weigh in favor of both a relatively short period after birth during which the mother can decide whether or not she wishes to retain her parental status and, if she does, an accelerated custody trial.

81. 405 U.S. 645 (1972).

82. Quilloin v. Walcott, 434 U.S. 246 (1978); Caban v. Mohammed, 441 U.S. 380 (1978); Lehr v. Robertson, 463 U.S. 248 (1983).

83. Lehr v. Robertson, 463 U.S. 248 (1983).

84. Quilloin v. Walcott, 434 U.S. 246 (1978); Lehr v. Robertson, 463 U.S. 248 (1983).

85. Caban v. Mohammed, 441 U.S. 380 (1978).

86. 463 U.S. 248 (1983).

Procreative Liberty and the State's Burden of Proof in Regulating Noncoital Reproduction

John A. Robertson

The growing popularity of noncoital solutions to infertility has raised questions about the need for public policies to regulate these techniques. While surrogacy has dominated public attention, controversy has also surrounded in vitro fertilization (IVF), embryo freezing, and gamete donation.

The policy concerns arise from the potential impact that the means of noncoital reproduction—embryo manipulation or use of gamete donors and surrogates—could have on offspring, collaborators, the family, and gender-based reproductive roles. For example, IVF techniques involving the creation and manipulation of human embryos may harm embryos and the offspring to which they lead. Noncoital techniques involving gamete donors and surrogates raise issues of offspring welfare, the interests of collaborators, exploitation of women, and effects on the family and society generally.

A basic question for public policy is the scope of private discretion over noncoital means of forming families. Should the state prohibit or regulate use of these techniques, or should their use be left to the free choice of infertile couples, collaborators, and physicians? Since state limits on re-productive choice are necessarily problematic, the issue is whether non-coital reproduction poses risks so significantly different from coital reproduction that regulation is justified. Although major toxicity from their use appears to be absent, at the present time it is not easy to answer this question with certainty. In the early stages of a technology, data about empirical effects will be lacking. However, many people object to some or all of the procedures in question. The policy choice is complicated by the strong emotions and fantasies about life, death, sexuality, and reproductive roles that noncoital reproduction inevitably stimulates.

In such a situation, the degree of freedom or regulation may depend upon the party bearing the burden of proof. If the state need establish only a low threshold of potential harm to regulate, then a great deal of regulation, including restrictions based on moralistic concerns, will be possible. On the other hand, if the state has the burden of showing that substantial harm will occur, then considerably more private discretion over use of these techniques will remain, with empirical uncertainties resolved in favor of individual choice.

How should the burden of proof concerning noncoital reproductive technologies be allocated? Of central importance is the connection between these techniques and the procreative and family privacy of infertile couples. Noncoital reproduction involving embryos, gamete donors, and surrogates enables infertile married couples to rear children who are biologically related to one if not both rearing partners. As such, use of these techniques would appear to deserve the same protection against state restriction that coital reproduction by married couples would receive. Thus the state should have the burden of showing that particular noncoital techniques threaten substantial harm if it is to limit private discretion in forming families. Unfortunately, advocates of regulation have often ignored or misunderstood the implications of procreative liberty for public policy regarding noncoital reproduction.

This article presents the constitutional argument for limiting state regulation or restriction of noncoital reproduction to cases of serious harm. It then briefly discusses the implications of this position in several areas of policy concern, addressing at greater length the question of paying surrogates and donors for their contributions. It closes with criticism of the New Jersey Supreme Court's handling of these issues in the Baby M case.

Procreative Liberty and Noncoital Reproduction

Western societies place a high priority on private discretion and choice in reproductive matters. In the United States the right to avoid reproduction by contraception and abortion is now firmly established. Whether single or married, adult or minor, a woman has a right to terminate pregnancy up to viability, and both men and women have the right to obtain and use contraceptives.[1]

The right to procreate—to bear, beget, and rear children—has received less explicit legal recognition. Because the state has never tried to prevent married couples from reproducing by coital means, no cases (with the possible exception of *Skinner v. Oklahoma*)[2] turn on the recognition of such a right. However, dicta in cases ranging from *Meyer v. Nebraska* to *Eisenstadt v. Baird* clearly show a strong presumption in favor of marital decisions to found a family.[3] One may reasonably conclude that a married couple's decision to have children coitally would have fundamental-right status as part of marital liberty or privacy. The state would have the burden of showing the extreme circumstances of great harm to others—compelling state interests not achievable by less restrictive means—that would be necessary to justify state limitation on the formation of families coitally.

What then about married couples who cannot reproduce coitally? Their need and interest in forming a family may be as strong as fertile couples. Furthermore, coital infertility does not render a couple inadequate as childrearers. The values and interests that undergird the right of coital reproduction clearly exist with the coitally infertile. Their interest in bearing, begetting, or parenting offspring is no less than that of the coitally fertile.

It follows that restrictions on noncoital reproduction by an infertile married couple should be subject to the rigorous scrutiny that would be accorded restrictions on coital reproduction. Restrictions on noncoital means of reproduction should meet the strict standards for limiting coital reproduction, not a looser standard. Only serious harm to the interests of others, not avoidable by less restrictive means, should justify interference with such a fundamental choice, with the state having the burden of establishing the requisite degree of harm.[4]

Consider the analogous effect of blindness on the First Amendment right to read books. Surely a blind person has the same right to acquire information from books that a sighted person has. The inability to read visually would not bar the person from using other means, such as braille or recordings, to acquire the information contained in the book. Because receipt of the information in the book is what the First Amendment protects, the means by which the information (sight or braille or audio) is received does not itself determine the presence or absence of First Amendment rights. Restrictions on the use of braille, for example, should be subject to the same scrutiny as restrictions on the publication of printed books.[5]

Thus if bearing, begetting, or parenting children is protected as part of marital privacy or liberty, those experiences are no less important when they are achieved noncoitally with the assistance of physicians, donors of gametes and embryos, or even surrogates. Reproduction matters not because of the coitus (though that has its own independent importance) but because of what the coitus makes possible. The use of noncoital techniques, including the assistance of willing collaborators, should thus be constitutionally protected.

The result is that coitally infertile married couples (and others accorded a right of coital reproduction)[6] should have the same liberty to choose noncoital means of reproduction that they would have to reproduce coitally if they were fertile. Moral condemnation of the separation of sex and reproduction or speculative fears of a slippery slope should not suffice to restrict such techniques, since such views would not suffice to restrict coital reproduction, to ban abortion, or to suppress speech. Only serious harm to the interests of others, not avoidable by less restrictive means, should justify interference with such a fundamental reproductive choice.

Of course, noncoital techniques may be regulated if they pose special problems to others not present in coital reproduction. But since the noncoital means are essential if reproduction is to occur, the legitimacy of the regulation should be measured by the rigorous standard that would be applied to state regulation of coital reproduction. The burden of proof should be on the state to show the compelling state interest necessary to interfere with fundamental rights of procreative choice. Indeed, permitting regulation of noncoital reproduction on lesser scrutiny would unfairly discriminate against infertile married couples.

In sum, the burden of proof for justifying interference with the use of noncoital reproductive techniques by coitally infertile couples should fall on the state. The state's burden is to present clear and convincing evidence that significant harm will befall important state interests unless a proposed restriction that interferes with procreative choice is passed. It may be that protection of offspring or valid interests of collaborators or others will justify some particular restrictions on use of these techniques. But moral condemnation or speculation about exploitation, commercialism, and slippery slopes alone should not justify interference with fundamental decisions about family formation.

APPLICATION OF THIS FRAMEWORK TO PUBLIC POLICY

If the state's power to regulate noncoital techniques must take the privileged status of procreative choice into account, then the range of policy options is narrower than occurs with less privileged decisions. Total prohibition of their use may not be an option. However, many types of regulation will still be possible, depending on the burdens imposed on procreative choice and the risks of the technique. In general, the state will be limited in imposing restrictions based on moralistic or symbolic concerns aside from actual harm.

While many concerns have been raised about noncoital reproduction, I will briefly discuss the calls for restriction or regulation that aim to protect embryos, offspring, reproductive collaborators, and moral views of how reproduction should occur.

Embryo Manipulations

An important part of noncoital reproduction involves the creation, manipulation, storage, and transfer of extracorporeal embryos through IVF, embryo freezing, embryo donation, and related techniques. Since these maneuvers will often be essential for an infertile couple to form a family biologically related to one if not both of the spouses, they would prima facie be a protected part of procreative liberty. Yet many persons have objected to some or all of these techniques because of their impact on embryos.

The validity of concerns about embryo manipulation depends in the first instance on whether the embryos in question will be transferred to a uterus for implantation and possible gestation and birth. If so, the interests of future offspring who could be harmed by the pretransfer activities is at stake. Protection of offspring against prenatal harm occurring at the extra-corporeal stage is a valid cause of concern and regulation.[7]

If no transfer is planned, however, the ground for concern must rest on a notion that embryos have a right to be transferred, or to be treated in a certain way even if not transferred. I have argued elsewhere that the only tenable grounds for respecting embryos that will not otherwise be trans-ferred are symbolic rather than rights-based.[8] Such symbolic concerns are not sufficient to trump the procreative rights of infertile couples. However, restrictions on the disposition of embryos and regulation of embryo re-search may not always conflict with procreative liberty.[9] Whether the sym-bolic gains justify the cost imposed on nonprocreative interests will depend on the specific restriction.

Preventing Harm to Offspring

A major concern with noncoital reproduction is the possibility of harm to offspring. If noncoital techniques harmed offspring, the argument for ban-ning them and directing infertile couples to the adoption market would be strong. Yet the concept itself of harm to offspring from techniques that make their birth possible needs clarification. Some harms to offspring can be avoided consistent with the birth of the child, while other harms can be avoided only by avoiding the birth altogether. In the latter case, pre-venting use of the technique at issue will prevent the very existence of the child whose protection is sought.

To illustrate this point, consider the possibility of psychosocial problems from use of collaborative techniques of family formation. Gamete donation and surrogacy have been singled out as especially troublesome because of the risk that offspring will be genetically confused or bewildered by the separation of genetic, gestational, and social parentage that these tech-niques entail.[10] Could gamete donation and surrogacy be banned to protect offspring from genetic confusion or later conflicts?[11]

The difficulty with this justification for banning third-party collaborative techniques is that the child would not be born but for the technique causing the concern. Banning the technique to prevent harm to the child hardly benefits the child, for the child loses the only existence that she could have.

The psychosocial problems of split parentage surely are not so great as to render the child's life a net loss to the child. If the child's life were truly wrongful, the proper remedy would be to cease all sustaining care, so that the child might die forthwith and thus be saved from any further burden of living.[12] Protecting the child from harm is thus not an adequate reason for discouraging use of these techniques.[13]

The state, however, may regulate transactions in which children will be born to assure that they are born in a reasonably healthy way. An important area for state regulation to protect the welfare of offspring is to assure that children born of collaborative transactions with donors and surrogates may obtain information about their genetic or gestational parents, if not also their actual identities. The split of genetic, gestational, and social parentage may be psychologically significant for many offspring. Although the situation is not exactly akin to adoption, enough shared elements exist to suggest that information about genetic and gestational identity may take on great importance for the offspring. It is less clear that offspring also need to know that they were conceived by IVF or resulted from frozen and thawed embryos.

While a strong argument in favor of permitting offspring to know or learn their genetic and gestational heritage can be made, the law has progressed slowly in making such information available to adopted children.[14] Because collaborative offspring will be born before this issue has been definitively settled, it is important that records be kept, so that offspring might have access to them at a later time if public policy or the original parties later permit access. Laws assuring access to some information should also be considered.

But laws allowing offspring access to parental information may discourage some persons from serving as gamete donors and surrogates. At present many programs involving donors and surrogates require anonymity and pledges of confidentiality. Collaborators may assert the right to be kept anonymous, thus conflicting with the offspring's need to know their genetic forebears. Yet the state's interest in assuring that children who are born have certain information concerning their identity would properly outweigh the privacy concerns of participants.[15] Infertile couples have no right to form families in ways that would harm offspring, when the offspring can be born free of the harm at issue. Thus laws assuring offspring access to parental information would be within state power.

Regulation to Protect Participants in Collaborative Reproductive Transactions

The greatest policy need may be for regulation to assure that participants will receive quality services, with certainty about legal effects, as a result of informed and knowing choices about use of their reproductive capacities.

Since regulations aimed at this goal will generally not interfere with or prevent noncoital family formation, the state will not have to meet the heavy burden of proof necessary for substantial interference or limitations on access. A rational basis test can easily be met when the state's efforts are directed at assuring good quality services, certainty of contracts, and knowledgeable contract formation.

Several types of public policy protections would thus clearly fall within state power.[16] Regulations designed to assure a minimum level of quality of care for consumers of these services would doubtlessly be valid. Quality control, through licensing and regulation of the health professionals, storage banks, and other parts of the system, would seem to be within state power. Informing consumers of actual success rates may also be desirable.[17]

A second regulatory area would be devices to assure that participants (gamete donors, recipients, and surrogates) in collaborative reproduction and in embryo and gamete storage make informed and knowing decisions about the consequences of their choices. In many cases a full and adequate informed consent procedure at the time of production, deposit, storage, or donation of gametes and embryos—including written statements communicating options and specifying the parties' wishes concerning rearing rights and duties and future decision contingencies—will suffice.[18] Whether more formalized procedures are needed to assure consent will depend on experience and the problems that arise. For example, some have proposed making surrogate contracts binding when the contract has been reviewed by a court to assure informed consent.[19] Because such procedures enhance autonomy and reproductive choice, they are easily reconciled with the demands of procreative liberty.[20]

A third area of acceptable public policy regulation is legislation or regulation that gives explicit legal recognition to use of noncoital techniques, so that infertile couples and collaborators have certainty about the legal effects of their decisions to proceed. For example, greater legal certainty about the rearing rights and duties towards offspring born of donor gametes or surrogacy or after posthumous thawing and transfer will enhance the likelihood that people will choose these techniques of reproduction. Predictable rearing outcomes will encourage financial and emotional investment in these reproductive alternatives.

Clarifying legislation is also desirable to resolve uncertainties and disputes in advance, and thus avoid painful custody battles such as the one that arose in the Baby M case. However, persons who have moral objections to embryo technology or collaborative techniques may oppose clarifying legislation because of the legitimacy it appears to give to those practices.[21]

The most controversial issue is, of course, the substance of such clarifying legislation. The major choice here is whether to give effect to the preconception or pre-implantation agreements of the parties concerning rearing rights and duties. Agreements to exclude gamete donors from later rearing are most easily accepted, since this has been the experience with donor sperm and has received legislative recognition in thirty states.[22] Agreements to exclude egg donors should be treated similarly.[23] Whether pre-conception agreements to exclude the surrogate from later rearing will also be enforced has been more hotly contested. A strong argument can be made that failure to enforce surrogate contracts, if only by damages, would violate the procreative rights of the infertile couple, though the New Jersey Supreme Court in the Baby M case took a different view.[24]

Interference on Symbolic Grounds: Paying Money

An important feature about demands for regulation of noncoital reproductive technologies is that explicitly or upon closer scrutiny many of the objections amount to moralistic or symbolic concerns that have no direct connection with actual harm to others. The Vatican's objections to all forms of IVF, for example, appear rooted in a moralistic view that separating sex and reproduction is per se immoral and to be discouraged.[25] Similarly, the Vatican's opposition to gamete donation because it is "contrary to the unity of marriage and the dignity of the procreation of the human person" is clearly a symbolic or moralistic judgment.[26] While the claim is often made that such immoral conduct will ultimately affect the welfare of offspring, the parents, the family, and society, nonspeculative evidence of harm sufficient to satisfy the state's burden of proof for restricting family formation by infertile couples is missing. Laws that prohibited IVF and gamete donation on this basis would be highly suspect, and would most likely be found unconstitutional.[27]

Another kind of symbolic objection appears in proposals to ban payments to gamete donors and surrogates. The concern with paying donors for their gametes and embryos seems to be symbolic or moralistic, for the chance of coercion or exploitation seems slight. The gamete donors would be selling renewable tissue usually obtainable without the bodily intrusion that sale of kidneys would entail (though some egg donors might undergo surgical removal with moderate risk).[28] At bottom the concern is that there is something denigrating or dehumanizing about trafficking in human embryos or gametes.[29]

In evaluating such claims, we must distinguish personal moral views and practices from public policy. Persons are clearly free to donate gametes or embryos without compensation because they find it dehumanizing to be paid. But should they also be free, through state power, to ban payments to persons who are willing to receive them? If a ban on payments for gametes and embryos would interfere with the ability of infertile couples to obtain needed gametes or embryos, then the privileged status of procreative liberty would place on the state the burden of showing substantial harm from paying donors. But it is difficult to show harm from payment, other than harm to a moral conception or view of dignity and commodification—a view that is disparately and not necessarily widely held. The desire of some to make a symbolic statement or express a moralistic judgment by banning payments would not be sufficiently compelling to justify this infringement of procreative choice.[30]

Paying surrogates might seem to be a different matter because of the greater gestational burden involved and the greater risk of coercion or exploitation of poorer women. Prof. Margaret Radin, for example, argues that paying surrogates could make both women and children "completely monetizable and fungible objects of exchange," alienating them from their personhood in a way that brings about "an inferior conception of human flourishing."[31] In the view of many, including the New Jersey Supreme Court in the Baby M case, such concerns about commodification are good grounds for legal prohibition of paid surrogacy.

Such concerns may well inform private sector efforts and individual choice. Persons are free not to participate in surrogacy arrangements or to participate altruistically without fee. However, a ban on payment will probably make it impossible for many couples to obtain the surrogate assistance they need to achieve their reproductive goals. Although motivated by a complex of factors, most surrogates will want to be paid for their considerable efforts.[32] Indeed, it is only fair to pay them for their labor, especially when sperm donors and all sorts of other physical laborers are paid.

Are fears about commodification of sufficient weight to justify state prohibition on payment which will prevent infertile couples from recruiting surrogates? The case for banning paid surrogacy would be stronger if coercion or exploitation of women clearly resulted. But financial inducements are not alone coercive. Surrogates surely have other ways of obtaining food, shelter, and other necessities, and in most cases will have alternative employment opportunities. A choice about how to use one's reproductive capacity is not coerced just because it is motivated in part by a desire for money. Also, it is unclear how surrogates are any more exploited than men and women who decide to join the military, be professional athletes, work in the petrochemical industry, or labor in the Texas sun—activities that impose risk and use the body in varying ways.

In short, the offense of paid surrogacy is largely symbolic. The concern is less with actual harm to the surrogates than with harm to a particular conception of how reproduction should occur and how a woman should use her gestational capacity. According to Radin, the danger is that all women and children will be seen as paid gestators or as commodities. But it is also possible that surrogates will be viewed as worthy collaborators in a joint reproductive enterprise from which all parties gain, with money being one way that the infertile couple pays its debt or obligation to the surrogate.[33] Given the multiple meanings that can be found in paid surrogacy and the speculative nature of fears about commodification of women and children, one particular moral-symbolic view of the transaction should not be sufficient to trump the fundamental procreative rights of infertile couples.

The key point for public policy regarding noncoital technology is that the community has no right through prohibition to express its moral views concerning intimate matters that are allocated to private discretion. This point is firmly established in the abortion context. A moral view about the worth of the early fetus and the immorality of abortion is not sufficient to override the right to have an abortion.[34] Nor can fears about commodifying the destruction of human life justify bans on paying doctors who perform abortions or on advertisements of their services.[35] Similarly, moral objections to the dehumanizing effects of profiting from the sale of sexually explicit material does not justify interfering with constitutional rights to read such material. If moral objections or speculation unrelated to actual harm would not justify interfering with contraception, abortion or coital reproduction, they should have no more weight in barring access to noncoital reproductive techniques dependent on payments, such as surrogacy.

THE NEW JERSEY SUPREME COURT AND PROCREATIVE LIBERTY

As public policy attempts to grapple with noncoital reproduction, the points discussed above need to be kept clearly in mind. Yet legislators and courts have often ignored or misunderstood the heavy burden that state regulation or restriction of these techniques must satisfy. An example of such confusion is the New Jersey Supreme Court's handling of these issues in the Baby M case.

In *Baby M* the New Jersey Supreme Court wrote a careful and craftsmanlike opinion interpreting New Jersey adoption statutes as excluding paid and enforceable surrogacy contracts. Although the statutes were not written with paid surrogacy in mind, the court was making a traditional juristic move in finding that existing adoption laws also applied to the new but distinguishable situation of surrogacy.[36]

Yet the opinion is quite cursory and superficial in discussing the constitutionality of the statutes that it interpreted to bar paid or enforceable surrogacy. The gaps and errors in its analysis are worth pausing over, for they show the need for policy-makers to pay closer attention to the procreative rights of infertile couples.

The New Jersey Supreme Court deals with the infertile couple's constitutional claim to paid, enforceable surrogacy contracts as a claim of a "right to procreate."[37] In rejecting this claim, the court gives "procreation" a very narrow definition that overlooks the infertile couple's interest both in conceiving and in rearing offspring, i.e., in forming a family that is biologically related to at least one of the parents (or both where the surrogate provides gestation of the embryo created by the couple). The court states without analysis or explanation:

> The right to procreate very simply is the right to have natural children, whether through sexual intercourse or artificial insemination. It is no more than that. Mr. Stern has not been deprived of that right. Through artificial insemination of Mrs. Whitehead, Baby M is his child. The custody, care, companionship, and nurturing that follow birth are not parts of the right to procreation: they are rights that may also be constitutionally protected, but that involve many considerations other than the right of procreation. . . .
>
> We conclude that the right of procreation is best understood and protected if confined to its essentials, and that when dealing with rights concerning the resulting child different interests come into play.[38]

The major problem here is the court's artificial separation of conception or begetting from rearing—the result that makes conception itself so worthy of protection. Perhaps genetic transfer or the begetting of biologic offspring without rearing itself deserves constitutional protection (a matter that remains to be elucidated by the Supreme Court).[39] But genetic transfer with intended rearing—the essence of procreative liberty—is another matter. Since genetic transfer for rearing is worthy of protection when achieved coitally by a married couple, genetic transfer for the purpose of rearing achieved noncoitally should also be protected. In *Baby M*, Mr. Stern's interest in hiring a surrogate is precisely to conceive a child whom he will then rear. His efforts should thus receive the same protected status that coital efforts to form a family with biologic offspring would receive.

Yet the court severs his interest in conceiving and rearing by posing a conflict between the right to rear of one biologic parent and the right to rear of the other biologic parent:

> To assert that Mr. Stern's right of procreation gives him the right to custody of Baby M would be to assert that Mrs. Whitehead's right of procreation does not give her the right to the custody of Baby M; it would be to assert that the constitutional right of procreation includes within it a constitutionally protected contractual right to destroy someone else's right of procreation.[40]

But this passage misdescribes the scope of procreative liberty to form families with biologically related offspring. Of course, each biologic parent (or procreator) has an equal claim to rear their biologic offspring. The question is how to arbitrate if there is a conflict, and either parent is a fit child-rearer. In that case neither the father's nor the mother's claim should automatically trump the other. The decision must be made on some other basis. A strong argument based on the autonomy of couples and surrogates can be made that the preconception agreement of the parties, which made the very existence of the child possible, should prima facie be determinative, just as it would be with sperm or egg donors.

The court further states:

> There is nothing in our culture or society that even begins to suggest a fundamental right on the part of the father to the custody of the child as part of his right to procreate when opposed by the claim of the mother to the same child.[41]

The statement repeats this error by overlooking the pre-conception agreement of the mother to be inseminated and to relinquish the resulting child. It simply is unclear why that agreement, if knowingly and freely made, should not control in those circumstances. The question to be analyzed is whether the surrogate's disappointment constitutes the compelling state interest necessary to override the infertile couple's right to form a family (e.g., procreate) noncoitally.

By failing to focus clearly on the protected status of the couple's use of noncoital means of family formation, the court avoids assigning the proper weight to the couple's need, and consequently to the necessity of weighing more closely the asserted reasons for overriding that interest. The court should have recognized the infertile couple's right to produce children noncoitally and then analyzed the reasons why the surrogate's change of mind did or did not justify overriding that right. When arrayed against the fundamental right of the couple, the concerns of the surrogate who knowingly chooses this role may turn out to be less weighty than they did to the court.

The policies behind criminal prohibition of paid surrogacy should also have been analyzed in this light. Absent a strong certainty of actual harm to the participants, a ban on payment serves symbolic or moralistic concerns. While these concerns provide a rational basis for state action, they would appear to be insufficient to trump the couple's need to hire a surrogate to found their family. Once again the court's analysis is flawed because it fails to analyze how a prohibitive statute impinges on the ability of infertile couples to form families, thus relieving the state of satisfying the heavy burden of proof for interfering with an infertile couple's use of noncoital reproductive techniques.

The incoherence of the court's approach emerges in other statements. For example, it states that its conclusion "illustrat[es] that a person's rights of privacy and self-determination are qualified by the effect on innocent third persons of the exercise of those rights."[42] It amplifies this point in a footnote, which after citing cases on abortion and forced treatment for the sake of third parties, states:

> In the present case, the parties' right to procreate by methods of their own choosing cannot be enforced without consideration of the state's interest in protecting the resulting child, just as the right to the companionship of one's child cannot be enforced without consideration of that crucial state interest.[43]

Of course, one cannot quarrel with this broad principle. Fundamental rights are not absolute and can be limited to protect innocent third parties from substantial harm. Noncoital techniques could be restricted to protect offspring or others from substantial harm. But the possibility of restriction does not speak to the level or certainty of harm that must be met to justify such restriction. When dealing with fundamental rights, more than a rational basis for restriction is' necessary. Mere speculation about harm to third parties will not do, yet the court relies on such a flimsy basis in banning paid surrogacy.[44] Indeed, banning paid surrogacy to protect offspring will simply prevent their coming into being. This hardly protects them, since being born to an enforced and paid surrogacy agreement hardly amounts to wrongful life.[45]

The deficiencies in the New Jersey Supreme Court's discussion of procreative liberty show how far the courts are from developing a coherent framework of analysis for public policy decisions concerning noncoital technologies. The desire of infertile couples to form biologically related families implicates constitutionally protected interests. It may be that state interests justify interference with those decisions in some cases, but such interests should be evaluated by the strict standards that would be applied to coital reproduction.

A Comment on Professors Capron and Radin

Legal and ethical commentators also have difficulty in seeing how a married couple's procreative liberty is implicated in surrogacy and other noncoital reproductive arrangements. In a later chapter of this book two respected legal academics argue that paid surrogacy should be prohibited and surrogate contracts should not be enforced.[46] In making their argument, however, Professors Capron and Radin overlook several key points about the constitutional status of procreative liberty.[47]

One error they make is to interpret the claim of a constitutional right to hire a surrogate as the claim of a right to proceed free of any regulation at all. But the claim presented here is not an argument "that there is an absolute right to paid surrogacy," as Professors Capron and Radin assert.[48] Rather, the argument is that because bans on paid surrogacy will prevent many infertile married couples from rearing children biologically related to one if not both rearing partners, they should be tested by the same rigorous standards that would be applied to bans on coital reproduction.

When that test is applied, regulations designed to assure the free, knowing choice of the parties and access of offspring to information about parentage may well be valid. On the other hand, prohibitions on paid surrogacy (and related activities such as advertising or for-profit surrogacy brokers) will fail if their purpose is to prevent a perception—not universally shared—that women and offspring are thereby "commodified," or that payment to surrogates is somehow inconsistent with human dignity. In any event, the claim is not to an absolute right but to a presumptive right, with the state bearing the heavy burden of showing compelling grounds for preventing infertile couples from forming biologically related families by the means in question.[49]

A second error is their rejection of a presumptive constitutional right to enforcement of surrogate (and other collaborative reproductive) agreements on the ground that such a claim "fails to distinguish negative from positive freedom."[50] It is true that substantive due process rights of liberty or privacy are negative rights against state interference, not rights to have the state provide the resources needed to exercise the right in question. As *Maher v. Roe* makes clear, the right to abort is a right to obtain the service without state interference.[51] It is not a right "to state aid in effectuating"[52] the choice to abort when the aid desired is the cost of the abortion itself.

But *Maher* and its structure of negative and positive rights is not apposite to the issue of surrogate or donor contract enforcement. The comparable situation with infertility would be a claim to state funds for indigent persons to hire a surrogate or to pay the costs of IVF. Failing to fund indigent access to noncoital techniques does not interfere with procreative liberty any more than failure to fund abortions does.

Seeking state enforcement of surrogacy agreements is not a claim for state funding of surrogacy for the indigent. Since funding of the infertility remedy itself is not at issue, characterizing access to contract enforcement as a negative or positive right is not determinative. Although the claim to enforcement is to a government service, it is a claim to a service unavailable privately and which is generally provided to all persons who make legal contracts. Thus denial of generally available contract remedies to reproductive collaborators functions like state interference with the negative right of procreative liberty.

A claimed right to enforcement of donor and surrogate contracts may also be posited in terms of equal protection. Excluding reproductive collaborators from remedies available to enforce other legal contracts treats reproductive collaborators unequally. Since this differential treatment may discourage infertile couples from making the donor or surrogate contracts essential to form families, the state's reasons for the differential treatment should be strictly scrutinized.[53] If a compelling reason for the unequal treatment is necessary, protecting human dignity or preventing surrogate disappointment may not be sufficient to deny access to the courts.

An analogy to abortion will help to clarify the point. Suppose a state, to avoid lending its resources to abortion, refuses to enforce all contracts arising from or related to the performance of abortion, including suits by physicians to collect the fee for the abortion, or suits by employees of an abortion clinic for payment of wages.[54] Such a law could be viewed as an interference with the right to abort (abortions will be harder to obtain if such contract remedies are unavailable). It could also be viewed as a violation of equal protection in access to the courts, requiring more than a rational basis justification because of its impact on abortion. A view that supporting abortion in this way is demeaning to human dignity or amounts to recognizing a claim of "freedom to" rather than "freedom from" state interference would not justify such exclusion.[55]

Professors Capron and Radin may overlook this point because of their mistaken assumption that recognizing a presumptive right to donor and surrogate contract enforcement would "generate an affirmative duty on the part of the state to enforce all arrangements through which people seek to form a family . . . including paying money for any adoption."[56]

But as previously noted, it does not follow that all such contracts would have to be enforced—only those for which the state has no compelling reason to override. For example, protecting the welfare of the resulting offspring might justify overriding the rearing arrangement in a particular case, as it might with pledges of confidentiality. On the other hand, if both surrogate and hiring couple are fit childrearers, the later disappointment of the surrogate might not be a sufficient reason to overcome her freely made, informed preconception agreement. Reproductive rights are not absolute. But they do put the burden on the state to show the compelling need to override them.

Nor would it follow that paying money for adoption would also be constitutionally protected. I have been discussing the status of offspring biologically related to at least one, if not both, rearing partners (as with gestational surrogacy or IVF). The claim is not to acquire any child to rear, but to acquire a biologically related child. Because of the traditional psychosocial meanings that attach to biologic kinship, that connection may be protected even if the right to form families with nonbiologically related offspring is not. Although accepting my position might set up a strong case for recognizing the latter as well, forming families with nonbiologically related offspring raises independent issues. The right to hire surrogates to bear biologically related offspring does not necessarily entail a right to pay women to relinquish offspring for adoption.

Conclusion

Public policy efforts to deal with noncoital reproduction must recognize the strong presumption in favor of private choice that use of these techniques necessarily requires. Because noncoital means may be essential for couples to form families, the use of IVF, gamete donors and surrogates should occupy a privileged position vis-à-vis state power, akin to the position occupied by coital reproduction. The Constitution, in short, has preempted many questions of public policy by allocating primary choice over use of noncoital techniques to infertile couples seeking to rear children biologically related to at least one of the parties.

As a result, the state must carry the burden of showing actual harm from use of these techniques, if it seeks to regulate them in a way that will substantially interfere with access by infertile couples. The moralistic or symbolic concerns that have figured so largely in public controversy over these techniques will not satisfy this burden. Policy-makers should pay attention to these principles if they wish to respect the freedom of infertile couples while protecting important state interests that arise in reproduction by infertile couples.

References

1. Bellotti v. Baird, 443 U.S. 622 (1979); Carey v. Population Servs. Int'l, 431 U.S. 678 (1977); Planned Parenthood v. Danforth, 428 U.S. 52 (1976); Roe v. Wade, 410 U.S. 113 (1973); Eisenstadt v. Baird, 405 U.S. 438 (1972); Griswold v. Connecticut, 381 U.S. 479 (1965).

2. 316 U.S. 535, 541 (1942).

3. For quotations from these cases and the applicable citations, see John Robertson, "Procreative Liberty and the Control of Conception, Pregnancy and Childbirth," *Virginia Law Review*, 69 (1983): 405, 414, n. 23.

The right involved here may be formulated either as the couple's right to reproduce or as a right to form a family. The latter formulation may be more desirable, since it is the couple's experience of rearing offspring biologically related to one or both of them that seems essential, rather than transmission of genes alone without rearing. However, since reproduction often leads to the rearing experiences at issue, talk of a right to "reproduce" or "procreate" is also accurate.

4. The need for the assistance of physicians, donors, and surrogates does not make noncoital reproduction a less protected aspect of marital privacy. Abortion is protected as part of procreative privacy even though it occurs under the gaze of and with the assistance of physicians and nurses. The personal importance of a decision or activity, rather than its secrecy from the gaze of others, determines its status as part of protected privacy (or liberty, to be more precise). In fact, the use of donors and surrogates will often occur "privately," with no one other than the couple and physician aware of the anonymous provision of missing reproductive factors.

40 SURROGATE MOTHERHOOD

5. For example, printing braille may necessitate the use of chemical and metallurgical processes that threaten environmental or physical harm to persons, just as use of donors and surrogates may be thought to threaten the welfare of offspring or the family. In either case, however, state action should be subject to the strict scrutiny that would be applied to restrictions on buying books or on coital reproduction. Technological aids to overcome physical disability may implicate different state interests, but they do not diminish the importance of the end being sought.

6. Robertson, "Procreative Liberty," supra note 3, at 427–33. See also John Robertson, "Embryos, Families and Procreative Liberty: The Legal Structure of the New Reproduction," *Southern California Law Review*, 59 (1986): 939, 957–62.

7. Robertson, "Embryos," supra note 6, at 987.

8. Id.: 974–75.

9. For example, the symbolic gain of showing respect for all human life by requiring donation of unwanted embryos may be outweighed by the psychosocial harm to gamete sources who wish no genetic offspring. Similarly, the symbolic gains from prohibiting the creation of embryos for research purposes may be outweighed by the loss of knowledge that results from this limitation on research. Id.: 980–85.

10. Noncoital techniques involving IVF may pose the threat of physical harm as well, but the evidence to date does not suggest a higher rate of physical defects in offspring from external conception. Id.: 991–92.

11. It should be noted that such offspring will have a biologic tie with at least one of the rearing parents and thus may be in a more favorable rearing situation than are adopted children.

12. Robertson, "Embryos," supra note 6, at 988–89.

13. Harm to offspring is to be distinguished from harm to others who must bear the costs of rearing offspring born as a result of these techniques. But this is a different basis for regulation than preventing harm to offspring, and should be evaluated like any other restrictions on reproduction enacted in order to prevent the imposition of rearing burdens on others. Id.: 989–90.

14. Id.: 1015–18, and authorities cited therein.

15. The result of such laws may be to discourage some collaborative births from occurring. But this result would not violate the rights of the children not then born, for no person exists with rights to be violated. The unborn have no right to be born. See id: 1018.

16. For a fuller discussion of these policy issues see, gen., id.

17. IVF programs have been notorious for giving patients inaccurate and overly optimistic estimates of likely success from use of the technique, when many IVF programs have had no or few live births. Soules, "The in Vitro Fertilization Pregnancy Rate: Let's Be Honest with One Another," *Fertility & Sterility*, 43 (1985): 511–12.

18. John Robertson, "Ethical and Legal Issues in the Cryopreservation of Human Embryos," *Fertility & Sterility*, 47 (1987): 371, 373–74.

19. A New York legislative committee proposed such a bill, which has received much favorable attention. New York State Senate Judiciary Committee, *Surrogate Parenting in New York: A Proposal for Legislative Reform* (Dec. 1986).

20. Planned Parenthood of Missouri v. Danforth, 428 U.S. 52 (1976) (requirement of written consent for abortions permissible even though no such consent is required for other medical procedures).

21. Robertson, "Embryos," supra note 6, at 1039.

22. For citations to these statutes, see Congress of the United States, Office of Technology Assessment, *Infertility Treatment and Prevention* (April 1988).

The enforceability of agreements to include the donor in rearing have not received legislative support, though some courts have given effect to such arrangements with donor sperm. See Robertson, "Embryos," supra note 6, at 1005–6.

23. John Robertson, "Technology and Motherhood: Ethical and Legal Issues in Human Egg Donation," *Case Western Reserve Law Review*, forthcoming.

24. See below for a critique of this decision.

25. Magisterium of the Catholic Church, *Instruction on Respect for Human Life in Its Origin and on the Dignity of Procreation: Replies to Certain Questions of the Day*, 25 (Feb. 22, 1987). See also "Dissenting Statement of Father Richard McCormick," *Fertility & Sterility*, 46 (1986), Supp. App. A, 82S.

26. Magisterium, supra note 25.

27. Robertson, "Embryos," supra note 6, at 965–67.

28. Robertson, "Technology," supra note 23, at 25.

29. George Annas, "Redefining Parenthood and Protecting Embryos: Why We Need New Laws," *Hastings Center Report*, 37 (Oct. 1984): 50–52.

30. The question of what is a sale also arises with payments for donation of embryos. The question of payment is most likely to arise when the recipient or transferee of an embryo is asked to pay a fee to cover acquisition and storage costs. Because creation of embryos is expensive ($700 to $1,000 per embryo in many American programs) and cryopreservation charges will arise, it is not unreasonable to ask the recipient of an embryo donation to share production and storage costs. Recoupment of costs can be distinguished from payments that reflect "profit" or other monetary gain from embryo donation.

The parallel to organ donation is instructive. The recipient of an organ transplant, rather than the donor family, pays the costs of maintaining brain dead cadavers and surgically removing donated organs. Such payments are consistent with a policy against the buying and selling of organs, and are explicitly recognized in the National Organ Transplant Act of 1984, 42 U.S.C.A. #274e (West Supp. 1987). A similar policy with embryo donations might permit the recipient to share the costs of embryo production and storage.

31. Margaret Radin, "Market-Inalienability," *Harvard Law Review*, 100 (1987): 1849, 1921–36. Whether my argument against a ban on payment of surrogate salaries would also invalidate laws against buying babies or paying fees beyond medical expenses for adoption is beyond the scope of this paper. See Robertson, "Embryos," supra note 6, at 961, n. 69.

32. Other motivations include a wish for attention, the desire for pregnancy and reproduction without the burdens of rearing, and the opportunity to relive and master a previous incident of relinquishing a child. Parker, "Motivation of Surrogate Mothers: Initial Findings," *American Journal of Psychiatry*, 140 (1983): 117.

33. For a discussion of the obligation to repay gifts, see Marcel Mauss, *The Gift* (1967); see also Murray, "Gifts of the Body and the Needs of Strangers," *Hastings Center Report*, 17 (1987): 30–35.

34. Roe v. Wade, 410 U.S. 113 (1973).

35. Bigelow v. Virginia, 421 U.S. 809 (1975).

36. An important difference between surrogacy and adoption is that the father has a genetic connection with the child—he is the father—that is missing in adoption.

37. 537 A.2d 1227, 1253 (N.J. 1988).

38. Id.

39. The United States Supreme Court has been willing to terminate a father's rearing rights when he played no rearing role for some period after birth. See Lehr v. Robertson, 463 U.S. 248 (1983); Parham v. Hughes, 441 U.S. 347 (1979).

The validity of mandatory embryo donation laws in lieu of discard also remains to be determined. See Robertson, "Embryos," supra note 6, at 979–81.

40. 537 A.2d 1227, 1254 (N.J. 1988).

41. Id.

42. Id.

43. Id.

44. Id: 1241–42.

45. Indeed, the state's concerns in *Baby M*, according to the court's interpretation of the adoption statutes, were not protection of the child's welfare but protection of the mother against exploitation and her later change of mind. These are not concerns about innocent third parties, but about the interests of adults who knowingly participate in the surrogate arrangement and then change their mind. It is not clear that their interests deserve the same protection as that of "innocent third parties."

46. A. M. Capron and M. J. Radin, "Choosing Family Law over Contract Law as a Paradigm for Surrogate Motherhood."

47. Id. The New York State Task Force on Life and the Law has recommended a public policy remarkably close to the result reached in the *Baby M* case—*Surrogate Parenting: Analysis and Recommendations for Public Policy* (1988). Its analysis of the constitutional issues is also flawed. To take one example, it states that "neither existing caselaw nor the underlying principles of the cases involving the right to privacy can logically be extended to provide constitutional protection to surrogate parenting" (id). But as this article makes clear, it is precisely the underlying logic of procreative liberty that gives infertile couples the presumptive right to form biologically related families with the use of surrogates or donors, or of other noncoital techniques.

48. Capron and Radin.

49. Thus there is a substantive constitutional right to pay donors and surrogates for their assistance in overcoming a married couple's infertility, just as there is a right to pay doctors for assistance in treating infertility, in childbirth, or in abortion. If payment is necessary to form the family, it will not do to assert that "there is no substantive constitutional guarantee for people's choices to commodify reproductive capacities or children" (Capron and Radin). One can as easily rail against paid abortion on the ground that it "commodifies" fetuses because they are killed for money.

50. Capron and Radin.

51. 432 U.S. 464 (1977).

52. Capron and Radin.

53. I assume that lack of contract remedies will discourage infertile couples from pursuing these alternatives.

54. If nonenforcement has little effect on their willingness to proceed, then there may be insufficient burdening or interference with procreative choice to call forth the higher standard of scrutiny that I have argued for. See, e.g., Whalen v. Roe, 429 U.S. 589 (1977).

55. One could make the same point, albeit not involving contract enforcement, with a law that denied abortion clinics police protection, in order to prevent the state "dirtying its hands" by support of or association with abortion.

56. Capron and Radin.

Fairy Tales Surrogate
Mothers Tell

George J. Annas

How did surrogate motherhood evolve from a "harebrained, fly by night" idea of the late 1970s into one that had at least some mainstream, middle-class support in the mid-1980s? Many explanations have been suggested. Although the rate of infertility has not increased,[1] infertility is no longer a secret, and there are major public support groups, like RESOLVE, that advocate for infertile couples. New and powerful techniques like IVF (in vitro fertilization) have been developed, and although they help very few people,[2] they have been widely publicized and approved. And babies are fashionable again. As one movie critic put it: "Men and women do not fall in love with each other in the movies anymore. They fall in love with babies. Babies are the new lovers—unpredictable, uncontrollable, impossible and irresistible."[3]

These explanations all have some merit. But the core of surrogate motherhood lies in the modern fairy tale that babies can properly be viewed as a consumer product for those with money to purchase them, and that by permitting this transaction we will all live happily ever after. As a product babies have been hyped by slick, white, middle-class professionals and advertised in the free-market environment of the 1980s. We are asked not to look behind the resulting children to see their lower-middle-class and lower-class mothers. But the core reality of surrogate motherhood is that it is both classist and sexist: a method to obtain children genetically related to white males by exploiting poor women. While it is promoted as simply supplying babies for those who "desperately" want them, in fact it subverts any principled notion of economic fairness and justice, and undermines our commitment to equality and the inherently priceless value of human life.

We all have myths to comfort us when reality is unacceptable. Surrogate motherhood is just one such myth. But the myth of surrogate motherhood is no longer sustainable, and without its fairy tale veneer, surrogate motherhood, as we now know it, cannot long survive. This brief article will argue that the death of commercial surrogacy should not be mourned. Instead, our attention should turn to planning for the future, to avoid the commercialization of human embryos, the degradation of pregnancy, and the further exacerbation of class distinctions and economic violence that the use of embryos genetically unrelated to the "surrogate mothers" who bear them could bring.

THE BIRTH OF "SURROGATE MOTHERHOOD"

Attorney Noel Keane, the self-proclaimed "father of surrogate mother-hood," first got the idea when Jane and her husband Tom visited him in September 1976.[4] Tom had "this harebrained idea of finding another woman to carry a child for them" (Jane was infertile) but didn't know how to go about it. He had ruled out adoption:

> Maybe it's egotistical but I want my own child. Adoption leaves me cold. I guess for some women, as long as they have a child, it's fine. But for me, it's like if I see my child do something, I need to know that he's *really mine*.[5]

Tom had met Jane during the Vietnam War. He had seen a lot of men get killed, and told Keane:

> [S]ay, if a woman had a couple of children and her husband was killed in the war, and, say, she needed a few extra dollars for the family, well, then maybe she could help someone out who couldn't have children. *The Lord intended women to have children and I thought maybe one would want to do what came naturally* and maybe help somebody else out while helping herself and her family. Like I say, *it's just a fly-by-night idea* I had.[6]

Tom needed an attorney because he wanted anonymity; otherwise, he said, "I could just go out and look for a woman." While Keane was thinking it over, an article appeared in the *San Francisco Chronicle* about a man who had successfully advertised to find a woman to bear a child for him through artificial insemination. He had paid $7,000 to the woman and another $3,000 in legal and medical expenses. The child was born September 6, 1976. Shortly thereafter a medical newspaper reported the story, headlining it: " 'Surrogate Mother' Is Recruited by Ad for Artificial Insemination." Noel Keane made his decision: "I had never done as much as an adoption, but if they can do it in California, I thought, what the hell, we can do it here."[7]

Tom and Jane eventually made a deal with Carol to be inseminated. There was no fee involved, because Keane had been properly advised by a probate court judge that fees were illegal in Michigan. Carol, who was divorced, recalls making the decision with her three sons. "I told them what good parents Tom and Jane would be, and, from the start, we agreed we would call *it* Tom and Jane's baby, *never mother's baby.*"[8] When Carol became pregnant, Jane recalls: "*I wanted to put Carol under a glass bowl.* You know, don't do this, don't do that. Are you eating right? Are you drinking enough? Are you taking your vitamins?"[9] The contract that Tom and Jane signed with Noel Keane stated, explicitly, "[I]f a surrogate is found and is, in fact, inseminated, there is no assurance she will give up the child."[10]

Carol did give up the child. But Keane's first case illustrates most of the problems and pitfalls of so-called "surrogate motherhood" that remain unresolved more than a decade later: the use of fairy tale language, the commodification of children, and the degradation of pregnant women.

THE REALITY BEHIND THE FAIRY TALES

Fairy tale language is not unique to surrogate motherhood. In the past year alone we have witnessed glitzy TV evangelists preach that they must have our money because God has demanded it, national security advisers surreptitiously trading arms for Iran-held hostages in the name of democratic values, and insatiable stock manipulators using inside information for personal gain in the name of free enterprise. Touted as family building for infertile couples, surrogate motherhood stems from the same greed that threatens the best impulses and values in our society. The truth about surrogacy's "family building" is that it can create one parent-child relationship only by destroying another parent-child relationship. As Elizabeth Kane, the country's first openly paid "surrogate mother," put it recently, "[S]urrogate motherhood is nothing more than the transference of pain from one woman to another."[11] Even its strongest supporters freely admit that if they could not pay women a large fee for giving up their children, they would be out of business. And the brokers, like Noel Keane, usually charge at least as much for their own services (approximately $10,000) as they are willing to pay women to undertake a pregnancy and give up their child. Nor is it "just like adoption." Adoption seeks to find rearing parents for children without them; surrogacy seeks a child for would-be rearing parents. Adoption places the interests of the child first; surrogacy places the interests of the adults first. The exclusive use of this method by rich and upper-middle-class white couples proclaims its economic class and racial characteristics. For example, although black couples are *twice* as likely as white couples to be infertile,[12] this method is not promoted for black couples, nor has anyone openly advocated covering the procedure by Medicaid for poor infertile couples.

The central deception, of course, is the name itself. The term "surrogate motherhood" seems purposely designed to dehumanize the mother and alienate her from her child. As Noel Keane put it in commenting favorably on the lower court *Baby M* decision, "She [the surrogate mother] has to realize she is carrying *their child*."[13] As the New Jersey Supreme Court noted simply and forcefully, in the Baby M case, "the natural mother [is] inappropriately termed the 'surrogate mother.' "[14] Whenever we decide not to give something its rightful, descriptive name (in this case, "mother" or "birth-mother"), it seems fair to assume that we are at least uncomfortable with the reality we are describing and want to believe some myth instead. In this case, the phrase "surrogate mother" actually comes from Harlow's monkey studies, in which newborn monkeys were separated from their mothers and placed in cages with a wire or a cloth-covered inanimate "surrogate mother" to test their responses.[15] Indeed, this identification of the "surrogate mother" as inanimate object is often complete, the so-called surrogate mother being referred to simply as the "surrogate," and sometimes as a "surrogate womb" or a "surrogate uterus."

Finally, although an attempt is almost always made to conflate "surrogate motherhood" with new science and technology, and with "new reproductive techniques," in fact the only thing new about this method is the introduction of attorneys into human reproduction. And the lawyer's role itself is inherently deceptive. Drafting a contract all parties sign, the lawyer usually assures them that it is "not enforceable"—but nonetheless accepts a very large fee for his draftsmanship. It seems overtime to ask why it's not legal malpractice and fraud for attorneys to charge clients large fees to draft contracts they publicly describe as unenforceable.[16] But, of course, it is not the role of contract-drafter that the lawyer actually plays—that's just another fairy tale for the adults. The lawyer's real role is that of procurer, obtaining a woman willing to bear a child for the couple and give it up to them upon birth. As Barbara Katz Rothman has noted, although debate on surrogate motherhood and prostitution continues among feminists, "There is virtual unanimity [among feminists] on the inappropriateness of other people selling our bodies." She goes on to term the brokers "the pimps" of the surrogacy business.[17] Like all pimps, their main motivation is greed, and their primary concern about women is how much money they can make by using them.

The reality of "surrogate motherhood" is that a lawyer-broker agrees, for a fee, to locate a woman who will agree to be inseminated with the sperm of a man, have a baby, and for a fee, agree to give the child up to the father (or relinquish her parental rights to the child) upon birth. This is artificial insemination coupled with baby-selling. But what's wrong with baby-selling?

BABY-SELLING

Baby-selling comes complete with its own fairy tale, the Grimms' "Rumpelstiltskin." Having agreed to give her first-born to Rumpelstiltskin if he would spin a roomful of straw into gold for her (a feat that helped make her queen), the queen changed her mind upon the birth of her son, and sought to get out of the contract. Rumpelstiltskin gave her a way out: three days to discover his name. Fortunately for her she did, and Rumpelstiltskin was so distressed to lose the child that "he tore himself in two." The Grimms' sympathy was obviously with the mother, even though she was rich, had entered into the contract voluntarily, and had profited greatly by it. So is the sympathy of most readers. But the baby brokers (and even some women) have argued that "a deal is a deal" and that the women—almost always poor women—who have agreed in advance to sell their babies at birth should be forced to go through with the deal so that the ability of women to enter contracts is not compromised.

Must we force women who change their minds to sell children they desperately want to raise in order to satisfy some unrealistic and nonlegal notion of specific performance? This is economic violence at its starkest and is properly labeled economic brutality. The simple answer might be that since we have outlawed the sale of human kidneys (and other organs) because of the degrading prospect of having the rich live off the body parts of the poor, it follows a fortiori that the sale of children should also be outlawed. If and when uterine transplants become feasible, it is doubtful we would (or should) permit fertile women to sell their uteruses to women who need them to become pregnant and give birth. But many would treat children with less respect than kidneys or uteruses, or at least are willing to permit fathers to buy the mother's interest in rearing the child from her and give that interest to their own wife. Should this be permitted? Sale was not involved in Carol's case, but was the key to the much more celebrated case of Mary Beth Whitehead (*Baby M*).

In that case, the New Jersey Supreme Court had no problem in concluding (as did the Michigan judge whom Noel Keane consulted more than a decade ago) that payment to place a child for adoption (even with the spouse of the child's father) violated the state's adoption laws. The court declared that "the evils of baby bartering are loathsome for a myriad of reasons."[18] There is coercion, lack of counseling, and exploitation of all parties (including desperate infertile couples), as well as the fact that "the child is sold without regard for whether the purchasers will be suitable parents"[19] and the lack of any protection of the natural mother. Making money takes precedence even over predictable human suffering. For example, the broker in the Baby M case failed to make further inquiry when a psychological evaluation of Ms. Whitehead revealed that she might change her mind. In the court's words: "It is apparent that the profit motive got the better of the Infertility Center. . . . To inquire further might have jeopardized the Infertility Center's fee."[20]

The selling of babies, which has been so slickly glazed over by others, properly disgusted the court. The court noted that the originator of this scheme to circumvent the law by private contract is "a middle man, propelled by profit" who "promotes the sale. . . . [T]he profit motive predominates, permeates, and ultimately governs the transaction."[21] What's wrong with profit and using money as the sole measure of the value of children? The court did not hesitate to say:

> There are, in a civilized society, some things that money cannot buy. . . . There are . . . values that society deems more important than granting to wealth whatever it can buy, be it labor, love, or life.[22]

Not the least of these values is the protection of children from the vicious exploitation that treating them as commodities would bring, exploitation of the poor by the rich, and the demeaning of pregnant women by treating them as breeders indentured to their "employers."

There has been much confusion about constitutional rights in the surrogacy arrangement. The only real rights at stake are those involving the rights to custody of a child resulting from an unwed pregnancy, and in this contest the rights of the child properly take precedence. There is no constitutional right to purchase a child, even your own. And whatever "procreation" rights might be raised to a constitutional level in the area of custody, the rights of the mother must be at least as strong as those of the father. Indeed, they are stronger, since fertile men need a nine-month commitment on the part of a woman to procreate, whereas fertile women only need sperm to procreate.

The constitutional right to privacy is founded on liberty interests in intimacy and freedom of association, and notions of self-identity and self-expression. Privacy is *not* a technocrat's toy, and does not require the government to keep its hands off any method of procreation that inventors can devise. Treating men and women equally in the realm of noncoital reproduction may require that egg donation be treated like sperm donation; but no principled argument can equate (as the trial judge in *Baby M* did) nine months of gestation and ultimate childbirth with sperm donation. As the U.S. Supreme Court has ruled, states cannot even permit husbands to prohibit their wives from having abortions, since, among other things, "it is the woman who physically bears the child and she is the more directly affected by the pregnancy."[23] An Oklahoma court has also noted that husbands have no right to prevent their wives from becoming sterilized. In the court's words:

> We have found no authority and the plaintiff has cited none which holds that the husband has a right to a childbearing wife as an incident to their marriage. We are neither prepared to create a right in the husband to have a fertile wife nor to allow recovery for damage to such a right. We

find the right of the person who is capable of competent consent to control his own body paramount.[24]

If husbands have no constitutional right to fertile wives, it follows that they have no constitutional right to contract with unrelated women for purposes of reproducing themselves. Although the *Baby M* court saved for another day the question of whether a woman can irrevocably waive her constitutional right to the companionship of her children by a pre-conception contract (assuming such a contract is "legalized" by future legislation), there would seem to be no basis that would allow the courts to enforce such an agreement. Even the lower court *Baby M* judge, for example, recognized that a woman could not irrevocably waive her right to terminate her pregnancy under the U.S. Constitution because judicial enforcement of such an agreement would be an intolerable burden on the woman.[25] The argument against permitting an irrevocable prebirth waiver of maternal rearing rights seems at least as strong. Both decisions are so intimately related to the individual's personhood and human dignity that it would be an intolerable violation of personal integrity to force compliance with either. This is because pregnancy and childbirth may predictably and radically change self-image and self-fulfillment aspirations that are central features of identity and personhood.

The *Baby M* court could have gone further. It did not, for example, even discuss the images of slavery inherent in enforcing contracts in commercial surrogate motherhood. Selling children conjures up the indignity and degradation of selling any human being; but more than that, specifically enforcing contracts that lead to the involuntary breakup of a family unit is at the heart of what many Americans found most repulsive about slavery prior to the Civil War. As James McPherson, one of the war's great historians, has noted: "This breakup of families was the largest chink in the armor of slavery's defenders."[26]

McPherson tells us that one of the most powerful "moral attacks" on slavery was Theodore Weld's *American Slavery as It Is*. First published in 1839, it was made up mainly of newspaper excerpts and advertisements. An example:

> NEGROES FOR SALE.—A Negro woman 24 years of age, and two children, one eight and the other three years. Said negroes will be sold separately or together as desired.[27]

He also notes that the influential *Uncle Tom's Cabin* was itself based on the forced breakup of the family: "Eliza fleeing across the ice-choked Ohio River to save her son from the slave-trader and Tom weeping for children left behind in Kentucky when he was sold South are among the most unforgettable scenes in American letters."[28] Surrogacy is not slavery. But our inability to seriously discuss the relevance of selling children and forcibly removing them from their mothers to one of the core aspects of nineteenth-century American slavery indicates our preference for dealing with fairy tale versions of surrogacy.

Since the sale of children can lead to their commodification or reification,[29] and since this will devalue all children and put all children at risk, it is quite reasonable to outlaw the sale of children, even to their fathers. But if greed is the real root of evil, isn't surrogacy motivated by love rather than by money (as in the case of Carol) acceptable?

THE DEGRADATION OF PREGNANCY

Margaret Radin has noted that whether surrogacy is paid or unpaid it may still involve "ironic self-deception." In her words:

> Acting in ways that current gender ideology characterizes as empowering might actually be disempowering. Surrogates may feel they are fulfilling their womanhood by producing babies for someone else, although they may actually be reinforcing oppressive gender roles.[30]

She goes on to note that would-be fathers can also be seen as oppressors of their wives, who, believing it is their duty to mother their husband's genetic child, "could be caught in the same kind of false consciousness and relative powerlessness as surrogates who feel called upon to produce children for others."[31]

These arguments seem intuitively correct: another key to surrogate motherhood is the traditional (and oppressive) female role it reinforces. The male's right to have a child is seen as paramount, and any interest the mother might have in their child is subordinated to it—even though a male has no more right to have a child than he does to have a fertile wife or to prevent his wife from being sterilized or from having an abortion. Men simply don't have this power over women, and we do not advance sexual equality by promoting a scheme that subordinates females so completely to male interests.

The "surrogate mother" is asked not only to perform this "service" for the male, but also to engage in purposeful self-deception. Like Carol, she is asked to pretend that the child she is carrying is not her own, but only the father's. The country's most famous surrogate mother, Elizabeth Kane, told her fairy tale simply during her pregnancy: "It's not my baby, it's the father's. I'm just growing it for him."[32] Another has declared on national television: "Motherhood is not biological."[33] Nor is the father's wife unaffected. As one infertile wife announced in support of surrogacy, "The most rewarding thing a woman can do is raise her husband's child."[34] The supposition that the women in surrogacy are involved in a "liberating" experience is akin to the supposition that selling one's kidney gives one the freedom to control one's body.

But surrogacy involves more than just fairy tale-like self-deception. It involves real degradation of the pregnant woman by proclaiming that the most important concern is not her welfare but that of the fetus she is carrying. And this is what makes this "harebrained" idea both so offensive and so potentially important symbolically for women. The lower court judge in the Baby M case, for example, termed surrogacy a "viable vehicle" to help deliver a baby to the Sterns; and the Sterns' expert witness termed Ms. Whitehead simply a "surrogate uterus."[35] The contract Noel Keane drafted, and which she signed, gave rights over her activities and body during the pregnancy to the father (William Stern), who could not only require that she undergo amniocentesis but also that she abort a handicapped child at his demand. If she refused, his contract obligations ended.[36]

This untenable proposition—that a pregnant woman's life is not her own but, rather, that others should be able to determine her activities based on what they think is in the best interests of the fetus she is carrying—underlies surrogacy. The contract attempts to get the mother to fantasize that she is simply a container carrying a precious cargo that she dare not injure. Since surrogacy does not take place in a vacuum, other physicians and courts have adopted the view that pregnancy is just for the fetus, and have ordered women to submit to Cesarean sections for the sake of their fetuses.[37] In one outrageous case (since vacated), a court even ordered a dying woman to undergo emergency surgery against her will, to deliver a fetus that was of questionable viability.[38] I have argued elsewhere that these cases were wrongly decided.[39] But they are consistent with the notion that pregnant women are not fully human and can properly be viewed as containers; and it is of at least passing interest that even the *Baby M* court cited the worst of these cases with apparent approval.[40]

The New Jersey Supreme Court is on solid ground in holding that surrogate mother contracts can never be specifically enforceable and that women must have the right to change their minds and assert their maternal rights to rear their children, at least up to the time after birth provided by the state's adoption statute.[41] The New Jersey Supreme Court also seems correct in decreeing that when the woman does assert her maternal rights, she should retain custody during the legal battle over permanent custody, a decision that ultimately must be based on the best interests of the child.[42] Arguing that we should try to prevent such custody battles by contract is tangential: the way to prevent them entirely is simply not to engage in this type of arrangement. Objecting to making decisions after birth in the child's best interests, and ignoring the interests of the child before birth, simply exposes the fact that the surrogacy arrangement *never* considers the child's welfare, only the welfare of the contracting parents. Nor is the argument that the child is always better off existing than not existing sufficient to justify surrogacy from the child's perspective.[43] Unconceived children have no "right to exist," and we do not harm them by not conceiving them or by prohibiting such practices as polygamy. We do, however, harm *real* children by commodifying them, forceably separating them from their natural mothers, and setting up situations that predictably lead to unstable and uncertain family relationships.

What Should Be Done?

I understand those who would prohibit not just commercial surrogacy, but voluntary surrogacy as well. But just as we permit organ donations among living family members, we may also wish to permit relatives (especially sisters) to have children for each other. My own preference is for legislation aimed at what has been mistermed "full surrogacy," the hiring of a woman to carry a fetus to whom she is not genetically related. This will involve "high tech" IVF and embryo transfer (and probably freezing), and could become more popular since the resulting child will be the genetic child of both the husband and wife (assuming they supply the gametes). Use of this technology could much more radically alter our notions of pregnancy and motherhood.

To prevent the gross exploitation of poor women, to prevent pregnant women from being viewed simply as vessels, to recognize the greater contribution of gestation to the child, and to ensure that the child is protected by having at least one parent with responsibility for it available at birth, the gestational mother should be irrebuttably considered the rearing mother for all legal purposes. She could give the child up to the genetic mother and father after birth, but only by acting in conformity with the state's adoption laws. Permitting the gestational presumption to be modified by contract would make *all* pregnancies and *all* births suspect. No one would know who the newborn's "mother" was until contracts were examined and genetic testing performed. This "suspended motherhood" model is (or should be) societally insupportable, since it endangers all mothers and children. A statute that irrebuttably presumes the gestational mother to be the child's legal mother for all purposes would protect both mothers and children, and should be enacted in all states.[44]

The second statute I endorse is one that would outlaw the sale of human embryos. A few states have already enacted legislation to do this. Embryo freezing is just beginning in the U.S., but it will not be long before it is commonplace. The attempted commercialization and sale of frozen embryos will not be far behind. Like children, embryos will be bought and sold in the belief that they will produce a healthy child, and probably one of a certain physical type, IQ, stature, and so on. All of these characteristics will command a specific market price—thereby monetizing the characteristics of all live children.[45] Because of this, and the fact that selling human embryos brings with it almost all of the problems and evils of selling children, their sale should be prohibited by statute.[46]

Commercial "surrogate motherhood" deserves the death without dignity that Rumpelstiltskin suffered. Legislation to try to resuscitate it and put it on temporary life-support systems would not be in the best interests of children, families, or society. But it has given us the opportunity to anticipate and plan for the next generation of issues brought to us by real science. We should act now to support economic and sexual equality, and to protect future children and families from commercial exploitation. We should work for a future in which pregnant women retain their personhood, a future of economic and social justice, rather than a future based on economic violence and social inequality. The fairy tales surrogate mothers tell must not be taken seriously.

REFERENCES

1. G. John et al., "Infertile or Childless by Choice? A Multipractice Survey of Women Aged 35 and 50," *British Medical Journal*, 294 (1987): 804; W. D. Mosher and W. F. Pratt, "Fecundity and Infertility in the United States, 1965–82," *NCHS Advance Data*, 104 (Feb. 11, 1985): 1; Mosher, "Reproductive Impairments in the United States, 1965–82," *Demography*, 22 (1985): 415; C. P. West, "Age and Infertility," *British Medical Journal*, 294 (1987): 853; J. Menken, J. Trussell, and U. Larsen, "Age and Infertility," *Science*, 233 (1986): 1389.

2. There have been fewer than 2,000 IVF births in the U.S. to date, compared with more than 4 million U.S. births annually.

3. D. Ephron. "In This Year's Movies Baby Knows Best," *New York Times*, March 13, 1988, A&L sec., p. 1. See also A. Kohn, "Parenthood Pabulum," *Psychology Today* (July/Aug. 1988): 64–65.

4. N. Keane and D. Breo, *The Surrogate Mother* (New York: Everest House, 1981), 27.

5. Id.: 29–30. Emphasis added.

6. Id.: 30. Emphasis added.

7. Id.: 37.

8. Id.: 79. Emphasis added.

9. Id.: 82. Emphasis added.

10. Id.: 53.

11. E. Kane, *Birthmother* (New York: Harcourt Brace Jovanovich, 1988), 275. And see P. Chesler, "What Is a Mother?," *Ms.*, May 1988, 26–39.

12. S. Aral and W. Cates, "The Increasing Concern with Infertility: Why Now?," *Journal of the American Medical Association*, 250 (1983): 2327.

13. J. Barron, "Views on Surrogacy Harden After Baby M Ruling," *New York Times*, April 2, 1987, Sec. B2, p. 1. Emphasis added.

14. In the Matter of Baby M, 537 A.2d 1227, 1234 (N.J. 1988).

15. H. F. Harlow, "The Nature of Love," *American Psychologist*, 13 (1958): 673;

Harlow, N.C. Blazek, and G. E. McClearn, "Manipulative Motivation in the Infant Rhesus Monkey," *Journal of Comparative Physiology & Psychology*, 14 (1956): 44.

16. G. J. Annas, "Death Without Dignity for Commercial Surrogacy," *Hastings Center Report*, 18, 2 (April/May 1988): 21, 23.

17. I. Peterson, "Feminists See Unfair Maternal Norm in Baby M Case," *New York Times*, March 20, 1987, at 13.

18. *Baby M*, supra note 14, at 1241. And see Surrogate Parenting Assoc. v. Kentucky, 704 S.W.2d 209 (Ky. 1986) (dissenting opinion).

19. Id.

20. Id.: 1247.

21. Id.: 1249.

22. Id.

23. Planned Parenthood of Central Missouri v. Danforth, 428 U.S. 52 (1976).

24. Murray v. Vandevander, 522 P.2d 302, 304 (Okla. App. 1974).

25. G. J. Annas, "Baby M: Babies (and Justice) for Sale," *Hastings Center Report*, 17, 3 (June 1987): 12, discussing In the Matter of Baby M, 217 N.J. Super. 313, 525 A.2d 1128 (1987).

26. J. M. McPherson, *Battle Cry of Freedom: The Civil War Era* (New York: Oxford University Press, 1988), 38.

27. Id.

28. Id.: 38–39. For a modern retrospective on how slavery destroyed families, see Toni Morrison's Pulitzer Prizewinning *Beloved* (New York: Knopf, 1987).

29. See M. J. Radin, "Market-Inalienability," *Harvard Law Review*, 100 (1987): 1849.

30. Id.: 1930.

31. Id.: 1931; and see G. Corea, *The Mother Machine* (New York: Harper & Row, 1985), 221–24.

32. Ms. Kane has since repudiated her role. See Kane, supra note 11.

33. *Geraldo*, "The Happy Surrogates," aired Sept. 29, 1987.

34. Id.

35. *Baby M*, supra note 25.

36. *Baby M*, supra note 14, at 1268 (contract clause 13).

37. V. E. B. Kolder, J. Gallagher, M. T. Parsons, "Court-Ordered Obstetrical Interventions," *New England Journal of Medicine*, 316 (1987): 1192. And see Note, "Maternal Rights and Fetal Wrongs: The Case Against the Criminalization of 'Fetal Abuse,' " *Harvard Law Review*, 101 (1988): 994.

38. In re A. C., 533 A.2d 611 (D.C. App. 1987), *vacated* 539 A.2d 203 (D.C. App. 1988). And see G. J. Annas, "She's Going to Die: The Case of Angela C.," *Hastings Center Report*, 18, 1 (Feb./March 1988): 23–25.

39. G. J. Annas, "Protecting the Liberty of Pregnant Patients," *New England Journal of Medicine*, 316 (1987): 1213; and see G. J. Annas, *Judging Medicine* (Clifton, N.J., 1988), 119–25.

40. *Baby M*, supra note 14, at 1254, n. 13. The entire note 13 is irrelevant to the *Baby M* opinion itself, and is seriously flawed as a matter of constitutional analysis.

41. Id.: 1244–46. See also S. Wolf, "Enforcing Surrogate Motherhood Agreements: The Trouble with Specific Performance," *NYLS Human Rights Annual*, 4 (1987): 375.

42. *Baby M*, supra note 14, at 1257–61.

43. See, e.g., J. Robertson, "Embryos, Families, and Procreative Liberty: The Legal Structure of the New Reproduction," *Southern California Law Review*, 59 (1986): 939, 995–1000.

44. S. Elias and G. J. Annas, *Reproductive Genetics and the Law* (Chicago: Yearbook Medical Publishers, 1987). On the centrality of birth to motherhood, see K. A.

Rabuzzi, *Motherself: A Mythic Analysis of Motherhood* (Bloomington: Indiana University Press, 1988).

45. Cf. Radin, supra note 29, at 1925–26.

46. G. J. Annas, "Making Babies Without Sex: The Law and the Profits," *American Journal of Public Health*, 74 (1984): 1415, 1417.

LEGAL STATUS

Choosing Family Law over Contract Law as a Paradigm for Surrogate Motherhood

A. M. Capron and M. J. Radin

Among the many new forms of human reproduction,[1] none raises more problems of public policy and of law than the practice of what is known, rather inaccurately, as "surrogate motherhood" or "surrogacy."[2] The central policy issue is settling on the paradigm that should govern surrogate motherhood, a model of family relations (adoption) or of contractual relations (sale of a product or service). And the central legal issue is whether any restrictions on personal choice that follow from the policy selected—and especially from a rejection of the contractual model with its implication of free choice—are constitutionally permissible.

We conclude that surrogate mother arrangements should be handled from the perspective of adoption. As recent judicial decisions have demonstrated, existing law on parents and children is largely adequate, and the emergence of surrogacy as a social practice does not require major "law reform" efforts. Furthermore, neither these rulings nor legislation proposed in many jurisdictions to ban commercialized surrogacy intrude impermissibly on the range of choices about reproduction protected by the Constitution of the United States. Although we conclude that commercialized surrogacy may be prohibited, we think the weight of any legal sanctions should be concentrated against those who arrange such transactions for profit rather than against the parties (parents and would-be parents) themselves. And we believe that unpaid surrogacy should be permitted.

The Family Law Model

Existing Policies and the Values on Which They Rest

Families in our society take many forms and may take even more as single people or couples who are not legally married, including gays and lesbians, assume the role of parents in increasing numbers. Under existing family law, a great deal of latitude is allowed in "private ordering" without state interference, and we believe that it is beneficial for society to take a liberal view of "the family" when framing family law, especially rules governing adoption and reproduction.

Certain core values are recognized, however, as matters of legitimate concern for the state. Among these are the protection of children's welfare and interests (especially through encouraging responsible behavior by parents), the maintenance of accurate records of vital statistics and family status, the promotion of human wellbeing, and the prevention of human exploitation. In light of concern for these values, the states have adopted laws about parentage, usually through provisions in the codes on civil law and evidence.

Presumptions of Parentage

California's laws are typical. The evidentiary laws provide that the woman who gives birth to a child—its natural mother—and that woman's husband are presumed to be the parents of that child.[3] In the case of artificial insemination by donor (AID), California follows the Uniform Parentage Act and holds that a husband who consents to AID of his wife by a physician is the legal father of the child.[4] Although such rules are often analyzed from the vantage point of the adults involved—"What rights do I have over this child?"—it is also essential to be alert to their beneficial effects for children, especially newborns.[5] In most cases, the persons identified and regarded by society as the parents of a child can be expected to provide care for the child and otherwise to behave responsibly toward it. Indeed, there are many means in society—cultural and social as well as official—to assist, to encourage, and if necessary even to force them to do so.

These legal rules serve children's interest in having clearly identified people recognized from the moment of birth as their legal parents, with all the obligations and expectations consequent to this role. If the status of adult parties in relation to a newborn child is dependent on any contracts or other agreements they may have reached, then this status—and the rights and responsibilities that flow from it—may be thrown into doubt when contractual terms are unclear or when the contract is disavowed due to alleged breaches or other disagreements.[6]

The interests of society, as well as those of parents and children, are also served by the laws on parentage. The state's interest in achieving certainty on this subject arises primarily from its parens patriae role as protector of minors and others who are unable to defend their own interests. The state also has interests in the certainty and reliability of records and in simplicity and economy in making determinations. These interests are well served by the existing law, which presumes the birth mother and her husband (if she is married) to be the parents. The resulting designations are seldom subject to dispute or litigation.

Adoptions and Foster Placement

Of course, the state has had to recognize that children also need protection when their parents die or are unable or unwilling to fulfill the parental role. All states have responded by creating procedures for transferring custody and control (either to temporary custodians or permanently to adopting parents) of children who are orphaned, abused, neglected, abandoned, or relinquished voluntarily for adoption.

The legal rules of greatest immediate relevance to the present topic are those on adoption. In many states, agreements to relinquish parental rights are not permitted prior to the child's birth.[7] Further, the statutes typically provide for a "change of heart" period after the agreement to release a child, although the standards for revoking one's choice vary.[8] Such provisions aim to balance several interests. On the one hand, the child needs unqualified acceptance and stability in its surroundings. This need is fostered by ensuring the people who are serving as caregivers and who intend to adopt the child that they will be able to keep it. On the other hand, permitting the birth mother to reclaim a child manifests society's traditional respect for biological ties. It also recognizes that circumstances may propel some women to make a decision before or immediately after the birth of a child that does not reflect their true wishes and the depth of the bond they feel to the child. Consequently, for some (usually brief) period, a parent who has consented to transfer custody and permit adoption of a child may reverse this choice, after which time an affirmative showing of unsuitability in the child's new home is usually necessary to reverse the choice.

The standards applicable to this area of the law seem—perhaps inevitably—vague and imprecise. In many cases—including those in which the parents' rights and responsibilities are suspended or revoked involuntarily, on grounds of abuse or neglect of the child—a child protective services agency or other state officer assumes responsibility for a child, subject to supervision by the family court or comparable judicial body. Regrettably, such agencies are woefully underfunded and the rules and standards they apply often seem arbitrary, especially in cases of temporary suspensions of parental rights and placement of children in foster homes. Such problems have badly tarnished the "best interests" standard applied by these agencies and the judicial officers who have ultimate control in such cases.

Although many adoptions are handled by agencies operated or licensed by the government, "private adoptions" are also permitted and are especially sought when the supply of children that couples want to adopt falls below the demand, causing lengthy delays and much frustration. Even when an adoption is privately arranged (by a family member, physician, lawyer, or the like), the official step of transferring parental rights and obligations is subject to state supervision. This will typically involve a social worker or comparable person inquiring into the background of the prospective parents and the suitability of their home. The results of such inquiries are then evaluated by a judge to ascertain that the placement is in the child's best interests.

Laws Against a Market in Children

Many states have forbidden "baby selling"—specifically, the paying or receiving of any money or other valuable consideration in connection with the placement of a child for adoption. The prohibition applies both to the transfer of already existing children and to the commissioning of pregnancy specifically for the release of the child for adoption (commissioned adoption). Moreover, it extends to those who arrange the adoption as well as to the natural and adoptive parents, except that reasonable medical expenses may be paid for the delivery and care of the child. Since such laws usually except the payment of the administrative fees of a state-approved adoption agency,[9] it is apparent that they are aimed especially at payments for privately arranged adoptions.

The prohibition on payments may be understood as protecting several important values. First, it may protect women—especially poor, single women—from being exploited.[10] Plainly, the concern that women not become paid "breeding stock," like farm animals, attaches at all points in reproduction. The view that women's reproductive capacities should not be placed into a market context is at least as offended by the choice of a woman who seeks to become pregnant in order to produce a salable product as it is by a much less free choice made by a woman who, after a birth, concludes that she should give up her child because she is unable to raise it.

The role of paid breeder is incompatible with a society in which individuals are valued for themselves and are aided in achieving a full sense of human well-being and potentiality. The fact that there are other impediments to human flourishing in contemporary society is no reason why the state cannot act—as it has in restricting payment for adoptions—to protect people from the dehumanizing pressures that would arise were reproductive capabilities removed from a private, and uniquely personal, sphere and turned into items of commerce. One such dehumanizing pressure on women—especially poor women—would be social pressure either to relinquish children for paid adoption or to create children for others for a price, in order to support their families.

The prohibition on paid adoptions serves the value of human personhood from another vantage point as well. It not merely restricts the freedom of women (and men) to sell their reproductive capabilities, but it also restricts the creation of a market in the products of those capabilities. Society has a legitimate interest in these goals, not the least because a market in reproductive services and babies would have adverse effects on all persons, not simply on those who choose to enter that market. All personal attributes of ourselves as well as our children (sex, eye color, predicted IQ and athletic ability, and so forth) would be given a dollar value by the market, whether or not we wanted to regard ourselves and our progeny in these terms.

What is probably most remarkable about the debate over surrogate motherhood is that it has necessitated defending a claim that was previously taken as self-evident: namely, that society has an interest in people being regarded as intrinsically valuable, not as monetized units in a marketplace. It oversimplifies matters to think of monetization as enslavement. In the adoption context, some of the rationale in support of the Thirteenth Amendment—that it is wrong for one group of people to treat another as chattel whom they are free to exploit (to the point of death)—is inapposite. The fact that adopting parents have paid for a child does not mean they will fail to incorporate it as a full family member. To worry that paying for babies will have the effect of "commodifying" them is not to suggest that parents will treat the children of paid, commissioned adoptions or commercial surrogacy as trivial objects to be discarded at will, like a magazine or a blouse. Many material objects, after all, are treated with respect and kept for a long time; but they are objects nevertheless.[11]

Moreover, even if a child once incorporated into a family is never again thought of as something acquired in an expensive transaction, the fact remains that during the *process* of the transaction the child was a thing. People had a transferable ownership interest[12] in it and bargained over it in a market in which other "products" were also for sale and in which other potential buyers may also have been bidding. In the townhouse outside Detroit where Michigan lawyer Noel Keane conducts his commercial surrogacy business, couples circulate among the rooms where surrogates wait their scrutiny. After each interview, the couple is encouraged to make its selection before the surrogate is snatched up by someone else.[13] Likewise, during the *process* of commissioning a pregnancy, the woman becomes a breeder to be bargained over in a market that will place a specific dollar value on personal traits that she may pass on to her offspring.

To demonstrate the unacceptability of commercial reproduction and transactions in children, one need only imagine the market carried to its natural conclusion (that is, to the point at which it would display its greatest strengths): an open, structured process of offering children of all ages to the highest qualified bidders (even markets may have entrance requirements).[14] In such a setting, advertising would play a large role. Buyers would seek protection in implied warranties of merchantability and in express warranties based on any claims of special attributes. And, to ensure market liquidity and responsiveness, participants would have to be free to resell what they had bought, either depreciated (like a used car) or appreciated on account of changes in the market or improvements made in the product since it was purchased (like real estate).

Transfers associated with the marketplace are simply very different both in their subjective connotations (that all things can be given a dollar value) and in their legal expectations (that people have special rights regarding things that they have purchased) from gifts and other nonmarket transfers. Thus, the intuition that baby-selling is simply wrong and ought to be prohibited reflects the view that the market model inherently misdescribes the reason that we value people[15] and wrongly suggests that they are fungible goods. Moreover, by undermining the relationship between personhood and social context, a market in babies would interfere with individuation and self-development and hence would detract from the ideal of human flourishing that society should seek to foster.[16]

Applying Existing Rules to New Reproductive Methods

We believe that the interests of the children and adults involved, as well as collective interests, mandate applying the same rules to surrogacy as to other arrangements involving the transfer of parental rights and responsibilities.

Enforcement of the anti-baby selling law will not prevent surrogacy, merely paid surrogacy. To further discourage paid contracts, and to remove the most distasteful aspects of a "market in babies," it is necessary to go a step beyond the United Kingdom's Surrogacy Arrangements Act 1985. That act prohibits individuals and organizations from engaging on a commercial basis in such activities as making lists of potential surrogates or negotiating or advertising surrogacy arrangements. However, it permits the parties to a surrogacy arrangement to agree on, pay, and receive money or other valuable consideration. The proposed 1986 amendments would have prohibited all paid surrogacy while continuing to allow unpaid surrogacy. Because the dangers of commodification are posed more imminently by those who organize and implement a market in babies than by parents and would-be parents themselves, the statute should be designed so that the weight of legal sanctions is brought to bear on those who attempt to create such a market (for example, lawyers who act as commercial brokers).

To protect both the children in surrogate arrangements and the women who bear them, the law should not differentiate women who are impregnated pursuant to surrogate mother contracts from those who bear babies under other circumstances. Thus, the normal rules of adoption would apply to the transfer of parental status to the woman who will raise the child that is biologically her husband's (though legally probably the child of the surrogate's husband, if the surrogate is married). Any element of uncertainty created by restricting specific performance and allowing "change of heart" by the natural mother will merely serve to underline the need for caution by all parties involved.[17]

Moreover, because there is no relevant distinction between a surrogacy contract and an ordinary commissioned adoption, the laws against baby-selling should be enforced when a "surrogate mother" (and her mate, if any) relinquish a child for adoption by its biological father (and his mate, if any). The claim that the payment to the "surrogate" is merely for "gestational services" is plainly just a pretense, since payment is made "upon surrender of custody" of the child and for "carrying out . . . obligations" under the agreement. These obligations include taking all steps necessary to establish the biological father's paternity[18] and to transfer all parental rights to the biological father and his mate.

Although language isn't everything (and an ingenious lawyer might find a subtler way to disguise the truth), the pretense of the contract-for-services can be seen in the Baby M case. The contract signed by William Stern, the biological father, and by Mary Beth Whitehead, the biological mother, and her husband, Richard, provided in part:

> $10,000 shall be paid to MARY BETH WHITEHEAD, surrogate, upon surrender of custody to WILLIAM STERN, the natural and biological father of the child born pursuant to the provisions of this Agreement for surrogate services and expenses in carrying out her obligations under this Agreement; . . .
>
> . . . MARY BETH WHITEHEAD, surrogate, and RICHARD WHITE-HEAD, her husband, agree to surrender custody of the child to WILLIAM STERN, Natural Father, immediately upon birth, acknowledging that it is the intent of this Agreement in the best interests of the child to do so; as well as institute and cooperate in proceedings to terminate their respective parental rights to said child, and sign any and all necessary affidavits, documents, and the like, in order to further the intent and purposes of this Agreement. . . .
>
> . . . MARY BETH WHITEHEAD and RICHARD WHITEHEAD agree to sign all necessary affidavits prior to and after the birth of the child and voluntarily participate in any paternity proceedings necessary to have WILLIAM STERN'S name entered on said child's birth certificate as the natural or biological father.

Bringing surrogacy arrangements within the usual rules of adoption will also mean that the state—through social workers and eventually through the court that approves the adoption—will be involved in the process, in order to ensure that the transfer will be in the child's best interests. The mere fact that a couple is willing to pay a good deal of money to obtain a child does not vouchsafe that they will be suitable parents; the mere fact that a child is born to a "surrogate mother," rather than to a woman who wishes to give the child up to a man who is not its father and to that man's wife, does not diminish the state's obligations toward that child. In the United Kingdom, where surrogacy is recognized as falling within existing family law expectations, local authorities have been reminded that when they know

> that a baby has been, or is about to be, born in its area as a result of a surrogacy arrangement it will wish to make enquiries . . . so as to be satisfied that the baby is not, or will not be, at risk as a result of the arrangement.[19]

Beyond reiterating the conclusion that "surrogate mother" arrangements are governed by the usual provisions of the parentage and adoption laws, the state should also regularize the process of record-keeping in such arrangements and in AID generally. As in adoption, this would preserve confidential records with accurate information about a child's biological origins, should such information later be needed for medical (especially genetic and diagnostic) reasons.[20]

The noncommercial treatment of surrogacy that we have in mind is illustrated by the judgment of Latey, J., in *In Re Adoption Application (Payment for Adoption)*,[21] handed down in the Royal Courts of Justice in London on March 11, 1987. In that case, the court approved an adoption by the child's father and his wife, Mr. and Ms. A, of a girl (then aged two years and four months) who had been conceived through sexual intercourse of the father and Ms. B, with whom Mr. and Ms. A had made "a surrogacy arrangement," as the court termed it. Initially, the parties had agreed that Ms. B would receive £10,000 to cover her expenses and loss of earnings during the pregnancy. In the end, the couple paid £5,000 and the surrogate refused to accept the balance.[22]

The question for the court was whether the adoption could be approved in light of statutes against baby-selling. Justice Latey accepted Ms. B's position that "I did not go into the arrangement for commercial reasons." Identifying commercial activities with profit-seeking, he concluded, "[T]here was nothing commercial in what happened." Although monetization and commodification can exist even without profit-seeking, adoption statutes do permit the payment of expenses in supervised settings. More important, the court was at pains to emphasize that what was involved was not commercial in the sense of involving a contract but was merely an arrangement. "There was no written contract or agreement; no lawyers were consulted until after the baby was born. The arrangement was one of trust which was fully honoured on both sides."

CONSTITUTIONAL IMPLICATIONS

We believe that policies on surrogate motherhood should—and can—be properly framed as issues of social policy, not constitutional law. Nevertheless, some commentators have attempted to "constitutionalize" the debate about the appropriate regulation of reproduction and adoption.[23] We will here reply briefly to the assertion that the states are constitutionally required to give effect both to commercial surrogacy contracts and to unpaid arrangements. Stated conversely, does a public policy that disfavors surrogacy unconstitutionally burden the rights of people[24] to establish a family by the use of methods—such as contracts that *are* worked out by lawyers and then honored by courts—to provide themselves with stronger assurance of a favorable outcome when trust breaks down and an arrangement to transfer a child is *not* "fully honoured on both sides"? We believe that limitations on surrogacy that arise from applying the family law model rather than the contracts model do not unconstitutionally burden any rights under present or ideal interpretations of the three doctrines of primary relevance—equal protection of the laws, substantive due process, and the right to privacy in family and reproductive choices.

Equal Protection

Equal protection claims rest on an assertion that a particular group has been disadvantaged by the law as compared with other groups. With whom should those who wish to use surrogacy—typically couples with female infertility—be compared? Were the comparison made with people generally, it would suggest that not just infertility but *any* barriers to founding a family, such as those caused by advanced age, low intelligence, poverty, and so forth, would be legally suspect—a dubious conclusion. Consequently, the comparison for surrogacy is usually framed in terms of the rules that govern AID, the principal procedure designed to overcome infertility.

So long as AID is legal—and, indeed, is facilitated by laws that make a consenting husband the legal father of the child and remove any parental rights or responsibilities from the man from whom the semen came—must surrogate motherhood contracts also be legally protected, lest couples with male infertility be favored over couples with female infertility? More specifically, if payments to semen "donors" are permitted, is commercial surrogacy—rather than just unpaid surrogacy (which we would allow)—constitutionally protected on equal protection grounds? An initial response is that the law does not differentiate the reasons people have for using one form of "assisted reproduction" or another. Indeed, surrogacy itself typically involves AID, except that the source of the semen does not view himself as a "donor" but as a "lender" or "beneficiary" who is making use of the services of a woman to produce a child whom he will then claim. On a formal basis, then, the laws adopted for AID can, and should, be applied to surrogacy. The woman who bears a child, and her mate, if any, are presumed to be the parents of the child, until the presumption is overcome or until they give up their parental rights and responsibilities to the biological father and his mate, if any. Thus, legal acceptance of AID is facially neutral among couples with different types of infertility.

Of course, the argument is then made that taken as a whole, AID (in which the child will stay with the woman who bore it) and surrogacy (in which the child will go to its genetic father) are different procedures, regardless of the use of artificial insemination in the latter. Yet even assuming that the equal protection clause would require that two procedures affecting somewhat different infertile populations must be treated symmetrically, AID and surrogate motherhood are simply not equivalent. First, the biological parallel fails: the female procedure that is comparable to (though more complex than) AID is egg or embryo donation. Second, the biological difference matters: the physical risk and labor of surrogacy, to say nothing of the emotional attachment of a surrogate mother to the child she carries and bears, is incomparably greater than the risk, labor, and attachment of a semen donor to the child or children who may be produced by inseminations with his ejaculate.[25]

Furthermore, the assumption of formal symmetry in the law as applied to men and women is itself questionable. Equal protection arguments turn on what counts as equal treatment of different groups, a much debated issue especially for feminist legal theorists. Some writers define equality between women and men as symmetrical treatment, whereas others argue that equality requires asymmetrical treatment because of the power imbalance that flows from gender bias and hierarchy.[26] It would be wrong to claim that equal protection rigidly requires that men and women be treated with formal symmetry in matters involving reproduction.[27]

A possible example of legitimate asymmetry can be found in the present custom of paying a small amount ($25–$50 in most cases) to semen "donors" (actually, vendors). Even if the law continues to permit women to pay for sperm for AID, it does not follow that it would be a denial of equal protection to prohibit men from paying surrogates to bear and turn over children to them. Paying women to deliver children to genetic fathers may pose a greater risk of commodifying women than paying men for sperm poses of commodifying men because, given the current gender structure, these payments may have different social significance. The desire to carry on the male line through the use of surrogates is more likely to render women fungible than is the desire to carry on the female line through the use of sperm donors likely to render men fungible.

Nevertheless, for the reasons already advanced, market transactions in human beings are troublesome. To the extent that semen partakes of humanness—especially because the semen may be valued deferentially for the genetic traits it is believed to transmit[28]—then its sale for amounts more than that which is appropriate payment for the costs of "harvesting," testing, storing, and distributing should be discouraged or perhaps even prohibited. Of course, the same policy should be applied to the female equivalent of AID—obtaining eggs and embryos from women.

As stated earlier, we reach such conclusions on policy, not constitutional, grounds. But an equal-protection argument against banning paid surrogacy because it discriminates against men should fail, because, at least in the current context of gender hierarchy, the state has a stronger interest in protecting women against exploitation. In other words, in the view of some feminists, the major issue of inequality associated with surrogate motherhood is the preference it seems to display for enabling men to continue their genetic lineage through an oppressive use of women as breeders, deprived of any involvement with the offspring they have produced on contract.

Yet if, as some feminists also urge, men should share equally in parenting—on the psychological and spiritual levels as well as on the material—then social policy should not devalue a man's desire to rear a child. Nor should it disparage his desire to have (if possible) a genetic as well as a social link with the child, even if the ideal of human flourishing would suggest that a genetic connection should not be the basis for psychological and spiritual interrelationships with one's children. Thus, although the *preference* for the male connection to the child manifested in the trial court opinion in the Baby M case[29] is improper, the law probably ought not to make it more difficult for a man without a fertile female partner to create a child of whom he is the biological parent than it is for a woman without a fertile male partner[30]—provided, in all cases, that one person's fulfillment of her or his wishes does not come at the expense of another person's rights (whether defined symmetrically or asymmetrically).

Substantive Due Process, Privacy, and Reproductive Freedom

Rather than making the equality argument that paid surrogacy must be permitted in a social context in which AID is permitted, some would argue that there is an absolute right to paid surrogacy. Such an argument would be based upon a claim of substantive due process, more plausibly upon its modern reincarnation in the constitutional right to privacy.

The claim that the government infringes liberty if it denies people the right to make enforceable contracts of exchange about anything they wish, children included, rests on a discredited view of the due process clause.[31]

If the government has good reasons for declaring something off-limits to the market, there is no absolute right to market-liberty that can trump regulation.[32] In the context of commissioned adoption and paid surrogacy, the good reason for enforced noncommodification is to protect the fundamental rights of women and children to be treated as unique persons not subject to monetization.

The more powerful claim under modern constitutional doctrine is that a ban on paid surrogacy violates the right to privacy (in certain reproductive and family matters) fashioned by the Court in recent years. It has been suggested that the failure of a state to enforce surrogacy contracts, or laws that restrict any agreements people desire to make to enable themselves to obtain children, would violate the right of privacy recognized in the contraception and abortion cases.[33] We think this claim fails because it rests on a misinterpretation of the rationale and effect of the privacy decisions.

The heart of the privacy doctrine developed by the Supreme Court has been to shelter individuals from governmental intrusion into the choices they make about selected intimate matters including abortion, contraception, and family living. As the Court stated in *Eisenstadt v. Baird*, the doctrine is particularly relevant to decisions about offspring:

> If the right of privacy means anything, it is the right of the *individual,* married or single, to be free from unwarranted governmental intrusion into matters so fundamentally affecting a person as the decision whether to bear or beget a child.[34]

The right to be *free from* interference is what Sir Isaiah Berlin terms a negative liberty,[35] rather than a positive liberty. In this instance it would amount to an obligation on the part of the state to ensure that individuals have the *freedom to* achieve the family they desire. How does the family law-oriented analysis for which we have argued here relate to either type of liberty, negative or positive?

Freedom From

The right of privacy gives wide scope for liberty of the former type—that is, freedom from undue governmental interference with decisions about reproduction—but it certainly does not preclude all types of state regulation. Requirements for accurate record-keeping, for example, are accepted without legal challenge. Their application to surrogacy (such as by requiring adoption procedures that result in confidential court records) are not an undue or discriminatory burden here. Furthermore, such rules and procedures are justified by state interests that are not merely legitimate but that may even be "compelling" to the extent that such records are necessary to protect the health and well-being of the children produced.

Indeed, regulations that go well beyond record-keeping requirements could be legitimate even if they precluded total freedom in reproductive choices. The interests of the state in protecting the health of the public would justify many forms of regulation of third parties who offer reproduction-related services. Sperm banks or in vitro clinics, for example, could be regulated to ensure compliance with at least minimum standards of safety and efficacy, as well as truthful advertising of services.

Freedom from governmental interference is itself subject to limitation on constitutional grounds. As one civil liberties group has concluded, the exercise of a person's fundamental right to have a family "[d]oes not embrace any right, nor permit any person, to treat a child as property."[36] The claim that the right to privacy protects surrogacy may be more plausible for noncommercial than for commercial surrogacy; even if the Constitution should be understood as including a right to bear a child for someone else, it should not be interpreted as including a right to be paid for it.

Because there is no substantive constitutional guarantee for people's choices to commodify reproductive capacities or children, there can be no constitutional objection to a state's choosing to prohibit commercial surrogacy agencies or other commercial reproductive brokerage. Moreover, despite the Supreme Court's recent propensity to treat commercial speech in the same fashion as noncommercial speech for First Amendment purposes, there is no objection on free speech grounds to prohibiting advertising by commercial surrogacy agencies or other brokers, as an aid to prohibitions on baby-selling.

Freedom To

The thrust of our argument, however, has not been toward prohibiting all surrogacy. Rather, we have urged only that paid surrogacy be prohibited and that other surrogacy arrangements not be regarded as legally binding. Arrangements made by individuals that are carried out voluntarily could continue to be accepted, provided that they accord with the usual rules on adoption (e.g., no payment, no agreement before a child's birth to give up custody, opportunity for the birth mother to change her mind, and protection against custody or adoption that is not in a child's best interests). People are thus free to choose unpaid surrogacy but cannot expect the state to enforce completion of the arrangement if disagreements arise.

Proponents of "procreative liberty" may claim that this result is unacceptable because the state is required by the constitutional right of privacy at least to enforce unpaid surrogacy arrangements. According to settled contract-law doctrines, however, promises without consideration are unenforceable. Moreover, the argument fails to distinguish negative from positive freedom. In finding a broad (albeit not unlimited) freedom from state interference in personal choices, the Supreme Court has declined to recognize a corresponding right to state aid in effectuating those choices.[37]

Moreover, declining to order specific performance of a surrogacy arrangement seems, in the language of *Eisenstadt*, less an "unwarranted governmental intrusion" into the would-be parents' reproductive liberty than the intrusion into the surrogate mother's rights that would occur were the state to enforce the arrangement.[38] The Court has been very specific in restricting state regulation of the reproductive choices of women and their *physicians*,[39] but it has never suggested a comparable obligation of the state to enhance the "contractual rights" of couples and their *lawyers* (or other *brokers* of children).

One need not agree with the current Court's emphasis on negative liberty to conclude that the protection of bodily integrity and consequently of the reproductive process encompassed within the right of privacy simply does not generate an affirmative duty on the part of the state to enforce all arrangements through which people seek to form a family. To hold otherwise would lead to the conclusion that all means by which people decide to obtain children are allowable, including paying money for any adoption (not just adoptions involving surrogates). In light of the strong connotations of commodifying all human beings were buying and selling permitted in our social context, this is an untenable proposition, and one that is clearly not compelled by the Court's decisions on the right of privacy.

In the end, we believe that whether or not the state must—or, indeed, may permissibly—provide enforcement machinery for arrangements regarding reproduction and children must be considered separately for each type of arrangement. For so-called surrogate motherhood, the weight of protected "procreative liberty" rests with the biological mother who changes her mind and decides to keep her child. Hence, arguments about procreative liberty cannot support constitutionalizing a requirement that states provide laws and mechanisms to enforce such arrangements. Indeed, we have argued in favor of a public policy that denies that states may permissibly maintain such legal rules and procedures.

REFERENCES

This article is adapted from testimony presented at a "Hearing on Surrogate Parenting" before the Senate Committee on Health and Human Services of the California Legislature on December 11, 1987.

1. See, gen., Alexander Morgan Capron, "Alternative Birth Technologies: Legal Challenges," *U. C. Davis Law Review*, 20 (1987): 679.

2. The term "surrogate mother" is inaccurate because in ordinary parlance one would say that a surrogate is someone who raises another's offspring, not a child's birth mother who then releases it to the wife of its biological father. The better term would be "surrogate wife" or "breeding mother." If the pregnancy results from an ovum that has come from the woman who plans to raise the child, the appropriate term might be "surrogate womb."

The use of the term "surrogacy" as shorthand for the practice adds further confusion, since the term has established legal connotations associated both with decisionmakers who are legally authorized to act on behalf of incompetents and with the courts that are responsible for the welfare of incompetents. Similarly, in the bioethics literature, much attention has been paid in recent years to the use of surrogate decisionmakers for those who are incapable of making medical decisions for themselves and particularly to the advantages for competent patients of executing a durable power of attorney to name a surrogate to make decisions if and when the patient becomes incapacitated. See, e.g., U.S. President's Commission for the Study of Ethical Problems in Medicine and Biomedical and Behavioral Research, *Making Health Care Decisions* (Washington, D.C.: U.S. Gov't Printing Office, 1982): 158–60.

3. Cal. Evid. Code §621 (West 1966). See also Cal. Civ. Code §7004 (West 1983), which extends the presumption in certain special circumstances (death, annulment, or divorce within 300 days of a child's birth; attempted but invalid marriages; subsequent marriage; holding out as natural child; etc.).

4. Cal. Civ. Code §7005 (West 1983).

5. See Capron, supra note 1, at 690–94.

6. As, for example, in the Malahoff-Stiver "case" that was worked out on the "Phil Donahue Show" in 1983, or the dispute over an early attempt at in vitro fertilization at Columbia University that was litigated in Del Zio v. Presbyterian Hosp., 74 N.Y. Civ. Ct. (S.D.N.Y. Nov. 14, 1978) (memorandum decision).

7. See, e.g., N.Y. Dom. Rel. Law §11–1 (c) (McKinney 1977); Lori Andrews, *New Conceptions: A Consumer's Guide to the Newest Infertility Treatments*, rev. ed. (New York: St. Martin's, 1985), 207; S. Green and J. Long, *Marriage and Family Law Agreements* (1984), 311 n. 693.

8. The standards vary from revocation at will to requiring proof of fraud or duress. Susan M. Wolf, "Enforcing Surrogate Motherhood Agreements: The Trouble with Specific Performance," *New York Law School Human Rights Annual*, 4 (Spring 1987): 375, 382–83.

9. See, e.g., N.J.S.A. 9:3–54b (West Supp. 1984–85) (exempts stepparents).

10. We recognize that poor women themselves may, under some circumstances, think themselves not exploited but, rather, empowered by an entitlement to sell babies. But poor women are caught in a double bind: it may be disempowering either to allow or to disallow "commodification" of children. If sales are disallowed, poor women remain in circumstances they perceive to be worse than becoming paid baby-producers; but if sales are allowed, poor women and their children are in danger of degrading their personhood by becoming fungible objects of exchange. See Margaret Jane Radin, "Market-Inalienability," *Harvard Law Review*, 100 (June 1987): 1849, 1915–36.

Sometimes an "incomplete commodification" may be the best pragmatic solution to this kind of dilemma. For example, prostitution (commodification of sexuality) may be best handled by criminalizing pimping or other forms of brokering of sexual services, while allowing prostitutes themselves to receive money for their services as long as they do not seek state enforcement of broken promises to pay. See id.: 1921–25. On balance, however, we do not think an analogous "incomplete commodification" would be appropriate for surrogacy, at least while other forms of commissioned adoption are treated as prohibited baby-selling. See id.: 1928–30.

11. See Margaret Jane Radin, "Justice and the Market Domain," in John W. Chapman, ed., *Markets and Justice* (NOMOS XXXI) (New York: New York University Press, forthcoming). Whether or not babies could be priced and yet not be inappropriately commodified depends on how risky allowing buying and selling would be, given the degree to which people in our society conceive of things that are purchased as fungible commodities. Even though there can be nonmarket aspects to much of what we buy and sell (for example, the personal care and concern we hope for between physician and patient), in our nonideal world, the mere fact that money changes hands might be rightly treated as having bad implications, or at

least bad possibilities, for an especially sensitive case like the sale of babies, in which complete commodification would deeply undermine personhood as we conceive it.

12. The notion of an ownership interest was strongly expressed in the trial court opinion in In re Baby M, 217 N.J. Super 313, 372, 525 A.2d 1128, 1157 (1987), in which Judge Sorkow ruled the anti-baby-selling provisions of the adoption law inapplicable because Mr. Stern "cannot purchase what is already his." It is also notable that in the trial court's view, the property right apparently resides with the biological father.

13. Anne Taylor Fleming, "Our Fascination with Baby M," *New York Times Magazine*, March 29, 1987, p. 32.

14. But see William Landes and Richard Posner, "The Economics of the Baby Shortage," *Journal of Legal Studies*, 7 (1978): 323 (speculating on the possibility of a thriving market in infants).

15. Of course, sometimes—for reasons of deterrence as well as of compensation—the legal system places a "dollar value" on human life. Yet in doing so—even when factors such as the emotional loss to survivors or the "loss of life's pleasures" by the deceased enter the calculation of damages—the tort system acknowledges that the money is no substitute for the person. In a social system in which families are dependent on their members' earning power to obtain a decent standard of living, some compensation for the loss of earning power of a family member is just. The existence of tort remedies is of more dubious value in deterrence terms, however. While the threat of liability may deter individuals from unduly risky behavior, the existence of the system—in which the loss of human life is "compensated" by the payment of money—may encourage more life-risking activities than would occur were such losses to lie beyond the scope of the tort system, in the realm of individual revenge or societal disruption and disharmony.

16. See Radin, supra note 10, at 1903–21.

17. The child's interests would, however, be protected because when a surrogacy agreement is held invalid or is "breached" (by a mother's refusal to turn over the child), *both* natural parents are bound by "the statutory rights and obligations [that] exist in the absence of contract," including custodial disposition based on the child's best interests. Surrogate Parenting v. Com. ex rel. Armstrong, 704 S.W.2d 209, 213 (Ky. 1986). The New Jersey Supreme Court likewise concluded that determining Baby M's custody on the basis of her best interests rather than automatically returning her to her mother would not embolden people to use surrogacy because its holding that surrogate mother arrangements are "unenforceable and illegal is sufficient to deter such agreements." In re Baby M, 537 A.2d 1227, 1257 (N.J. 1988). The court also held for the future that, pending a court determination of the child's best interests, a woman who decides not to go through with a surrogate arrangement should be allowed to keep her child, absent proof that she is an unfit mother.

18. For example, Cal. Civ. Code §7006 (West 1983) provides that actions to establish a father and child relationship may only be commenced by the child, its natural mother, or the man presumed to be the child's father.

19. U.K. Department of Health and Social Security, "Responsibility of Local Authority Social Service Departments in Surrogacy Cases," *Local Authority Circular* (85)12 (3 May 1985).

20. U.S. President's Commission for the Study of Ethical Problems in Medicine and Biomedical and Behavioral Research, *Screening and Counseling for Genetic Conditions* (Washington, D.C.: U.S. Gov't Printing Office, 1983): 45–47, 68–70.

21. [1987] Fam. 81, [1987] All ER 826, [1987] 3 WLR 31.

22. The court states that the refusal came from the fact that Ms. B and a professional writer co-authored a book telling her story, from which she made money.

23. See, e.g., Ethics Committee of the American Fertility Society, "Ethical Con-

siderations of the New Reproductive Technologies," *Fertility & Sterility*, 46 (Supp. 1) (1986): 2S–6S; John Robertson, "Procreative Liberty and the Control of Conception, Pregnancy and Childbirth," *Virginia Law Review*, 69 (1983): 405.

24. Although the people who seek surrogate arrangements are today typically married couples, single persons—especially single men—might also seek to make such contracts. If "reproductive rights" apply here, that which is permitted to couples may apply to singles as well because the Supreme Court has made clear in other contexts that many privacy rights regarding reproductive decisions protect the unmarried equally with the married. See, e.g., Eisenstadt v. Baird, 405 U.S. 438 (1972). See also Note, "Reproductive Technology and the Procreative Rights of the Unmarried," *Harvard Law Review*, 98 (1985): 669, 684–85.

25. See Capron, supra note 1, at 699–700.

26. See Christine Littleton, "Reconstructing Sexual Equality," *California Law Review*, 75 (1987): 1279.

27. Cf. Laurence Tribe, *American Constitutional Law*, 2d ed. (Mineola, N.Y.: Foundation Press, 1988), 1582: "[A]n approach to the equal protection clause that is dominated by formal comparisons between classes of people thought to be similarly situated is inadequate to the task of ferreting out inequality when a court confronts laws dealing with reproductive biology, since such laws, by definition, identify ways in which women and men are definitely *not* similarly situated." The Supreme Court's attempts to deal with such problems have been seen by many commentators as unsatisfactory, whether its approach has been symmetrical or asymmetrical. See, e.g., Geduldig v. Aiello, 417 U.S. 484 (1974) (California's failure to cover pregnancy and childbirth in its disability insurance system did not violate equal protection, because it covered all "nonpregnant persons," both male and female); Michael M. v. Superior Court, 450 U.S. 464 (1981) (California's statutory rape law providing for criminal sanctions only upon the male participant in underage, nonmarital sex did not violate equal protection, because only women bear the risk of becoming pregnant). Recently the Court adopted an asymmetrical approach, albeit in a statutory context, in California Federal Savings & Loan Ass'n v. Guerra, 107 S.Ct. 683 (1987) (California statute requiring unpaid leave with guaranteed job reinstatement for pregnancy, but not for disabilities unrelated to pregnancy, is not preempted by Title VII of the Civil Rights Act of 1964, as amended by the Pregnancy Discrimination Act to require that employers treat pregnancy the same as any other disability, because the statute makes it possible for female as well as male workers to keep their jobs and also become parents). For a discussion of the debate on this issue within the community of feminist legal scholars, see Littleton, supra note 26.

28. Although the "Nobel Sperm Bank" plainly hoped to attract suitable female clients because of the perception that its sperm samples were genetically superior, it did not operate on a market basis. Yet it still serves as an illustration of the risk that the men from whom sperm are obtained could be treated like commodities were a true "sperm market" permitted to operate.

29. See *Baby M*, supra note 12.

30. The same argument applies when reasons other than infertility (such as genetic risk) preclude a person from being a biological parent.

31. Since the downfall of *Lochner v. New York* (198 U.S. 45 [1905])—which invalidated a state law setting a ten-hour daily maximum and sixty-hour weekly maximum for employment by bankers—there is no constitutional right to treat anything and everything as commodities in a laissez-faire marketplace. Tribe, supre note 27, summarizes this era in American legal history in Chapter 8, entitled "The Model of Implied Limitations on Government: The Rise and Fall of Contractual Liberty."

32. Substantive due process notions do still occasionally emerge in decisions in which the Supreme Court limits governmental restrictions of individual choices

about some fundamental matters. See, e.g., Moore v. City of East Cleveland, 431 U.S. 494 (1977) (plurality opinion voids city's attempt to zone for nuclear family residence).

33. See, e.g., John Robertson, "Embryos, Families, and Procreative Liberty: The Legal Structure of the New Reproduction," *Southern California Law Review*, 59 (1986): 939.

34. 405 U.S. 438, 453 (1972).

35. Isaiah Berlin, *Four Essays on Liberty* (Oxford: Clarendon Press, 1969).

36. American Civil Liberties Union of Southern California, *Policy # 262a (Surrogate Parenting)* §C(1)(b) (adopted March 18, 1987). The policy states that a child is being treated as property "if (a) her/his custody is conditioned on payment of consideration or vice versa or (b) consideration or custody is conditioned upon the child surviving for any fixed period of time, or upon the child's meeting specifications concerning fitness, health, race, gender, color, genetic identification, or other such criteria." Id.: §B(1).

37. In Maher v. Roe, 432 U.S. 464 (1977), for example, the Court denied the claim that a woman had a right to public funding of an abortion, even though the choice to abort is for the Court a cardinal instance of the right of privacy. Although *Maher* is thus a formidable doctrinal obstacle for those who would claim some positive right to enforcement of surrogacy contracts, we do not mean to endorse its rationale. Because state denial of freedom to choose abortion is, in the context of the current gender bias in economic and social power, a denial of equal opportunity to women, we think the right to choose abortion would be better analyzed as an equality right than as a privacy right.

38. As the ACLU of Southern California concludes, people may not exercise their right to form a family in a manner "that would compel the waiver or alienation of the fundamental rights of [a] surrogate." See ACLU, *Surrogate Parenting*, supra note 36, at §C(1)(a). In the *Baby M* decision, the New Jersey Supreme Court identified the surrogate's right to the companionship of her child as "a recognized fundamental interest protected by the Constitution" (subject, it said, to state regulation). In re Baby M, 537 A.2d 1227, 1255 (N.J. 1988). In contrast, it noted that the father's asserted right to procreate "very simply is the right to have natural children whether through sexual intercourse or artificial insemination." Id.: 1253. William Stern had a right to father Baby M but not to insist that she be turned over to him to raise or that the Whiteheads be forced to fulfill their promise to relinquish their parental rights to the Sterns.

39. For example, in *Roe v. Wade* the Court held that through the first trimester of pregnancy, "the attending physician, in consultation with his patient, is free to determine, without regulation by the State, that, in his medical judgment, the patient's pregnancy should be terminated." 410 U.S. 113, 147 (1973).

Surrogate Motherhood and the Best Interests of Children

Angela R. Holder

Commercial surrogacy presents complex legal issues; the problems that it does not present are those of "high tech" reproductive medicine. All the new techniques for overcoming infertility, such as in vitro fertilization and the like, are medically complex but—as long as they involve a married couple and no third-party donors—legally simple. Surrogacy is so medically uncomplicated that it can be done without any physician involvement, but it is the most legally complicated means of providing a baby for an infertile couple.[1]

From a time in England when fathers could sell their children into slavery[2] to a day in which the legal system supposedly protects "the best interests of the child," the common law increasingly respects the rights of children as individuals with constitutional rights and not as chattels of their parents. If the courts accept commercial surrogacy as a legitimate enterprise, it seems that we have again reverted to the concept of child as chattel.

ADOPTION

The nearest legal analogy to surrogacy is the law of adoption. Adoption law, of course, is directly relevant to surrogacy agreements, since in each case the father's wife will presumably seek to adopt the surrogate's child. Adoption was unknown at common law,[3] and thus in each American jurisdiction adoption is adjudicated under the authority of a specific state statute.[4] Although some states permit private adoptions (direct placement of the child by the mother or her intermediary, usually a lawyer or physician, without involvement by an agency) and other states permit private adoptions with strict supervision by agencies, some states forbid private adoptions altogether. All states, however, make it a criminal offense to sell one's child.[5] Some states' statutes forbid adoptive parents to pay any of the birth mother's expenses.[6] Others permit the couple to pay the mother's medical and hospital expenses and other provable necessary expenses, such as food and rent, incurred during her pregnancy. In no state may she receive a sum above those amounts.[7]

Thus, as the New Jersey Supreme Court ruled in *Baby M*,[8] any contract by which a surrogate is paid a fee above her expenses to gestate a child is unenforceable as a violation of the baby-selling statute in the state. The court said:

> The evils inherent in baby bartering are loathsome for a variety of reasons. The child is sold without regard for whether the purchasers will be good parents. The natural mother does not receive the benefits of counseling and guidance to assist her in making a decision that may affect her for a lifetime. In fact, the monetary incentives to sell her child may, depending on her financial circumstances, make her decision less voluntary. . . . Baby-selling potentially results in the exploitation of all parties involved.

In 1980, in the earliest reported surrogate mother case of which I am aware, the trial judge found the contract to be against public policy on the grounds that "[i]t is a fundamental principle that children should not and cannot be bought and sold."[9] That decision was upheld by the Michigan Supreme Court.[10] The Kentucky Supreme Court has held that the baby-selling law of that state is not violated by commercial surrogacy contracts, but to date it is the only state with such an appellate ruling.[11]

Proponents of commercial surrogacy argue that the fee the surrogate receives is payment for her time and for the risks and discomforts of pregnancy and childbirth. The contract[12] signed by Baby M's mother, Mary Beth Whitehead—which is apparently standard in that surrogate agency—provided that Ms. Whitehead would receive $10,000 if the baby was born alive but $1,000 if there was a stillbirth. Since the mother's time, risk, and discomfort are identical regardless of the condition of the baby, it seemed to the Supreme Court of New Jersey that at least $9,000 of the fee was to buy a live baby.

Many states' adoption statutes invalidate any adoption release executed by the mother before the birth of the baby.[13] This appears to be the case in New Jersey. Even in those states where prenatal surrenders are not absolutely void, they are voidable. The burden of proving the validity of a prenatal adoption surrender is on the party who wishes to uphold it.[14]

These restrictions on prenatal adoption surrenders are to protect the desperate, destitute pregnant woman from the situational coercion of being promised the necessities of life in return for her baby.[15] Since the surrogate signs the contract before conceiving, she is presumably not desperate and, at least in the cases that have been reported in the press, far from destitute as well. However, presumably the legislators who drafted these statutes also did not wish to envision a sheriff wresting a new baby from the mother's arms as if he were repossessing the family car.

Since 1852 all courts have held that there can be no order for specific performance of a contract of personal service. In that year, the English court heard the case of *Lumley v. Wagner*.[16] Johanna Wagner, a Prussian soprano, contracted with Mr. Lumley to sing at his London theater on certain days and not to sing anywhere else in England without his permission. A Mr. Gye, owner of a rival establishment, offered her more money and she sang there. Lumley sued her for specific performance and asked the court to order her to sing. The court refused. Bearing a child and then giving him or her away is clearly more of a "personal service" than is singing a concert.[17] Nine months of pregnancy, labor, delivery, and emotional involvement seem to be far more "personal" and much more of a "service" than two or three hours of singing.

Handicapped Newborns

If a surrogate's baby is born with serious birth defects, the legal issue may not be, as with Baby M, which parent eventually obtains custody. If the baby has severe problems, a court may find it necessary to decide who has to take the baby when neither parent wants him or her.

This has has already happened at least once. In 1982 a Michigan woman named Judy Stiver entered into a surrogate contract with Alexander Malahoff, a resident of New York. When Stiver's baby was born in January 1983, he had microcephaly and a strep infection. Malahoff, claiming that the contract gave him sole custody, refused consent to any treatment for the infection. The hospital obtained a court order to treat the baby. Malahoff then denied any responsibility for custody or support of the baby, but Stiver insisted that he take the baby, claiming that he had a contractual obligation to do so. The results of blood tests—which indicated that Stiver's husband, not Malahoff, was the biological father—were disclosed to the participants live on the Phil Donahue television show.[18] The Stivers eventually took the baby they did not want and placed him in a state institution.

In the usual situation of babies born with unexpected handicaps, parents may be shocked but they do not attempt to solve their problem by displacing custody onto anyone else. In the surrogate situation, however, the mother has doubtless attempted not to think of herself as the baby's "mother" or to become too attached, since she plans to surrender it for adoption. Thus it is certainly not surprising that, if a problem occurs, her response is, "Here, take it. I did what I was supposed to do, so give me my money." The father-by-contract, as well, having thought of the arrangement as placing an order for a baby, not surprisingly takes the position that there has been some sort of breach of warranty of quality and doesn't want the baby either. Regardless of obligation to support, the situation does not bode well for love and acceptance of the handicapped child.

Moreover, at least in the Baby M case, the contract stated:

> Mary Beth Whitehead further agrees . . . to undergo amniocentesis or
> similar tests to detect genetic and congenital defects. In the event said
> test reveals that the fetus is genetically or congenitally abnormal, Mary
> Beth Whitehead, Surrogate, agrees to abort the fetus upon demand of
> William Stern, natural Father, in which event the fee paid to the Surrogate
> will be in accordance with Paragraph 10 ($1,080.00). If Mary Beth White-
> head refuses to abort the fetus upon the demand of William Stern, his
> obligations as stated in this Agreement shall cease forthwith, except as
> to obligations of paternity imposed by statute.

Thus the surrogate who refuses to abort a fetus diagnosed as having a
defect will have to keep the child herself, presumably with minimal child
support. The mother clearly could expect no emotional or other non-fi-
nancial support from the father, who presumably is better situated economically than she to raise a handicapped child. Such a stipulation in the
contract may, however, force a potential surrogate to think carefully if she
would abort a fetus with serious problems. If she decides that she would
not, she may decide not to participate further.

The trial judge in the Baby M case found that the abortion provision in
the surrogacy contract was legally unenforceable as coercive. If it was freely
and knowingly agreed to, however, it would be difficult to find it coercive.
Coercion is defined as "compulsion by force or intimidation." Coercion
involves a threat that is designed to alter someone's behavior by making
the person's existing situation worse if she does not cooperate or comply.
Bribery is paying someone to do something that they would not otherwise
do. A person is not coerced into performing an action if she performs it
because someone has offered her something to induce her to do it; she is
bribed.[19] Mary Beth Whitehead, who was not pregnant when she signed
the surrogacy contract, was not "coerced" into agreeing to its terms, including the provisions for prenatal diagnosis and abortion. Thus it is somewhat puzzling that that was the sole provision the trial judge held to be
unenforceable.

In terms of the "best interests of the child," however, parenthood-by-
contract is generally not an efficacious way of providing a warm and loving
home for a child with handicaps, and it is unlikely that the child's best
interests will be promoted by that approach.

PROCREATIVE FREEDOM

In their argument to the Supreme Court of New Jersey, the Sterns argued
that Mr. Stern's constitutional right of procreative freedom would be violated if the surrogacy contract was not upheld. As the court noted in its

decision, however, the right to procreate does not extend to surrogacy arrangements. The right to procreate is the right to have natural children (or not to have children, as the case may be), but, as the court noted, this right does not include a constitutional right to custody of one's child.

The "right of privacy," of which the right of procreative freedom is a part, was first mentioned in 1890 in a *Harvard Law Review* article by Warren and Brandeis.[20] That article dealt with one's right not to be the subject of commercial advertisement without one's consent. The same concepts were applied in the 1920s, however, when the Supreme Court struck down a Nebraska statute prohibiting the teaching of foreign languages to young children[21] and also found unconstitutional an Oregon statute that required children to attend public, not private, schools.[22] In 1942 the Supreme Court struck down as invasive of privacy a statute providing for involuntary sterilization of those convicted for the third time of a "crime involving moral turpitude."[23] Several major Supreme Court criminal law decisions in the 1950s and 1960s involving Fourth Amendment protections against searches and seizures also involved the right of privacy—defined by the Court as the right to be let alone by the government.[24] In 1964, finally, the Supreme Court invalidated a statute denying United States passports to members of the Communist party, on the grounds that the right to travel is a fundamental aspect of privacy and liberty.[25]

Procreative freedom as a part of the right of privacy was defined by *Griswold v. Connecticut*,[26] *Roe v. Wade*,[27] *Loving v. Virginia*,[28] and other decisions establishing the right of a man and a woman to conceive and bear (or not) children without interference from the state.

In all of the privacy cases, courts frame the right as the right to be let alone—to attend to one's business without meddlesome intervention from the state. The right against interference does not, however, confer a right to demand positive assistance from the state—including access to the state's courts with standing to request a court order in an adoption case, a ruling determining custody of a child, or interpretation of a surrogate contract—to achieve one's desired goal. There is no constitutional right to positive state assistance to pay for abortion if one chooses not to have children,[29] and there is no constitutional claim to Medicaid funding for infertility treatment if one cannot afford in vitro fertilization on one's own.[30] There is not now in this country a positive constitutional right to demand assistance for any sort of medical care—even for life-threatening illness, which infertility is not.

Moreover, the "right to procreate" does not authorize anyone to hire a third party to assist in its fulfillment. A gynecologist, for example, does not have to offer access to artificial insemination or abortion.[31] It seems that the right to procreate is limited to the right to make private choices, and does not include the right to make contracts about reproduction and to ask the legal system to recognize or enforce them.

SURROGATE MOTHERHOOD

The Thirteenth Amendment

The trial judge in *Baby M* wrote, without further comment:

> The third argument is that to produce or deal with a child for money denigrates human dignity. To that premise, this court urgently agrees. The 13th Amendment to the United States Constitution is still valid law.[32]

The court noted in a footnote that

> opponents of surrogacy have put forth arguments based on the Thirteenth Amendment as well as the Peonage Act. We need not address these arguments because we have already held the contract unenforceable on the basis of state law.[33]

If one accepts the concept that surrogate agreements violate baby-selling statutes, it is difficult to understand why only one trial court has considered the effect of the Thirteenth Amendment on this practice. This amendment, apparently of interest nowadays only to legal historians, states:

> Neither slavery nor involuntary servitude, except as punishment for crime whereof the party shall have been duly convicted, shall exist within the United States, or any place subject to their jurisdiction.

A slave, by definition, is a person whose master "may sell and dispose of his person."[34] When a surrogate mother makes a contract to conceive a child and to transfer custody after birth in return for the payment of money, I have always thought that she is "selling and disposing of the person" of her child. Without regard to whatever rights a fetus may have, the child, once born, is clearly a separate being with the rights and privileges of citizenship. These rights and privileges presumably include a right not to be bought or sold.[35]

In a recent Michigan trial court case similar to *Baby M*, the mother had stated even before her twins were born that she had changed her mind and did not want to give them to the father and his wife. The trial judge held that surrogate contracts are void as against public policy and are therefore unenforceable. In commenting on that decision, the Supreme Court of New Jersey noted that

> [t]he court expressed concern for the potential exploitation of children resulting from surrogacy arrangements that involve the payment of money. The court also concluded that insofar as the surrogacy contract

may be characterized as one for personal services, the thirteenth amendment should bar specific performance.[36]

It is not clear whether the trial judge thought the mother or the twins were
protected by the anti-slavery amendment.

Moreover, from time to time the national press has a story about someone
who has tried to sell his or her young child or, in some instances, to trade
the child for a car. These situations are invariably prosecuted as criminal
violations of the child-selling laws and, as well, as child abuse. What logical
legal difference is there between selling a three-year-old and selling a newborn?

Those who do not think that the Thirteenth Amendment is applicable
to the surrogate situation base their views on the idea that the money is
paid not to purchase a child but, rather, for the surrogate to relinquish her
parental rights. As long as the amount varies according to the outcome,
however, that position seems untenable. Moreover, in ordinary divorce
proceedings, it is usually held to be against public policy for a custodial
parent to accept a lump-sum payment in return for the other parent's
agreement to hold him or her harmless for future child support and to
relinquish parental rights or any claim to custody or visitation rights.[37]

THE ETHICAL OBLIGATIONS OF THE LAWYERS

Most of the problems of the Baby M case could have been avoided if the
parties had had independent counsel. As the Supreme Court of New Jersey
pointed out, the surrogate agency—Infertility Center of New York, owned
by Noel Keane, the lawyer who has been involved in many of the disputed
surrogacy-contract cases—makes a profit if the deal goes through. As the
court put it, "It is apparent that the profit motive got the better of the
Infertility Center."

The only "independent" legal advice Ms. Whitehead received was from
a lawyer who had an agreement with Infertility Center to counsel prospective surrogates. Presumably if he counseled many to change their
minds, his agreement would no longer exist. The surrogacy contract the
Infertility Center provided included the abortion-on-request section, although it is hard to believe any practitioner would not know such a provision would be held unenforceable by any court. Thus one must assume
that the section was added to make the parties think certain rights existed
when any competent lawyer would know that they did not. If the Sterns
had also sought completely independent counsel, they might have discovered before the problems began how legally entangled these situations
may be.

If other states legislate approval of surrogate motherhood, I would hope that they would include a statutory requirement of *independent* counsel for each party involved in the transaction. Only when the lawyers involved have no financial motive for encouraging the arrangement, apparently, will the prospective father and mother and their spouses receive objective information about the possible legal hazards of the undertaking. Informed consent applies to the practice of law as well as to the practice of medicine.[38]

If a lawyer owns a surrogacy agency and provides the contract, he has an enforceable fiduciary obligation to both the prospective surrogate and the couple who wish to hire her. The *New York Times* of February 5, 1988, carried a brief story that Mary Beth Whitehead-Gould and her former husband, Richard Whitehead, agreed to a settlement of their federal fraud and negligence suit against the Infertility Center of New York, which had arranged the contract. The story said:

> The suit, pending since October, 1986, accused the Center and its Director, Noel P. Keane, a lawyer and surrogate broker from Dearborn, Michigan, of negligence for failure to exercise proper care in selecting Mrs. Whitehead Gould as a surrogate.

The amount of the settlement was not revealed.

In states where courts find that commercial surrogacy arrangements violate public policy, lawyers who broker these contracts will not be able to obtain malpractice insurance for their activities. Professional liability insurance, of course, like all types of insurance, does not insure against claims arising out of activities deemed to be in violation of public policy.[39]

THE SURROGATE'S OTHER CHILDREN

One aspect of the surrogate arrangement that does not appear to have engendered any interest is the effect of the surrogate contract on the surrogate's other children. Are these contracts in violation of the best interests of those children? Press reports indicate that the commercial surrogacy agencies will not hire surrogates who have not had children of their own— presumably on the theory that an uncomplicated obstetrical history bodes well for the surrogate undertaking. Thus most if not all of these women have children at home. A child whose half-sibling is sold might feel a certain amount of anxiety about his or her own future in the family. "If I am naughty, will Mommy sell me, too?" may be a real concern for such a child. No one has inquired if these situations could or do constitute emotional abuse for them. If surrogacy contracts continue to be written, it would seem a worthwhile area for exploration by child psychiatrists, psychologists, and social scientists.

As long as the adoption occurs in the state of the surrogate's residence, the court hearing the surrogate adoption would have *parens patriae* jurisdiction over the surrogate's other children. It is at least arguable that some court at some point may be interested in inquiring about the best interests of the other children in the family as well.

THE COMMODIFICATION OF CHILDREN

A contract of surrogacy seems similar to dealing in the futures market. For those who try to make the welfare of children an issue that politicians ignore at their peril, raising the sensitivity of the voters of this country to the needs of American children is the first step. I am deeply concerned that the mindset that finds it acceptable to view children as the subjects of contracts and commerce, ordered precisely as one orders a car or buys pork futures, will remain insensitive to the national failure to provide for children whose parents cannot or will not provide for their needs. Trying to convince voters that children are important is difficult at best. Trying to do so in a society that considers it "all right" to make contracts to buy children strikes me as impossible.

REFERENCES

1. See, for varying views on this topic, John Robertson, "Embryos, Families and Procreative Liberty: The Legal Structure of the New Reproduction," *Southern California Law Review*, 59 (1987): 939; Shari O'Brien, "Commercial Conceptions: A Breeding Ground for Surrogacy," *North Carolina Law Review*, 65 (1986): 1271. Most other countries that have considered the matter have banned the commercial aspects of surrogacy. See, e.g., Thomas Eaton, "Comparative Responses to Surrogate Motherhood," *Nebraska Law Review*, 65 (1986): 686. The British, for example, have outlawed commercial surrogacy. Surrogacy Arrangements Act, 1985, 49 Eliz II. See the report of the Warnock Commission, established by Parliament to study a variety of issues involving reproductive technology, fetal rights, and surrogacy. Department of Health and Social Security, *Report of the Committee of Inquiry into Human Fertilisation and Embryology*, Dame Mary Warnock, chairman (London: Her Majesty's Stationery Office, July 1984); and Mary Warnock, "Moral Thinking and Government Policy: The Warnock Committee on Human Embryology," *Millbank Memorial Fund Quarterly*, 63 (Summer 1985): 504.

2. Until the seventh century, English fathers could sell their sons until they were seven years old. Older boys had to consent to being sold. Sir Frederick Pollock, and Frederick Maitland, *The History of English Law*, 2d ed., (Washington, D.C.: Lawyers' Literary Club, 1959): 436.

3. Stephen Presser, "The Historical Background of the American Law of Adoption," *Journal of Family Law*, 11 (1972): 143.

4. Ruth-Arlene Howe, "Adoption Practice: Issues and Laws, 1958–1983," *Family Law Quarterly*, 17 (1983): 173.

5. See, e.g., Barwin v. Reidy, 307 P.2d 175, N.M. 1957.

6. See, e.g., A. v. C., 390 S.W.2d 116, Ark. 1965.

7. See, e.g., Hendrix v. Hunter, 100 S.E.2d 35, Ga. 1959.

8. In re Baby M, 525 A.2d 1128, 217 N.J. Super. 313 (Superior Ct. Chancery Div. 1987), *reversed on appeal*, 1988 West Law 6251 (N.J. Supreme Ct., Feb. 3, 1988).

9. Doe v. Kelley, 2 *Human Reproduction Law Rptr* 2A1, Circuit Court of Wayne County, Michigan, 1980; also published in Michael Shapiro and Roy Spece, *Bioethics and Law*, pp. 537–42.

10. Doe v. Attorney General, 307 N.W.2d 438, Mich. 1981.

11. Kentucky Parenting Associates, Inc. v. Commonwealth of Kentucky, 704 S.W.2d 209, 1986.

12. The contract is appended to the New Jersey Supreme Court opinion in the case.

13. See, e.g., Nev. Rev. Stats, section 127.070, Mass. Gen. Laws Ann. C. 210, section 2.

14. See, e.g., Adoption of McKinsie, 275 S.W.2d 365, Mo. 1955; Note, "Revocation of Parental Consent to Adoption: Legal Doctrine and Social Policy," *University of Chicago Law Review*, 28 (1961): 564.

15. See, e.g., Adoption of Ashton, 97 A 2d 368, Pa 1953.

16. Lumley v. Wagner, 1 De Gex, M & G 616, 1852.

17. Note, "Rumplestiltskin Revisited: The Inalienable Rights of Surrogate Mothers," *Harvard Law Review*, 99 (1986): 1936; Barbara Cohen, "Surrogate Mothers: Whose Baby Is It?," *American Journal of Law & Medicine*, 10 (1984): 234.

18. See Judith Areen, et al., *Law, Science and Medicine*, at pages 1313–14. See also *Newsweek*, February 14, 1983, page 76; *New York Times* January 23, 1983, page 19; *New York Times* February 7, 1983 page 8; *Washington Post* Jan 21, 1983, page A11, *Washington Post* February 3, 1983, page 8.

19. Robert J. Levine, *Ethics and Regulation of Clinical Research*, 2d ed. (Baltimore: Urban and Schwarzenberg, 1986), 278.

20. Samuel D. Warren and Louis D. Brandeis, "The Right of Privacy," *Harvard Law Review*, 4 (1890): 193.

21. Meyer v. Nebraska, 262 U.S. 390, 1923.

22. Pierce v. Society of Sisters, 268 U.S. 510, 1925.

23. Skinner v. Oklahoma, 316 U.S. 535, 1942.

24. See, e.g., Jones v. United States, 357 U.S. 493, 1958; Stanford v. Texas, 379 U.S. 476, 1965; Mapp v. Ohio, 367 U.S. 643, 1961.

25. Aptheker v. Secretary of State, 378 U.S. 500, 1964.

26. Griswold v. Connecticut, 381 U.S. 479, 1965.

27. Roe v. Wade, 410 U.S. 113, 1973.

28. Loving v. Virginia, 388 U.S. 1, 1967.

29. Harris v. McRae, 448 U.S. 297, 1980.

30. Matthew Eccles, "The Use of in Vitro Fertilization: Is There a Right to Bear or Beget a Child by Any Available Medical Means?" *Pepperdine Law Review*, 12 (1985), 1033.

31. PL 93–348, section 214 (d).

32. In re Baby M, supra note 8, at 70.

33. I was co-author of the amicus brief, filed on behalf of Odyssey Institute of Connecticut, in which that issue was raised. Prof. Cyril C. Means, Jr., of New York Law School was the primary author of the brief.

34. Civil Code of Louisiana, Article 35.

35. In Moss v. Sandefur, 14 Ark. 381 (1854), for example, a man fathered a child by a slave he had rented from her owner. The Supreme Court of Arkansas held that if he wanted his child, he had to buy it from the mother's owner.

36. Yates v. Keane, #9758 and #9772, slip op., Mich. Circuit Ct., Jan. 21, 1988 (less than two weeks prior to the *Baby M* decision.)

37. See, e.g., Barrow v. State, 74 S.E.2d 467, Ga. 1953; Walker v. Walker, 266 So.2d 385, Fla. 1972; State v. Bowen, 498 P.2d 977, Wash. 1972; Commonwealth v. Pewatts, 186 A.2d 408, Pa. 1962; Wilson v. Caswell, 172 N. E. 251, Mass. 1930.

38. E.g., Angela Holder, "Client Autonomy and Divorce Negotiations," *Family Law*, 17 (1977): 11.

39. E.g., Esmond v. Liscio 224 A.2d 793, Penn. 1966; Wilson v. Maryland Casualty 105 A.2d 304, Pa. 1954; Glesby v. Hartford Accident and Indemnity Co., 44 P.2d 365, Cal. 1935.

Legislative Approaches to Surrogate Motherhood

R. Alta Charo

By the beginning of 1988, nearly six hundred babies had been born through surrogate mothering arrangements. Although there have been a number of lawsuits concerning custody or challenging adoption laws that appear to prohibit payments to surrogates, the majority of surrogacy arrangements proceed without judicial involvement. Nevertheless, surrogate mothering has engendered considerable activity in state legislatures, as well as two bills in Congress to ban the practice (H.R. 2433 and H.R. 3264) and hearings by the House Committee on Energy and Commerce and the Subcommittee on Transportation, Tourism, and Hazardous Wastes. Most recently, the Congressional Office of Technology Assessment (OTA) released a report, *Infertility: Medical and Social Choices.*[1] That report included the results of a survey of surrogate-mother matching services active in the United States in late 1987 (see Table 1).

This article reviews the structure of surrogacy arrangements and summarizes the legislative and judicial responses to date, both here and abroad, drawing on the data collected in the 1988 OTA survey. The article concludes with the suggestion that while surrogacy arrangements ought not to be criminalized, they should not be enforceable either. Further, it suggests that payment beyond the actual and reasonable expenses associated with surrogacy ought to be prohibited, along with the professional services of surrogate matching services. Finally, to protect the reproductive autonomy of all women, it proposes that the federal government should recognize that there is nothing "surrogate" about surrogate mothering, and should enact legislation to define "mother" as a woman who carries a child to term, regardless of the source of the egg and sperm or her intentions with regard to custody.

The Structure of Surrogacy Arrangements

Who Hires a Surrogate Mother?

The overwhelming majority of those seeking surrogates are white, married couples in their late thirties or early forties, although agencies reported agreeing to hire a surrogate mother for five unmarried couples and nine single men, according to the OTA survey.[2] The number of homosexual individuals or couples who seek to hire a surrogate mother is consistently reported as no more than 1 percent, but three agencies have sought surrogates for a homosexual male couple, and one for a homosexual female couple. Approximately 25 percent are Catholic, a similar proportion are Jewish, and approximately 42 percent are Protestant. On average agencies report that about 25 percent of the couples are already raising a child. In one 1988 development, a family with several boys hired a surrogate in the hopes of obtaining a girl. When she conceived fraternal twins, one a boy and one a girl, the intended rearing parents accepted the girl but placed the boy in a foster home, from which his biological mother retrieved him.[3]

Those seeking to hire a surrogate mother are generally well off and well educated. Agencies reported that approximately 64 percent of their clients have a household income over $50,000, with an additional 28 percent earning $30,000 to $50,000 per year. Overall, the services reported that at least 37 percent of their clients are college-educated, while another 54 percent have attended graduate school.[4]

Who Becomes a Surrogate Mother?

Agencies report that the women waiting to be hired as surrogate mothers are generally non-Hispanic Protestant whites, twenty-six to twenty-eight years of age. Approximately 60 percent are married (see Table 1). Most have had a prior pregnancy, and approximately 20 percent have had either a prior miscarriage or an abortion. Generally fewer than 10 percent have previously relinquished a child through adoption, and fewer than 7 percent have been surrogates before.[5] One psychiatrist suggests that some surrogates offer this service as part of their personal effort to overcome the memory of a prior loss of a child or their own placement for adoption.[6] No study has yet confirmed this suspicion, however.

Surrogate mothers are less educated and less financially secure than those who hire them. Fewer than 35 percent of those waiting to be hired as surrogates had ever attended college, and only 4 percent had attended any graduate school. Thirty percent earn from $30,000 to $50,000 per year, but two-thirds (66 percent) earn less than $30,000.

Fees

As reported to OTA, the most common fee for a surrogate mother is $10,000 plus expenses for life insurance, maternity clothes, required transportation to the matching center or physician, necessary laboratory tests, and the delivery. That figure has not changed since 1984, although two agencies reported a fee of $12,000 and three stated that each fee is negotiated in-

TABLE I: Demographic Surveys of Surrogate Mothers

	OTA	Linkins	Hanifin	Parker 1	Parker 2	Franks
Sample size	>334[a]	34	89	30	125	10
Average age	27	28	28	25	25	26
Marital status						
Married	60%	73%	80%	87%	53%	50%
Single	40%[b]	18%	14%	10%	19%	40%
Divorced	—	9%	5%	3%	22%	10%
Unknown	—	—	—	—	6%	—
No. of children	N/A	1.8	2.0	1.9	1.4	1–3
Race/ethnicity						
White non-Hispanic	88%	N/A	85%	100%	100%	N/A
Hispanic	2%	N/A	14%	—	—	N/A
Black non-Hispanic	<1%	N/A	<1%	—	—	N/A
Asian	2%	N/A	<1%	—	—	N/A
Other	8%[c]	N/A	<1%	—	—	N/A
Religion						
Protestant	67%	N/A	74%	53%	55%	N/A
Catholic	28%	N/A	25%	47%	40%	N/A
Jewish	3%	N/A	<1%	—	1%	N/A
Other	2%	N/A	<1%	—	4%	N/A
Household income						
<$15,000	13%	N/A	N/A	N/A	N/A	N/A
$15,000–$30,000	53%	N/A	N/A	N/A	N/A	N/A
$30,000–$50,000	30%	N/A	N/A	N/A	N/A	N/A
>$50,000	4%	N/A	N/A	N/A	N/A	N/A
Average	N/A	$25,000	N/A	N/A	N/A	N/A
Range	N/A	$12K–$68K	N/A	N/A	6K–$55K	(modest to moderate)

						— (average for sample)
Education						
Some high school	61%[d]	12%	—	20%	18%[e]	—
High school graduate	—	38%	52%	53%	54%[e]	—
Some college	35%[d]	47%	24%	27%	26%[e]	—
College graduate	—	3%[f]	24%[f]	—	2%[e]	—
Some graduate school	4%[d]	—	—	—	—	—
Previously relinquished child by:						
Surrogacy	7%	N/A	N/A	N/A	N/A	N/A
Adoption	7%	N/A	1%	10%	9%	N/A
Abortion	18%	N/A	37%	23%	26%	N/A
Are themselves adopted	12%	N/A	1%	1%	1%	N/A

a. Data supplied by matching agencies, not by surrogates themselves.
b. Includes divorced.
c. May include Hispanics.
d. Includes graduates.
e. Includes only fifty women in sample.
f. Includes category "some graduate school."

Note: "N/A" means "not applicable" or "not available."

Sources:
Franks—D. D. Franks, "Psychiatric Evaluation of Women in a Surrogate Mother Program," *American Journal of Psychiatry*, 138 (1981): 1378–79.
Hanifin—H. Hanifin, *The Surrogate Mother: An Exploratory Study* (University Microfilms International: Chicago, 1984); H. Hanifin, "Surrogate Parenting: Reassessing Human Bonding," paper presented at the American Psychological Association Convention, New York, August 1987.
Linkins—K. Linkins, H. Daniels, and R. Richards, McLean Hospital, Boston, Mass., Jan. 8, 1988.
OTA—Office of Technology Assessment, U.S. Congress, 1988.
Parker 1—P. J. Parker, "The Psychology of the Surrogate Mother: A Newly Updated Report of a Longitudinal Pilot Study," paper presented at the American Orthopsychiatric Association General Meeting, Toronto, April 9, 1984.
Parker 2—P. J. Parker, "Motivations of Surrogate Mothers: Initial Findings," *American Journal of Psychiatry*, 140 (1983): 117–18.

dividually.[7] In addition, fees are paid to the commercial broker (commonly $3,000 to $7,000, but ranging up to $12,000); the physicians (from $2,000 to $3,000) and psychiatrists (from $60 to $150 per hour); and the attorneys (up to $5,000). The total cost of all these fees and expenses can be roughly $30,000 to $50,000, meaning that about $1 of every $4 actually goes to the surrogate mother herself.

At least thirty-six states make it illegal to induce parents to part with offspring or to pay money beyond medical, legal, and certain other expenses for a parent to give a child up for adoption. All the states, whether by statute or judicial decision, prohibit baby-selling.[8] Whether these laws apply to surrogate transactions depends upon judicial decisions in each state, as well as upon interpretations of state and federal constitutional protections of the right to procreate (see infra). The preconception agreement lacks the coercive pressures of unwanted pregnancy or recent childbirth that are at the root of many prohibitions on baby-selling.[9] Further, the baby is given over to another genetic parent, who is thereby buying exclusivity of custody, rather than the actual baby. Some contracts are written to pay the mother a monthly fee, rather than a lump sum upon relinquishment of the child, perhaps to enhance the impression that it is her services that are being bought, not the baby.[10]

On the other hand, a miscarriage or stillbirth often results in only a nominal fee being paid, ranging from nothing to $3,000.[11] At least two centers reduce or eliminate the fee if the surrogate is found to have behaved in a way that resulted in a health-impaired child. Finally, the hiring couple generally will pay no fee unless the mother will relinquish the child at birth.[12] The Kansas attorney general, considering this point, concluded, "[W]e cannot escape the fact that custody of the minor child is decided as a contractual matter" involving the exchange of funds, and thus violating public policy that "children are not chattel and therefore may not be the subject of a contract or a gift."[13]

If state laws prohibiting monetary inducements to adoption are applicable to paid surrogacy, they make payment of money to surrogates illegal baby-selling. This was the conclusion of courts in Indiana,[14] Michigan,[15] and New Jersey.[16] In contrast, courts in New York[17] and Kentucky[18] have held that their baby-selling prohibitions do not specifically address the situation created by surrogate motherhood, and that therefore payments are allowable until the state legislature decides otherwise.[19] Only Louisiana's and Nevada's legislatures have acted on this point. In 1987, amendments to Nevada's adoption law exempted "lawful" surrogacy contracts from the provisions of the statute prohibiting payment to a mother beyond her expenses.[20] Louisiana, on the other hand, found such contracts to be prohibited baby-selling, and made the arrangements void from their inception, as did legislatures in Indiana, Kentucky, and Nebraska.

Limitations on Behavior or
Medical Treatment During Pregnancy

Surrogacy contracts typically prohibit the mother from smoking, drinking alcohol, and taking illegal drugs. She must also agree to abide by physician's orders,[21] which may oblige her to undergo amniocentesis, electronic fetal monitoring, or a Cesarean delivery. Two-thirds of the agency contracts allow the client some control over whether the surrogate mother will undergo chorionic villi sampling, amniocentesis, or abortion, as well as the type of prenatal care she will receive.[22]

A practical problem with provisions such as these is the difficulty of enforcement. It is hardly feasible to follow a woman around to observe or control her behavior. Suits for breach of contract would also be of limited use: it is unlikely that any minor breach of these behavioral restrictions will lead to an identifiable health problem in a child, leaving it unclear how to assess damages. Even liquidated damages cannot be used, unless the figure set for the damages bears some reasonable relationship to the harm caused by the breach. Thus, both prenatal efforts to enforce the behavioral lifestyle restrictions or postnatal attempts to collect damages for their breach are difficult propositions.

Another enforcement mechanism is specific performance. However, that remedy could unconstitutionally interfere with individual rights to privacy, personal autonomy, and bodily integrity. Behavioral and medical restrictions in the contract may give the client more control over the surrogate mother's pregnancy, as it gives the client a basis upon which to seek an injunction to force her to comply or to seek damages should she refuse to comply. Yet principles of personal autonomy would probably prevent the enforcement of any requirement to undergo amniocentesis or abortion, and many proposed state laws would prohibit enforcement of such clauses. Once involved, however, courts might seek to require certain treatments on the basis of a noncontractual duty to the fetus.

A pregnant woman may possibly have a noncontractual duty to prevent harm to her fetus,[23] regardless of whether she intends to raise the child. This is a controversial and developing area of law, and a number of commentators have expressed concern that the identification of such a duty might unconstitutionally limit women's bodily autonomy.[24] A few courts have held that women may have an obligation not only to refrain from harmful behaviors—such as taking drugs—but also to take affirmative steps to prevent harm, such as undergoing Cesarean sections.[25]

Surrogacy arrangements could affect the development of this evolving area of law because the pregnant woman is often unrelated to the intended rearing parents of the child. The couple generally invest a great deal of time and money in trying to ensure that they will raise the child she bears. They have no recourse other than legal methods to try and control her behavior. A client might use the contractual arrangement with the birth mother and the evidence of intent to rear the child to argue that he and his partner have standing to seek an injunction ordering the mother to undergo a medical procedure such as a Cesarean section. This is particularly important in light of the controversy surrounding the use of court orders to force women to undergo Cesarean sections because their physicians or husbands disagree with their decision to forgo the procedure.[26] How the courts might react in the contractual surrogacy situation, however, is difficult to predict, as is the extent to which judicial decisions would be taken to apply equally to women who intend to raise the children they bear.

The Surrogate Mother's Rights to the Child

Surrogate contracts typically require the mother to immediately relinquish custody of the newborn baby. (Only three agencies do not use this provision, each reporting that it would appear to be unenforceable under their state law.) She is then required to sign papers terminating her parental rights.

The central issue in surrogacy is whether a contract can determine custody and parental rights when the surrogate mother refuses to relinquish either. Courts and attorney general opinions have consistently stated in dictum that a surrogate mother has the same rights to her child as does a mother who conceived with the intention of keeping her baby, and that the best interests of the child would dictate the court's decision regarding custody.[27] The courts reasoned that a surrogate motherhood contract, while not void from inception, is nevertheless voidable. This means that if all parties agree to abide by the contract terms, and the intended rearing parents are not found to be manifestly unfit, then a court will enter the necessary paternity orders and approve the various attorney's fees agreed upon.[28] If, on the other hand, the surrogate mother changes her mind about giving up her parental rights within the statutory time period provided by the applicable state law, then "[s]he has forfeited her rights to whatever fees the contract provided, but both the mother, child and biological father now have the statutory rights and obligations as exist in the absence of contract."[29]

ENFORCEABILITY OF SURROGACY CONTRACTS

Until the *Baby M*[30] and *Yates v. Huber*[31] cases, no custody dispute ever made it to trial in the United States. In both of these 1988 decisions, however, surrogate motherhood contracts were voided and held irrelevant to determining custody of a child wanted by both the surrogate mother and the genetic father. The New Jersey decision is particularly important because that state's nationally influential Supreme Court held that commercial surrogacy contracts are void (and possibly criminal), not merely voidable. Finding the contract void has several important consequences. First, as noted supra, it removes an important basis upon which a court could order a surrogate mother to relinquish a child to the genetic father pending resolution of a custody dispute. Second, it eliminates the contractual authority of a genetic father to control the behavior of a surrogate mother during pregnancy or to specify the conditions of her prenatal care and delivery. Finally, it makes a surrogacy contract unenforceable, so that courts would not be allowed to order even monetary damages for its breach. This complete lack of enforceability could be a tremendous deterrent to the further popularization of surrogate motherhood, although it should be noted that similar unenforceability with regard to prenatal independent adoptions has not eliminated that practice. Discussing the analogy of commercial surrogacy to prohibited baby-selling, the New Jersey Supreme Court acknowledged that the surrogate consents to adoption before conceiving the child, and therefore does not act under the duress of an unintended pregnancy.[32] Nevertheless, it stated:

> The natural mother is irrevocably committed before she knows the strength of her bond with her child. She never makes a totally voluntary, informed decision, for quite clearly any decision prior to the baby's birth is, in the most important sense, uninformed, and any decision after that, compelled by a pre-existing contractual commitment, the threat of a lawsuit, and the inducement of a $10,000 payment, is less than totally voluntary.

The idea of informed consent to engage in a surrogacy arrangement is made even more problematic in transnational surrogacy arrangements, where language barriers, absence of legal counsel, and immigration considerations may affect the transaction. For example, one surrogacy contract between an American couple and a Mexican cousin has resulted in a custody dispute complicated by allegations of misunderstanding and violations of immigration law. The surrogate understood that she was to undergo in vivo fertilization and embryo transfer, a commitment of several weeks. The couple asserts, however, that the handwritten contract and oral understandings always contemplated a full-term pregnancy, with the child relinquished to the genetic father and his wife at birth. In exchange, the couple was to provide clothing, medical care, food, and assistance in obtaining a visa for permanent residency in the United States.[33] The arrangement was complicated by the fact that it included providing housing in the United States for the Mexican mother, in violation of immigration regulations.

One proposed solution to the problem of ensuring informed and voluntary consent would require that surrogacy contracts be reviewed in a court before being signed by the parties. As described infra, several state bills, as well as recommendations by advisory bodies in the Netherlands and Ontario, Canada, have suggested that the contract be enforceable if a court has fully satisfied itself that it is not overreaching and that the parties are fully aware of the meaning of their promises. However, the problem of the inherent coercion created by economic need resulted in the Dutch proposal being limited to noncommercial arrangements, with commercial surrogacy still disapproved.

To date, only Indiana, Kentucky, Louisiana, and Nebraska have passed legislation specifically addressing enforceability. The Kentucky, Louisiana, and Nebraska statutes void all surrogacy contracts involving "compensation" or "consideration." As the term "consideration" was not defined, it remains somewhat unclear whether payment of a surrogate's actual and reasonable expenses would void a contract. Indiana's statute voids all surrogacy contracts, regardless of payment.

Nevada's legislation, which exempted "lawful" surrogacy from baby-selling prohibitions, does not speak to enforceability. Nevada law still invalidates a mother's consent to relinquish a child for adoption if made less than forty-eight hours after birth. It is not clear whether a surrogacy contract that commits the mother to relinquish the child is in and of itself a violation of the law, making the contract "unlawful" and therefore outside the provisions of this amendment. Further, the statute is not clear on how the courts should balance the competing provisions of the contract terms and the statutory forty-eight-hour cooling-off period, should there be a dispute. Although the intent of the amendment clearly seems to be to exempt surrogacy from the prohibitions on baby-selling, it is not clear whether the amendment is also intended to render surrogacy agreements fully enforceable.

Surrogacy Arrangements: Models of State Policy

Legislation related to surrogate motherhood has been introduced in over half the state legislatures since 1980[34]; many of these bills are still pending. Only seven states have passed legislation. Their approaches have differed: Arkansas endorsed surrogacy, Kansas simply exempted surrogacy from prohibitions on adoption agency advertising, and Nevada exempted it from its prohibition on baby-selling. Kentucky, Louisiana, and Nebraska, on the other hand, voided commercial surrogacy contracts, and Indiana voided all surrogacy contracts. The approaches taken by state legislatures may be broadly grouped into five categories: static, private ordering, inducement, regulatory, and punitive.[35]

The Static Approach

The static approach is basically one of inaction, an effort to maintain the status quo. To date, it has had mixed results. Several courts have so far declined to find that surrogates lose their rights of motherhood by virtue of their pre-conception agreement to relinquish parental rights. But most courts have at the same time agreed to enforce the paternity and fee-payment provisions of these contracts, at least when all parties to the agreement still desire its enforcement. In other words, although these courts have found surrogate agreements to be voidable, they generally have not found them to be void. A notable exception is the New Jersey Supreme Court, which held that these agreements are void.[36]

This socially and psychologically conservative approach seeks to minimize the impact of noncoital reproductive techniques upon the structure and relationships of the traditional family, mainly by refusing to recognize new parental configurations. "The family unit has been under severe attack from almost every element of our modern commercial society, yet it continues as the bedrock of the world as we know it. Any practice which threatens the stability of the family unit is a direct threat to society's stability," stated the dissenting justice in *Surrogate Parenting Association, Inc.*, the 1986 case finding that paid surrogate matching services are permissible under Kentucky law. This attitude is typical of the static approach, which aims to support traditional family configurations.

One legislative method for furthering this viewpoint would be to define "mother" as the woman who either gives birth to a child or who obtains a child through a legal adoption proceeding. Such a definition could guarantee surrogate mothers control of their pregnancy and at least those rights held by all mothers with respect to their children. However, given the economic and educational disparity between surrogates and those who hire them, merely having equal footing will not ensure that surrogates who wish to retain custody of their children will have success at least half the time. For example, Mary Beth Whitehead did not win exclusive or primary custody of Baby M, and Laurie Yates (of the *Yates v. Huber* case) relinquished custody of her twins to their biological father rather than proceed with a custody trial after the surrogacy agreement had been declared void. Ms. Yates and her husband were both unemployed, and despite the fact that the children had lived with them in the seven months since their birth, the Yates' success in a custody trial was far from assured.

Thus, although the static approach will undoubtedly slow the growth of surrogate motherhood as an industry, it will not eliminate it entirely. The expansion of these services since 1980, in the absence of judicial or legislative guidelines, demonstrates that this arrangement can be used when all parties abide by their original intentions. There can be some problems with the use of state laws and courts to manage birth certificate recordations and paternity orders. It is primarily when the parties change their minds, however, that state action becomes important and that the absence of governmental guidelines becomes an active barrier to the successful conclusion of the arrangement.

The Private Ordering Approach

The private ordering approach holds that government's primary role is to facilitate individual arrangements, and thus would compel recognition and enforcement of any conception and parenting agreement freely formed among consenting adults. Such an approach could accommodate commercializing the services of surrogate mothers.[37] Private ordering is, of course, subject to some limited constraints, such as those offering special protection to vulnerable parties in the transaction. Children are traditionally viewed as such vulnerable parties, and thus judicial intervention to ensure that custody is awarded to a fit parent would be consistent even with this approach of limited governmental intervention.

Examples of such private-ordering philosophy can be found in several of the bills introduced in state legislatures, such as the Nevada amendment that exempts surrogacy from prohibitions on baby-selling. Proposed legislation in Oregon would also follow this model, and another Oregon proposal goes further to specifically legalize paid and unpaid surrogacy, while providing for specific enforcement and damages as remedies for breach of contract. An early Rhode Island bill also aimed to make surrogacy contracts enforceable, stating that surrogate motherhood "is to be viewed as a business venture" and that the "rights of motherhood" do not apply to the surrogate mother.[38]

Without addressing the question of the enforceability of surrogacy contracts, an amendment to an Arkansas artificial-insemination statute explicitly contemplates surrogate arrangements. With respect to unmarried women at least, it allows an exception to the presumption that the woman who bears a child is its legal mother. The amendment states that in the case of surrogate motherhood, the child "shall be that of the woman intended to be the mother." The statute does not address questions of evidence, such as the kind of agreement necessary to demonstrate who was intended to be the mother or the enforceability of these arrangements. Nevertheless, it is the first statute in the United States of its kind. A Wisconsin bill calling for a presumption that the intended social parents are in fact more fit to raise the child also exemplifies the private ordering approach, but with some protection for the vulnerable child. Further, the bill attempts to ensure that if all the adult parties refuse custody, an adoptive home will be found for the child.

Consistent with the private ordering approach are state law provisions to ensure the informed and voluntary consent of all parties. A number of bills require that the surrogate and the intended rearing parents be represented by attorneys; many further specify that the parties be represented by separate counsel. Bills in at least five states require that the intended rearing parents review the results of medical, psychological, and genetic examinations of the surrogate mother before agreeing to hire her. Bills in Michigan and the District of Columbia propose that at least thirty days pass between the time that the contract is signed and the first insemination, to allow a cooling-off period.[39] It is unclear if such provisions could meet all the objections of the New Jersey Supreme Court, but the *Baby M* decision did say that state legislatures could legalize and regulate surrogacy, within constitutional limits.[40]

The private ordering approach can be inadequate if parties fail to agree to a contract that spells out all contingencies and their outcomes. For example, a contract might fail to specify a remedy if one or both of the intended social parents were to die, leaving it unclear whether the surrogate mother or the state is responsible for the child. Contracts may also fail to specify the medical tests to be performed during pregnancy, remedies for failure to abide by lifestyle restrictions, or the lines of authority for emergency medical decisions concerning the health of the newborn. In the absence of state guidelines that create presumptive responses to these situations, private contracts may lead to disagreement and confusion. Courts attempting to enforce the contracts and carry out the parties' intentions could find it necessary to decide on matters not explicitly contemplated under the contract, making even these arrangements unclear as to their outcome and highly variable from state to state.

The Inducement Approach

The inducement approach offers individuals an exchange. If the contracting parties agree to follow prescribed practices—such as judicial review of the contract, adherence to a model set of terms and conditions, or use of a licensed surrogate matching service—the state will facilitate legal recognition of the child born by the arrangement.[41] For example, a Missouri bill introduced in 1987 would require that judges approve surrogate contracts before insemination takes place. In exchange, the bill would automatically terminate the rights of the surrogate mother, thereby offering the intended rearing parents the certainty that they will be able to gain custody of the child. The penalty for failure to follow these practices might be that the contract is unenforceable under state law or that adoption proceedings are ineligible for expedited treatment. Of course, penalties that harm a baby's psychological, physical, or even legal well-being would probably be unacceptable. A preliminary draft by the National Conference of Commissioners on Uniform State Laws takes a similar approach.[42] A 1986 report by the independent Health Council of the Netherlands also endorsed this approach,[43] although only for noncommercial contracts and only with the proviso that a surrogate have three months following birth to change her mind about relinquishing custody. Commercial contracts were disapproved in the report.

Another form of this approach is to induce use of a particular approved procedure or agency by offering some governmental assurance of its quality. Thus, for example, government could license particular adoption agencies to operate as surrogate matching services. As a condition of licensing, the agency could agree to certain conditions, such as use of a standard contract or psychological screening of participants. The state would also ensure that the personnel of the agency meet certain minimum criteria, such as years in practice or professional training. Although there would be no penalty for failure to use the service, many participants would probably be interested in assuring themselves that the surrogates they hire have been screened for drug or alcohol abuse, that the persons for whom they bear children have been interviewed to identify the kind of home they plan to provide for the child, or that the contract they sign has been reviewed for fairness, completeness, and enforceability.

Any inducement approach that relies at least partly upon licensing surrogate matching agencies permits the government to prevent abuses without necessarily limiting the freedom of individuals who wish to pursue these agreements. For example, licensing could specify permissible and impermissible ways of recruiting surrogates and infertile couples, standardize the medical testing and screening of the participants and their gametes, require monitoring of the health of the baby, or set standard fees and expenses. To allow poorer couples access to surrogacy, licensing could provide sliding fee scales and agency-financing. Inducement or regulatory approaches may also, however, enable the government to specify who will be permitted to take advantage of the agencies. Agencies might, for example, be limited to serving married couples, thereby leaving unmarried couples, homosexual couples, and single persons without access to the advantageous state-approved method of surrogate adoption. Any such limitations would be subject to constitutional review, particularly to the extent that they are viewed as state interference in the right to privacy with regard to procreative decisions.

The Regulatory Approach

State regulation can also be used to create an exclusive mechanism by which an activity may be carried out. A number of proposals have been made to regulate surrogacy. Bills in Florida, Illinois, New Jersey, and South Carolina, for example, would permit only married couples to hire a surrogate. Bills in at least eight states would further specify that surrogates can be used only for medical reasons, such as inability to conceive or to carry a pregnancy to term.[44] A South Carolina bill would require extensive investigation of the intended parents' home, as is generally done prior to adoption. Bills also propose standards for potential surrogate mothers, such as excluding women who have never had children before.

Besides regulating who may participate in surrogacy arrangements, a number of bills specify that the surrogate and at times the intended parents undergo psychological screening or counseling, and bills would require the biological mother and father to be tested for sexually transmitted diseases. This latter point takes on particular importance after the report that one surrogate who was not stringently screened before she became pregnant bore a child who was seropositive for the human immunodeficiency virus. The biological father and his wife rejected the child.[45] Regulations have also been proposed in South Carolina to require the surrogate mother to follow physician's orders during pregnancy, to adhere to a particular prenatal care schedule, and to forgo abortion unless medically indicated.

Regulations have also been proposed to limit compensation to the surrogate mother, or to set forth pro rata schedules of fees in the event of abortion, miscarriage, or stillbirth. Some proposals have also been made to maintain state records of surrogacy arrangements, and in a few cases, to provide the child, at age eighteen, with information about his or her conception. State proposals have split on whether to allow the surrogate a period after birth in which to change her mind about relinquishing custody and on whether the remedy should she do so would be monetary damages or specific enforcement of the contract's custody provisions.[46]

The Punitive Approach

The punitive approach is hostile to surrogacy arrangements. To put an end to them, it prohibits the practice, or at least its commercial forms. An alternative mechanism is to make the contracts unenforceable.

Punitive measures may be directed at a variety of parties. Civil and criminal sanctions could attach to the professional matching services, to the physicians and attorneys who are involved in the arrangements, or to the surrogates or couples themselves.[47] Nevada's legislature, for example, is to consider a bill making surrogate matching a felony punishable by up to six years in prison. A Michigan bill also treats surrogate matching as a felony, making the penalties particularly stiff for any person who matches a couple to a surrogate who is not of legal age. The bill would make the participation by the surrogate and the genetic father a felony as well. However, the fact that surrogacy does not require the services of a physician or an attorney, and therefore is not easy to detect, means that prohibitive approaches are unlikely to completely eliminate surrogate arrangements, although they may drive them underground.

England's 1985 Surrogacy Arrangements Act bans commercial surrogacy, although without criminal penalty. The Spanish report, however, recommended criminal penalties for both commercial and noncommercial surrogacy.[48] The Surrogacy Arrangements Act in England, as well as regulations in France[49] and court decisions in the Federal Republic of Germany,[50] also outlaw the operation of surrogate matching services in those countries. In fact, with the exception of reports recommending limited approval of supervised, noncommercial surrogacy contracts in the Netherlands and in Ontario, Canada, every nation that has examined surrogacy arrangements has taken a punitive approach and concluded that they should be at the least unenforceable and, at the most, criminal.[51] The recommendations of the two approving reports have not yet been implemented, although they are under review in Canada.[52]

In the United States, the idea of prohibiting all forms of surrogacy, including those involving no compensation beyond direct expenses, raises the question of interference with the right to procreate. Such a prohibition would seem to interfere more with the ability of a couple to raise a genetically related child than with an individual's right to have a child, however. Limitations on surrogacy do not prevent the man from procreating (albeit outside marriage), nor do they affect his wife's inability to procreate. Rather, they interfere with their ability, as a couple, to raise a child genetically related to at least one of them. As such, prohibitions on surrogacy may invite judicial challenge but would probably be upheld.

The courts in *Doe v. Kelly*[53] and *Baby M*[54] characterized surrogacy as an effort to use contract law to further the statutory right to change the legal status of a child via adoption, rather than as an effort to exercise the right to procreate per se:

> The right to procreate very simply is the right to have natural children, whether through sexual intercourse or artificial insemination. It is no more than that. Mr. Stern has not been deprived of that right. Through artificial insemination of Mrs. Whitehead, Baby M is his child. The custody, care, companionship, and nurturing that follow birth are not parts of the right to procreation; they are rights that may also be constitutionally protected, but that involve many considerations other than the right of procreation.[55]

The question can be recast as: Is there a constitutional right to have custody of a biologically related child? No such right has been identified in the past:

> There is nothing in our culture or society that even begins to suggest a fundamental right on the part of the father to the custody of the child as

part of his right to procreate when opposed by the claim of the mother to the same child.[56]

Thus, prohibitions on surrogacy pose a somewhat attenuated threat to the right to procreate.

Short of prohibiting surrogacy, a state could take a punitive approach by making surrogacy contracts unenforceable. Thus, for example, a bill could prohibit payment of fees to surrogates, by stating that commercial surrogacy contracts are void and therefore unenforceable. This was the approach taken in the Kentucky, Louisiana, and Nebraska laws. Proposals in Alabama, Minnesota, and New York take this same approach. Proposals in Connecticut, Illinois, North Carolina, and Rhode Island would void even noncommercial contracts, an approach adopted into law in 1988 by Indiana. Voiding these contracts means that should the surrogate change her mind about relinquishing the child, she will stand on at least equal footing with the genetic father when she seeks permanent custody. In some states, if the surrogate is married, her husband will be presumed by law to be the child's father, leaving the genetic father with a difficult task should he seek custody of the baby.

A number of countries have taken this approach. Legislation, court cases, or regulations in South Australia and Victoria, Australia,[57] the Federal Republic of Germany,[58] France,[59] Israel,[60] Norway,[61] South Africa,[62] and the United Kingdom[63] state that surrogacy contracts, whether commercial or noncommercial, are unenforceable. Other countries, such as Spain[64] and Sweden,[65] have issued parliamentary reports recommending that these nations enact similar legislation, as has the Council of Europe's Ad Hoc Committee of Experts on Progress in the Biomedical Sciences (CAHBI)[66]; Quebec's Council on the Status of Women has also been highly critical of surrogacy.[67] Even if there were a constitutional right preventing states from prohibiting or criminalizing surrogacy, they could still refuse to enforce the contractual agreements. Although failure to enforce the agreements may constitute a significant interference with an extended interpretation of procreative freedom,[68] such unenforceability of prebirth adoption agreements has not prevented couples from using the technique for private adoption. Failure to enforce surrogacy contracts is not a sufficiently direct interference with the right to procreate or even with the privilege to adopt to be outside the limits of governmental authority.

Even if states were obligated to enforce the agreements, they would not necessarily be required to order the mother to relinquish custody of the child and to terminate her parental rights. Imposing monetary damages for breach of contract could be considered a sufficiently strong mechanism for ensuring the general regularity of these arrangements, and should meet any test of a state's obligation to facilitate the use of social arrangements for the formation of families. To announce a constitutional right to con-

tractually obtained custody of a child would deprive the surrogate mother
of the same constitutional right to custody. "It would be to assert that the
constitutional right of procreation includes within it a constitutionally protected contractual right to destroy someone else's right of procreation,"
said the New Jersey Supreme Court.[69]

THE DEFINITION OF MOTHERHOOD:
MODELS FOR POLICY

For many years, a woman who bore a child was clearly the mother of that
child: *mater est quam gestatio demonstrat*.[70] This relationship is no longer
unequivocal. The possibility of embryo transfer or egg donation separates
biological motherhood into genetic and gestational components. It opens
the door to fresh legal consideration of the definitive aspect of motherhood—whether genetics, gestation, or intention—that entitles a particular
woman to a priori rights to a child. "I always considered myself her aunt,"
said Linda Kirkman, gestational mother of a baby conceived with a sister's
egg and destined to live with the infertile sister and her husband.[70A] By
contrast, Carol Chan, who donated eggs so that her sister Susie could bear
and raise a child, said, "I could never regard the twins as anything but my
nephews."[70B] The two births occurred in Melbourne within weeks of each
other.

The dilemma of gestational surrogates, those who are not genetically
linked to the fetuses they carry and deliver, most clearly poses the question
of whether a genetic or gestational relationship, in and of itself, ought to
determine maternal parentage and legal rights. The determination of their
rights will in turn affect the definition of the rights of mothers who conceive
with the intention to relinquish custody. Ultimately, it might affect determination of the rights of those women now offering naturally conceived
children up for adoption.

The question of legal maternity and surrogacy has been addressed by
law in only two states. Arkansas Statute Section 34–721, touching on birth
certificates, declares:

> For birth registration purposes, in cases of surrogate mothers, the woman
> giving birth shall be presumed to be the natural mother and shall be listed
> as such on the certificate of birth, but a substituted certificate of birth can
> be issued upon orders of a court of competent jurisdiction.

Thus, even in Arkansas, a court order is needed to issue a birth certificate
with the name of a woman other than the one giving birth. Whether a
court would issue such an order based upon genetic maternity or contractual intent to take custody is not clear.

One approach is to mimic the law of paternity, by providing that genetic parentage is definitive. This would mean that a genetic mother could apply to a court for a prebirth ruling that she is the legal mother of a child being carried to term by another. Such a ruling has been issued at least twice,[71] although in those cases the orders were made with the consent of all the parties involved and in furtherance of their stated intentions. A similar request was made in 1987 by a Massachusetts couple who had a Virginia woman carry their genetic child to term and relinquish the infant at birth, with a court decision expected in 1988.[72] The very need to resort to a court order, however, implies a de facto presumption that the birth mother is the child's legal mother. In many ways this is analogous to the determination of paternity, in which a presumption exists that the husband of a pregnant woman is the father of her child, with the presumption rebuttable by evidence that another man is the genetic father.

Recent regulations issued by the Israeli Health Ministry follow this sort of genetic model of maternity.[73] A woman who accepts a donated ovum but gives birth herself must nonetheless formally adopt the child she bore. Although the regulations forbid all forms of surrogacy, thereby making them irrelevant to the question of legal rights for surrogate gestational mothers, they do reflect the Ministry of Health's intention to consider genetic connections to be determinative of parentage, pending a legal change of status.

Another approach is to enforce the surrogacy agreements, regardless of the various genetic, gestational, and intended social arrangements. In the case of gestational surrogacy, this would grant the parental rights of motherhood to a genetic mother who intends to rear a child brought to term by another. Such an approach was taken for the first time when the Wayne County Circuit Court in Michigan issued an interim order declaring a gamete donor couple to be the biological parents of a fetus being carried to term by a woman hired to be the gestational mother. The judge also held that the interim order would be made final after tests confirmed both maternity and paternity.[74] Upon the child's birth, the court entered an order that the names of the ovum and sperm donors be listed on the birth certificate, rather than that of the woman who gave birth. The gestational mother was termed by the court a "human incubator."[75]

One state law attempts to define motherhood in terms of contractually stated intentions for all surrogacy arrangements, not merely those involving ovum transfer. Arkansas Statute Section 34–721(B) states:

> A child born by means of artificial insemination to a woman who is unmarried at the time of the birth of the child, shall be for all legal purposes the child of the woman giving birth, except in the case of a surrogate mother, in which event the child shall be that of the woman intended to be the mother.

This provision avoids the complications of adoption by declaring the intended rearing mother to be the child's legal parent, without the usual elaborate procedures for home review.[76] Thus, if all parties agree to fulfill the contract terms, the surrogate mother's rights would be cut off in favor of those of the intended rearing mother, without the need to get a court order or approval.

The statute is unclear, however, on certain points. First, by its terms it applies only to unmarried women, leaving open the question of the child's legal parentage if the surrogate is married. (In 1987 a bill to extend the provision to married women was passed by the Arkansas legislature but vetoed by the governor.) Section 34–721(A) of the statute states without reservation that a child born by artificial insemination to a married woman is presumed to be her husband's child. Second, the statute concerns "presumptions" of legal parenthood. Unless clearly stated otherwise, presumptions are generally rebuttable. The statute does not address the problem of a surrogate mother changing her mind and deciding to retain parental rights, and it is unclear whether this statute would automatically cut off her rights should she choose to rebut the presumption. Artificial insemination statutes are similarly written in terms of "presumption of paternity," and those presumptions are rebuttable under certain circumstances—for example, if the husband can show that he did not consent to the insemination. The Arkansas law does not specify the reasons for which a surrogate mother can rebut the presumption of maternity.

A third approach is to consider the woman who bears the child as the legal mother, with any further changes in parental rights to be made as per agreement or, in the event of a dispute, as per court order. Such an approach implicitly asserts the primacy of the nine-month pregnancy experience as the key factor in designating a "mother." The approach has simplicity as one advantage. For example, hospital officials would always know at the time of birth the identity of the legal mother. This is also the approach taken in the Arkansas statute discussed previously, which addressed the use of birth certificates in the context of surrogate mother agreements.

The United Kingdom,[77] South Africa,[78] and Bulgaria[79] have explicitly adopted this approach, with legislation stating that the woman who gives birth is to be considered the mother of a child. In West Germany, an advisory Federal-State Parliamentary Working Group[80] and the national medical association[81] have recommended similar legislation, as has CAHBI.[82] The Swiss Academy of Medicine, and the Swiss public through referendum, expressed general hostility to the idea of using in vitro fertilization or embryo transfer in conjunction with surrogacy.[83]

One unusual gestational-surrogacy case involving a model of maternity has drawn international attention to South Africa. In 1987 a forty-eight-year-old grandmother bore triplets conceived in vitro from her daughter's ova and her son-in-law's sperm.[84] Experts disagreed on the legal status of the children, but tended to find that the daughter might have to adopt the children to protect her rights.[85] Nevertheless, the Department of Home Affairs registered the babies as children of their genetic parents. Had they been born after October 14, 1987, when the Children's Status Act came into operation, such registration would have been impossible. They would then have been deemed by law as the children of their birth mother.[86]

SUGGESTIONS FOR FEDERAL ACTION

Surrogacy arrangements are based upon principles of contract and family law, and therefore fall largely within the traditional domain of state legislative activity. With surrogacy an interstate business, Congress has the power under the Interstate Commerce Clause to enact regulatory legislation. Just as it does with interstate adoption activity, however, Congress may choose to leave this area primarily to state and local oversight. State legislators have not moved to coordinate their efforts as yet, with the exception of certain committees of the National Conference of Commissioners on Uniform State Laws and of the American Bar Association.

Absent federal direction, surrogate motherhood is likely to be the subject of extensive state legislative debate and action over the next few years. Statutes, when enacted, are likely to vary considerably, ranging from complete bans to only minimal oversight of contractual arrangements. This period of state legislative activity may be a useful experiment toward finding a workable legislative scheme for either banning or promoting the practice. But lengthy and complicated custody battles could ensue if courts must first decide choice-of-law questions. The problem can become particularly acute if the choice between using one state's law rather than another's could essentially decide the case. Lengthy custody suits are troubling because it becomes progressively more difficult to remove the child from his or her initial home, regardless of the merits of the case. Numerous custody battles may exact a heavy toll on the families and children involved.

Congress ought to step into this arena to accomplish four goals: to reduce the demand for surrogacy, to harmonize the state and transnational laws that govern the arrangement, to ban commercial surrogacy, and to define the legal uses of the term "mother," in order to protect the rights of all pregnant women.

Reduce the Demand for Surrogacy

To avoid the need for state and federal involvement, Congress should focus on preventing infertility and on facilitating adoption for those who are already infertile.

Reducing infertility is an exceedingly difficult task, but some progress might be achieved through more research, education, and data collection on the prevention of sexually transmitted disease.[87] Congress could also help by facilitating the integration of employment, career development, and reproduction, so that couples might be better able to have children during their peak fertility years.

Another path would be to facilitate adoption. The Adoption Assistance and Child Welfare Act of 1980, the Title IV funding of child welfare (including foster care) and adoption assistance under that act, and the 1978 Child Abuse Prevention and Treatment and Adoption Reform Act have produced results worthy of Congress' consideration. These programs have been used to develop a limited national database of adoptable children for use by couples seeking private adoption, as well as to remove barriers to the adoption of children with physical or mental handicaps, older children, or children of a different race. Much better use could be made of a national clearinghouse for adoptable children to make adoption a more manageable and successful, even if time-consuming, effort. Finally, Congress should improve the opportunities for domestic and international adoption, by offering couples the same economic benefits to finance this choice as they would receive in conjunction with childbirth (e.g., maternity and paternity leave) and by simplifying the search for adoptable babies.

Facilitate Harmonization of State Laws

To forestall fragmentation of state laws, Congress should at least exercise oversight of trends in those laws, in order to ascertain whether federal action is necessary. Topics of interest could include state legislation and case law on resolution of custody disputes; development of standard contract provisions, including provisions relating to a surrogate's choice of diet, medical care, and pregnancy continuance; fee structures; and protection for offspring in the event of the death or disability of an adult participant.

Further to this end, Congress could facilitate the development of state laws on surrogate motherhood. Congress could authorize the use of challenge grants to encourage states to explore approaches to surrogate motherhood. Funds could be used to finance studies of proposed legislation; to begin pilot projects for licensing of professional surrogate matching services or review of surrogate contracts; to determine the need for home studies of couples seeking a surrogate mother; or to carry out research concerning the psychological impact of surrogacy arrangements on a child, any siblings, and the adult participants.

Congress could also facilitate joint efforts by states to develop a uniform approach to surrogate motherhood. Congress could pass a joint resolution, for example, calling on the states to adopt one of the model laws now being developed by various professional groups, such as the American Bar Association and the National Conference of Commissioners on Uniform State Laws. Congress could also draft such a model law itself, to be published in the *Federal Register*, as was done in a 1981 effort to harmonize state laws on the adoption of children with special needs.

Although joint resolutions and model legislation are not binding upon the states, they could be used to express the sense of Congress concerning the use of surrogate motherhood. Congress could also encourage states to develop interstate compacts in order to avoid difficult choice-of-law problems in the event of a custody dispute surrounding an interstate arrangement, and to harmonize regulations concerning surrogate-mother matching and child placement. The Interstate Compact on Placement of Children provides a precedent for the use of such compacts in the area of family law, with respect, in that case, to placing children in foster care or adopting homes.

A particularly useful provision that Congress should encourage states to adopt would be to prohibit specific performance of lifestyle and medical care restrictions or of custody provisions. Thus, while allowing states to differ on whether surrogacy contracts should be criminal, void, voidable, or enforceable with monetary damages, uniformity on prohibiting specific performance would protect the personal autonomy of surrogate mothers and prevent child custody from being determined wholly or in great part by contractual terms.

Another topic for forceful congressional action is requiring that surrogacy brokers, if permitted to continue doing business, be licensed by their state. In lieu of federal licensing legislation or regulations, Congress could exercise its power to attach conditions to the receipt of federal funds to require states at least to license professional surrogate matching services, if they are not already outlawed in that state. For example, conditions could be attached to federal funding for Aid to Families with Dependent Children, family planning agencies, or adoption assistance programs. Some of these programs are heavily dependent on federal funding, and many states would probably feel compelled to pass the necessary legislation.

Another area of federal activity should focus on facilitating international agreements concerning transnational surrogacy arrangements. Already, in the brief history of commercialized surrogate motherhood, women of other countries have contracted with American women to act as surrogates, and vice versa. This may become more common in the future. Gestational surrogacy may also become more common. Affluent couples, for example, could hire women from developing nations, for whom a fee of far less than $10,000 would still constitute a considerable sum.

To ensure that there is no confusion concerning the rights of these women, and to avoid conflicts of national law concerning maternity and child custody in the event of a dispute, Congress could work to facilitate international cooperation and agreement on transnational surrogacy arrangements. This could be accomplished by submitting proposals to amend one of the existing child welfare agreements (e.g., the Hague Convention on International Parental Kidnapping), in order to state clearly who—at least initially—shall be considered the mother and the father of a child, and who shall have initial rights to physical custody.

Ban Commercial Surrogacy

Congress should enact legislation to ban for-profit surrogate motherhood, leaving individuals able to engage in the practice as long as no money changed hands, beyond actual expenses. Such a ban would probably have the effect of drastically reducing the scope of the practice. Alternatively, Congress could outlaw commercial intermediaries while leaving individuals free to make their own arrangements even if they involve payments to the surrogate. This too would probably reduce the scope of the practice.

The purpose of such a ban would be to ensure that children are not simply offered to the highest bidder. Parents cannot at this time sell their parental rights to strangers or to each other, even when they are estranged or divorced. Surrogacy should provide no exception to this rule. Further, the commercialization of pregnancy and childbirth creates a dangerous temptation to resort to courts to determine the limits of pregnant women's control over their own bodies, because the people waiting to take the baby home have nothing other than a commercial relationship with the woman to whom they have entrusted the gestation of this child. To prevent a dispute over a surrogate's refusal of fetal monitoring from becoming the test case for all women refusing fetal monitoring, it is probably best to remove commercial relationships from the delivery room.

At the same time, allowing individuals to pursue their own private, contractually unenforceable arrangements reduces the degree of possible interference with the right to procreate and form a family, as well as demonstrates respect for the ability of competent adults to make informed and voluntary choices. Further, it does not foreclose surrogacy entirely to those interested infertile couples with a willing friend or relative. In addition, criminalizing such private activities is unlikely to end surrogacy, but would merely drive it entirely underground.

A ban on commercialized surrogacy, however, would not only be consistent with the spirit behind the prohibitions on baby-selling in place in every state, but would also bring the U.S. in line with the unmistakable majority of other nations that have considered this issue. It would also prevent the U.S. from continuing to grow as a surrogacy haven, to which foreign couples come to arrange for a baby. One Michigan broker has made a number of such arrangements, and it may be only time before this practice leads to a painful transnational custody dispute.

Even if the states and the federal government could not ban all forms of surrogacy, they could prohibit its commercialization, based on the need to avoid encouraging individuals to view embryos, mothers, and babies as articles of commerce.[88] While commercialized surrogacy finally acknowledges the economic value of women's reproductive capabilities—i.e., that "labor" is labor—it also makes biological mothers into "workers on a baby assembly line, as they try to convert their one economic asset—fertility—into cash for their other children."[89] Other sales of the body, whether in prostitution, peonage, or slavery, are prohibited under law when there is broad social agreement that the sale violates basic principles of personhood. Unfortunately, surrogacy has a strong potential for leading to a view of women as childbearers for hire and of babies as articles of commerce.[90] As a commercial ban interferes only with an asserted right to pay for surrogacy, not with the right to procreate, and as women's self-reported motivations for becoming surrogates usually include noncommercial considerations, such as a desire to help other people,[91] a commercial ban should be upheld as a rational expression of state interest that does not unduly interfere with the right to procreate. This conclusion is shared by at least two state courts.[92]

Commercialized reproduction might also lead to the exploitation of certain women. Because of the considerable difference in average income and education between surrogates and those who hire them, some argue that there is an inherent element of coercion in surrogacy arrangements, even if the surrogate is free of the pressure of an unwanted pregnancy at the time she agrees to enter into the contract. A woman faced with an inability to feed her existing children may find herself making a choice that is, albeit autonomous, not genuinely free. Another consideration, beyond economic need, is that surrogacy may be the most efficient way for women with children to supplement the family income without having to leave home. With this consideration, commercial surrogacy may be viewed as a sinister relief from the situational coercion created by the widespread preference for in-home parental care of small children coupled with the small proportion of fathers willing to take on that responsibility. The New Jersey Supreme Court, while recognizing that surrogates consent to the arrangement before conception, nevertheless equated surrogacy with traditional baby-selling:

> The essential evil is the same, taking advantage of a woman's circumstances (unwanted pregnancy or the need for money) in order to take away her child, the difference being one of degree.[93]

While American society has long tolerated the idea that economic need and limited opportunity may lead people to give their children up for adoption or to relatives, and to work under unpleasant and even somewhat hazardous conditions, there has been little tolerance for the idea that such circumstances can be alleviated through the sale of children.

Of course, even as statements of "rational" state interest, arguments based on protecting public morality are generally weak, if only because the harms to society are usually speculative and attenuated. In this case, however, the state rationale is further supported by a history of prohibitions against buying adoptable babies, because it degrades human life and puts children at risk of being placed in inappropriate homes simply because the occupants were able to outbid a competing set of aspiring parents. The New Jersey Supreme Court's *Baby M* decision considered this a crucial point:

> There is not the slightest suggestion that any inquiry will be made at any time to determine the fitness of the Sterns as custodial parents, of Mrs. Stern as an adoptive parent, their superiority to Mrs. Whitehead, or the effect on the child of not living with her natural mother. This is the sale of a child, or, at the very least, the sale of a mother's right to her child, the only mitigating factor being that one of the purchasers is the father. . . . In surrogacy, the highest bidders will presumably become the adoptive parents regardless of suitability, so long as payment of money is permitted.[94]

Undoubtedly the ban on baby-selling in ordinary adoption makes it more difficult for some couples to raise a family, but the limitation has been tolerated in light of the need to protect the interests of the available children. Despite the fact that childlessness is an unhappy affliction for many, there has never been a recognized right to obtain custody of a child.

One leading proponent for the constitutional protection of commercial surrogacy has speculated that prohibitions on private, paid adoptions might indeed be affected if the courts were to find that there is a right to contract for reproductive services and custody of a child:

> Recognition of such a [surrogacy] contract right also raises the question of why contracts to adopt children made before or after conception but before birth would not be valid, nor why parties should not be free after birth to make private contracts for adoption directly with women who want to relinquish their children. The logic . . . is that *persons, at least if married, have a right to acquire a child for rearing purposes,* and may resort to the medical or social means necessary to do so. Although IVF and its variations preserve a genetic or gestational link with one of the rearing parents, the right at issue may not be so easily confined. It may be that the law of adoption needs to be rethought in light of the right to contract for noncoital reproductive assistance.[95]

Traditionally, prohibitions on paying for adoptable babies are based on a collective judgment that certain things simply should not be bought and sold. Prohibitions against buying human organs have been based on the same reasoning[96]; and no successful challenge has ever been mounted to the fact that this interferes with the rights of individuals willing to purchase organs without which they might die. The New Jersey Supreme Court, considering this point in the Baby M case, stated:

> There are, in a civilized society, some things that money cannot buy. In America, we decided long ago that merely because conduct purchased by money was "voluntary" did not mean that it was good or beyond regulation and prohibition. Employers can no longer buy labor at the lowest price they can bargain for, even though that labor is "voluntary," or buy women's labor for less money than paid to men for the same job, or purchase the agreement of children to perform oppressive labor, or purchase the agreement of workers to subject themselves to unsafe or unhealthful working conditions. There are, in short, values that society deems more important than granting to wealth whatever it can buy, be it labor, love, or life.[97]

Even if surrogacy fees purchased "services" rather than a baby, the overall transaction is one that has the potential to submerge biological ties and children's interests to monetary and contractual considerations. "The profit motive predominates, permeates, and ultimately governs the transaction," said the New Jersey Supreme Court. State regulations forbidding parents to buy and sell custody rights to each other have long been recognized as constitutional. Overall, commercialization of familial rights and duties is one area in which courts have consistently upheld the constitutionality of legislation based both on protecting the interests of the children involved and more generally on protecting society's morals.

Define the Term "Mother"

Finally, regardless of what else is left to state courts and legislatures, Congress should choose to set forth a national definition of the term "mother" for the purposes of all federal legislation, international agreements, and other areas under federal jurisdiction. Congress could enact a provision such as that in the United Kingdom, which defines a child's "mother" as the woman who was pregnant and gave birth.

While it could serve at times to defeat the interests of one or more interested persons, one advantage of this last choice is that it makes it easy to determine a child's mother. Hospitals, immigration services, and others would not need to enquire further into the circumstances surrounding the conception of a child in order to determine maternity. Pregnancy and childbirth would speak for itself. Legal maternity could change, as it does now, with formal adoption.

As discussed supra, the most important reason for this action is to protect the reproductive autonomy of pregnant women. Even if commercial surrogacy continues, and other parties have a legally cognizable interest in the child being carried by a woman, her undisputed legal status as mother of the child she carries may help to protect her from any efforts by the intended rearing parents to force her to undergo any treatment or delivery method she wishes to refuse.

Summary and Conclusions

The legal status of surrogate arrangements is still unclear. Despite activity in over half the state legislatures, only seven have enacted legislation either facilitating or inhibiting the arrangement. Kentucky, Louisiana, and Nebraska have voided commercial surrogacy contracts, and Indiana has voided all contracts regardless of payment. On the other hand, Arkansas has begun to regularize the legal parentage of the child. Nevada has exempted surrogacy contracts from its prohibition against baby-selling, and Kansas from its prohibition on adoption-agency advertising. With the exception of two advisory reports offering cautious approval of noncommercial forms of surrogacy, every other nation examining this issue has concluded that surrogacy arrangements are unenforceable and, at times, criminal. Several countries have implemented these findings in legislation, regulations, or judicial decisions.

State court decisions are sparse, but consistently find surrogacy contracts unenforceable in the event of a custody dispute, although the decisions do split on whether the contracts necessarily violate state adoption law. The 1988 Baby M case held that commercial surrogacy contracts are completely void and possibly criminal. This decision, coming from the highest court in that state, may well be influential in other state courts. Every judicial decision and legislative action by other nations examining this issue has resulted in making contracts unenforceable. Nevertheless, absent federal legislation or a federal judicial decision identifying constitutional limitations on state regulation in this field, state courts and legislators are likely to continue to come to different conclusions about whether these arrangements can or should be enforced, regulated, or banned.

The federal government ought to step into this arena to reduce the need to resort to surrogacy, to encourage states to harmonize their local laws on this topic and to prohibit specific enforcement of surrogacy contracts, to clarify procedures in the event of a transnational surrogacy dispute, to ban commercialized forms of surrogacy, and to define the legal meaning of the word "mother."

REFERENCES

The author served as legal analyst for the U.S. Congress, Office of Technology Assessment's report *Infertility: Medical and Social Choices,* and gratefully acknowledges the assistance of E. Blair Wardenburg in preparing the international and surrogate mothering surveys used in that report and discussed in this article. The opinions expressed here are those of the author, and do not necessarily reflect the views of the Office of Technology Assessment or of the project staff for the OTA report.

1. U.S. Congress, Office of Technology Assessment, *Infertility: Medical and Social Choices,* OTA-BA-358 (Washington, D.C.: U.S. Government Printing Office, 1988).

2. Id.

3. Associated Press, "Surrogate Mother Troubled by Lack of Regulation of Contracts," April 23, 1988.

4. OTA, *Infertility,* supra note 1.

5. Id.

6. Assoc. Press, supra note 3; P. J. Parker, "Motivation of Surrogate Mothers: Initial Findings," *American Journal of Psychiatry and Law,* 140 (1983): 1–4; P. J. Parker, "Surrogate Motherhood, Psychiatric Screening and Informed Consent, Baby Selling, and Public Policy," *Bulletin of the American Academy of Psychiatry and Law,* 12 (1984): 21–39.

7. L. B. Andrews, "The Stork Market: The Law of the New Reproduction Technologies," *American Bar Association Journal,* 70 (1984): 50–56; B. Dickens, "Surrogate Motherhood: Legal and Legislative Issues," in A. Milunsky and G. J. Annas, eds., *Genetics and the Law III* (New York: Plenum Press, 1985); OTA, *Infertility,* supra note 1.

8. OTA, *Infertility,* supra note 1.

9. A. Katz, "Surrogate Motherhood and the Baby Selling Laws," *Columbia Journal of Law and Social Problems,* 20 (1986): 1–53.

10. B. Dickens, University of Toronto, Faculty of Law, personal communication, Oct. 12, 1987.

11. M. Gladwell and R. Sharpe, "Baby M Winner," *The New Republic* (Feb. 16, 1987): 15–18; OTA, *Infertility,* supra note 1.

12. OTA, *Infertility,* supra note 1.

13. Kansas Attorney General Opinion No. 82–150, 1982.

14. Miroff v. Surrogate Mother, Marion Superior Court, Probate Division, Marion County, Indiana (Oct. 1986).

15. Doe v. Kelly, 307 N.W.2d 438, 106 Mich. App. 169 (1981); 122 Mich. App. 506, 333 N.W.2d 90 (1983).

16. In the Matter of Baby M, 525 A.2d 1128, 217 N.J. Super. 313 (Superior Ct. Chancery Division 1987), reversed on appeal, 537 A.2d 1227, 109 N.J. 396 (N.J. S. Ct. 1988).

17. In the Matter of Adoption of Baby Girl L. J., 505 N.Y.S. 2d 813, 132 Misc.2d 172) (Surr. Ct. Nassau Cty. 1986).

18. Surrogate Parenting Associates v. Commonwealth of Kentucky, ex rel Armstrong, 704 S.W.2d 209 (1986).

19. *Baby Girl L. J.,* supra note 17; *Surrogate Parenting Assoc.,* supra note 18.

20. Nevada Revised Statutes, ch. 127.

21. Andrews, "Stork Market," supra note 7; K. M. Brophy, "A Surrogate Mother Contract to Bear a Child," *University of Louisville Journal of Family Law,* 20 (1982): 263–91; OTA, *Infertility,* supra note 1.

22. OTA, *Infertility,* supra note 1.

23. J. A. Robertson and J. Schulman, "Pregnancy and Prenatal Harm to Offspring: The Case of Mothers with PKU," *Hastings Center Report,* 17, 4 (1987): 23–28.

24. R. B. Dworkin, "The New Genetics," in J. Childress et al., eds., *Biolaw* (Frederick, Md.: University Publishers of America, 1986); J. Gallagher, "The Fetus and the Law—Whose Life Is It Anyway?," *Ms. Magazine* (Nov. 1984); J. Gallagher, "Prenatal Invasions & Interventions: What's Wrong with Fetal Rights," *Harvard Women's Law Journal,* 10 (1987): 9–58; D. E. Johnsen, "The Creation of Fetal Rights: Conflicts with Women's Constitutional Rights to Liberty, Privacy and Equality," *Yale Law Journal,* 85 (1986): 599–625; D. E. Johnsen, "A New Threat to Pregnant Women's Authority," *Hastings Center Report,* 17, 4 (1987): 33–38.

25. N. Rhoden, "The Judge in the Delivery Room: The Emergence of Court-Ordered Cesareans," *California Law Review,* 74 (1986): 1951–2030.

26. V.E.B. Kolder, J. Gallagher, and M. T. Parsons, "Court Ordered Obstetrical Interventions," *New England Journal of Medicine,* 316 (1987): 1192–96; Rhoden, supra note 25.

27. *Baby Girl L.J.,* supra note 17; Kansas Atty General, supra note 13; Louisiana Attorney General Opinion No. 83–869, 1983; *Miroff,* supra note 14; Ohio Attorney General Opinion No. 83–001, 1983; *Surrogate Parenting Assoc.,* supra note 18.

28. *Baby Girl L.J.,* supra note 17.

29. *Surrogate Parenting Assoc.,* supra note 18.

30. *Baby M,* supra note 16.

31. Yates v. Huber, as reported by Associated Press, Sept. 2, 3, and 10, 1987; Jan. 22 and Apr. 14, 1988.

32. Katz, supra note 9.

33. Haro v. Munoz, as reported by Associated Press, June 10 and Nov. 29, 1987; U.S. Congress, House Committee on Energy and Commerce, Subcommittee on Transportation, Tourism, and Hazardous Wastes, Hearings on H. R. 2433 ("The Anti-Surrogacy Act of 1987"), Oct. 16, 1987.

34. American College of Obstetricians and Gynecologists, Governmental Affairs Division, personal communication, Nov. 23, 1987; L. B. Andrews, "The Aftermath of Baby M: Proposed State Laws on Surrogate Motherhood," *Hastings Center Report,* 17, 5 (1987): 31–40; A. Jaeger and L. Andrews, American Bar Foundation, personal communication, Nov. 24, 1987; Katz, supra note 9; National Committee for Adoption, personal communication, Oct. 13, 1987; W. Pierce, "Survey of State Activity Regarding Surrogate Motherhood," *Family Law Reporter,* 11 (1985): 3001.

35. Dickens, "Surrogate Motherhood," supra note 7; W. Wadlington, "Artificial Conception: The Challenge for Family Law," *Virginia Law Review,* 69 (1983): 465–514.

36. *Baby M,* supra note 16.

37. Dickens, "Surrogate Motherhood," supra note 7.

38. H.B. No. 83H-6132, 1983.

39. Andrews, "Aftermath," supra note 34.

40. *Baby M,* supra note 16.

41. Dickens, "Surrogate Motherhood," supra note 7.

42. R. C. Robinson, Chair, National Conference of Commissioners on Uniform State Laws, Committee on the Status of Children, Portland, Maine, personal communication, Oct. 17, 1987.

43. M. de Wachter and G. de Wert, "In the Netherlands, Tolerance and Debate," *Hastings Center Report,* 17, Supp. (1987): 15–16.

44. Andrews, "Aftermath," supra note 34.

45. W.R. Frederick et al., "HIV Testing on Surrogate Mothers," *New England Journal of Medicine,* 317 (1987): 1351–52.

46. Andrews, "Aftermath," supra note 34; Katz, supra note 9.

47. Dickens, "Surrogate Motherhood," supra note 7.

48. Spain, Congreso de los Diputados, Comisión Especial de Estudio de la Fecondación "In Vitro" y la Inseminación Artificial Humanas (Special Commission for the Study of Human in Vitro Fertilization and Artificial Insemination), "Informe," *Boletin Oficial de las Cortes Generales*, 166 (April 21, 1986): AD 38–1.

49. J. Cohen, Chief of Obstetrics and Gynecology Clinic, Hospital of Sevres, Paris, France, personal communication, Oct. 21, 1987.

50. Associated Press, "Court Orders U.S. Agency Promoting Surrogate Motherhood to Close," Jan. 1, 1988; W. Wagner, Medical Director, Duphar Pharma, Hannover, Federal Republic of Germany, Oct. 30, 1987.

51. OTA, *Infertility*, supra note 1.

52. G. J. Whitman, Counselor for Scientific and Technological Affairs, Embassy of the United States of America, Rome, Italy, personal communication, Oct. 7, 1987.

53. *Doe v. Kelly*, supra note 15.

54. *Baby M*, supra note 16.

55. Id.

56. Id.

57. Infertility Medical Procedures Act, Nos. 10122–71, 1984.

58. Deutscher Juristenag (German Law Association), "Beschluesse: Die kuenstliche Befruchtung Beim Menschen/Recht auf den Eigenen Tod (Resolution: On Artificial Human Fertilization)," *Deutsches Artzeblatt*, 83 (1986): 3273–76; Federal Republic of Germany, Bund-Länder Arbeitsgruppe (Federal-State Working Group), *Zwischenbericht: Fortpflanzungsmedizin* (Interim Report: Reproductive Medicine) (Bonn, 1987); Federal Republic of Germany, Bundestag (Parliament), Enquete-Kommission, *Chancen und Risiken der Gentechnologie* (Risk Assessment of Genetic Engineering) (Bonn: Wolf-Michael Catenhausen, Hanna Neumeister, 1987); G. E. Hirsch, Doctor of Jurisprudence, Augsburg, West Germany, Jan. 11, 1988; M. H. Kottow, Stuttgart, Federal Republic of Germany, personal communication, Oct. 10, 1987; H. M. Sass, "Moral Dilemmas in Perinatal Medicine and the Quest for Large Scale Embryo Research: A Discussion of Recent Guidelines in the Federal Republic of Germany," *Journal of Medicine and Philosophy*, 12 (1987): 279–90.

59. Cohen, supra note 49; Comité Consultatif National d'Ethique pour les Sciences de la Vie et de la Santé, *Journées Annuelles d'Ethique, Sommaire* (Paris and Lyons, 1986); Comité Consultatif National d'Ethique pour les Sciences de la Vie et de la Santé, *Lettre d'Information*, No. 9 (Paris, 1987).

60. American Medical News, "Israel Outlaws Practice of Surrogate Motherhood," June 12, 1987, p. 23, as cited in Childress et al., *Biolaw*, supra note 24.

61. Act No. 68 of June 12, 1987.

62. J.D. Battersby, "Woman Pregnant with Daughter's Triplets," *New York Times*, Apr. 9, 1987, p. 1; H. A. Bell, Office of Science and Technology Policy, Embassy of South Africa, Washington, D.C., personal communication, April 7, 1988.

63. United Kingdom, Department of Health and Social Security, *Legislation on Human Infertility Services and Embryo Research: A Consultation Paper* (London: H. M. Stationery Office, 1986).

64. Spain, supra note 48.

65. Sweden, Ministry of Justice, Insemination Committee, *Barn Genom Befrunktning Utanfor Kroppenmm* (Children Born Through Fertilization Outside the Body, etc.) (Statens offentliga utredningar) (Stockholm: Liber Allmnna Frlaget, 1985).

66. C. Byk, "The Developments in the Council of Europe on Reproductive Medicine," paper submitted to the Colloquium of the United Kingdom National Committee of Comparative Law, Cambridge, England, Sept. 15–17, 1987, reprinted in C. Byk, "Elements de Droit Comparé Relatifs à la Procréation Artificielle Humaine," in C. Byk, ed., *Procréation Artificielle: Analyse de l'Etat d'une Reflexion Juridique* (Paris:

Ministère de la Justice, 1987); Council of Europe, Ad Hoc Committee of Experts on Progress in the Biomedical Sciences (CAHBI), "Provisional Principles on the Techniques of Human Artificial Procreation and Certain Procedures Carried out on Embryos in Connection with Those Techniques," Secretariat memorandum, prepared by the Directorate of Legal Affairs, 1986.

67. Québec, Conseil du Statut de la Femme, *Nouvelles Technologies de la Réproduction: Questions Soulevées dans la Littérature Générale* (Québec: Gouvernement du Québec, Sept. 1985); Québec, Conseil du Statut de la Femme, *Nouvelles Technologies de la Réproduction: Analyses et Questionnements Feministes* (Québec: Gouvernement du Québec, March 1986); Québec, Conseil du Statut de la Femme, *Nouvelles Technologies de la Réproduction: Etudes des Principals Legislations et Recommandations* (Québec Gouvernement du Québec, March 1986); Québec, Conseil du Statut de la Femme, *Nouvelles Technologies de la Réproduction: Pratiques Cliniques et Experimentales au Québec* (Québec: Gouvernement du Québec, Jan. 1986).

68. J. A. Robertson, "Procreative Liberty and the Control of Conception, Pregnancy, and Childbirth," *Virginia Law Review*, 69 (1983): 405–64.

69. *Baby M*, supra note 16.

70. J. K. Mason and R. A. MacCall-Smith, *Law and Medical Ethics*, 2d ed. (London: Butterworths, 1987).

70A. R. Dixon, "Sisters Tell of Planning Their Special Baby," *The Age* (Melbourne, Australia), June 9, 1988, p. 3.

70B. F. Brennan, "A Sister's Priceless Gift—Twins," *Australian Women's Weekly*, 56 (May 1988): 14–15.

71. Smith v. Jones, CF 025653 (Los Angeles Superior Court, 1987); Smith & Smith v. Jones & Jones, 85–532014 DZ, Detroit, 3d Dist. (March 15, 1986), as reported in Childress et al., *Biolaw*, supra note 24.

72. Doe v. Roe, Fairfax County (VA) Circuit Court (Chancery No. 103–147), as reported by Associated Press, Aug. 16, 1987, and Jan. 12, 1988.

73. Israel, Ministry of Health, Public Health (Extracorporeal Fertilization) Regulations of 1987 (unofficial translation by A. Shapira, Tel Aviv University Law School, 1987).

74. P. King, "Reproductive Technologies," in Childress et al., *Biolaw*, supra note 24.

75. *Smith & Smith*, supra note 71.

76. National Committee for Adoption, *Adoption Factbook: United States Data, Issues, Regulations and Resources* (Washington, D.C.: 1985).

77. United Kingdom, supra note 63.

78. Bell, supra note 62.

79. C. Byk and S. Galpin-Jacquot, *Etat Comparatif des Règles et Juridiques Relatives à la Procréation Artificielle* (Paris: Ministère de la Justice, Ministère de la Santé et de la Famille, 1986).

80. Federal Republic of Germany, *Zwischenbericht*, supra note 58.

81. Federal Republic of Germany, Bundesministerium für Justiz and Bundesministerium für Forschung und Technologie (Ministry of Justice and Ministry of Research and Technology), *In Vitro Fertilisation, Genomanalyse und Gentherapie* (IVF, Genome Analysis, and Gene Therapy) (Munich: 1985).

82. Byk, "Developments," supra note 9; Council of Europe, supra note 66.

83. A. Campana, Servicio di Endocrinologia Ginecologica, Ospedale Distrettuale di Locarno, Switzerland, personal communication, Nov. 18, 1987; Questiones Familiales editorial/sommaire "Commission d'experts pour les questions de technologie génétique chez l'homme" (Bern: Dec. 1986 issue); S. Zobrist, M.D., Special Assistant for International Affairs, Federal Office of Public Health, Bern, Switzerland, personal communication, Nov. 5, 1987.

84. C. Erasmus, "Test-Tube Babies Common in South Africa," *Daily Nation* (Nairobi), Oct. 3, 1987, p. 2; M. C. Michelow et al., "Mother-Daughter in Vitro Fertilization Triplet Surrogate Pregnancy," *Journal of in Vitro Fertilization and Embryo Transfer*, 5, 1 (1988): 1–56.

85. Battersby, supra note 62.

86. Bell, supra note 62.

87. OTA, *Infertility*, supra note 1.

88. M. J. Radin, "Market-Inalienability," *Harvard Law Review*, 100 (1987): 1849–1946; P. Ramsey, *Fabricated Man: The Ethics of Genetic Control* (New Haven: Yale University Press, 1970).

89. M. A. Lamanna, "On the Baby Assembly Line: Reproductive Technology and the Family," paper presented at the University of Dayton conference "Reproductive Technologies and the Catholic Tradition," Oct. 30, 1987.

90. A. Goerlich and M. Krannich, "Summary of Contributions and Debates at the Hearing of Women on Reproductive and Genetic Engineering," *Documentation of the Feminist Hearing on Genetic Engineering and Reproductive Technologies*, March 6–7, 1986 (Brussels: Women's Bureau, European Parliament, 1986).

91. H. Hanifin, "Surrogate Parenting: Reassessing Human Bonding," paper presented at the annual meeting of the American Psychological Association, Aug. 1987; Parker, "Motivation," supra note 6; Parker, "Surrogate Motherhood," supra note 6; J. Sutton, paper presented to the Pennsylvania State Legislature on behalf of the National Association of Surrogate Mothers, 1987.

92. *Doe v. Kelly*, supra note 15; *Baby M*, supra note 16.

93. *Baby M*, supra note 16.

94. Id.

95. J. A. Robertson, "Embryos, Families and Procreative Liberty: The Legal Structure of the New Reproduction," *Southern California Law Review*, 59 (1986): 939–1041. Emphasis added.

96. U.S. Congress, Office of Technology Assessment, *New Developments in Biotechnology: Ownership of Human Tissues and Cells*, OTA-BA-337 (Washington, D.C.: U.S. Government Printing Office, 1987).

97. *Baby M*, supra note 16.

ETHICS

Surrogate Motherhood as Prenatal Adoption

Bonnie Steinbock

The recent case of "Baby M" has brought surrogate motherhood to the forefront of American attention. Ultimately, whether we permit or prohibit surrogacy depends on what we take to be good reasons for preventing people from acting as they wish. A growing number of people want to be, or hire, surrogates; are there legitimate reasons to prevent them? Apart from its intrinsic interest, the issue of surrogate motherhood provides us with an opportunity to examine different justifications for limiting individual freedom.

In the first section of this article, I examine the Baby M case and the lessons it offers. In the second section, I examine claims that surrogacy is ethically unacceptable because it is exploitive, inconsistent with human dignity, or harmful to the children born of such arrangements. I conclude that these reasons justify restrictions on surrogate contracts, rather than an outright ban.

Baby M

Mary Beth Whitehead, a married mother of two, agreed to be inseminated with the sperm of William Stern and to give up the child to him for a fee of $10,000. The baby (whom Ms. Whitehead named Sara, and the Sterns named Melissa) was born on March 27, 1986. Three days later, Ms. Whitehead took her home from the hospital and turned her over to the Sterns.

Then Ms. Whitehead changed her mind. She went to the Sterns' home, distraught, and pleaded to have the baby temporarily. Afraid that she would kill herself, the Sterns agreed. The next week, Ms. Whitehead informed the Sterns that she had decided to keep the child, and threatened to leave the country if court action was taken.

At that point, the situation deteriorated into a cross between the Keystone Kops and Nazi stormtroopers. Accompanied by five policemen, the Sterns went to the Whitehead residence armed with a court order giving them temporary custody of the child. Ms. Whitehead managed to slip the baby out of a window to her husband, and the following morning the White-heads fled with the child to Florida, where Ms. Whitehead's parents lived. During the next three months, the Whiteheads lived in roughly twenty different hotels, motels, and homes to avoid apprehension. From time to time, Ms. Whitehead telephoned Mr. Stern to discuss the matter: he taped these conversations on advice of counsel. Ms. Whitehead threatened to kill herself, to kill the child, and to falsely accuse Mr. Stern of sexually molesting her older daughter.

At the end of July 1986, while Ms. Whitehead was hospitalized with a kidney infection, Florida police raided her mother's home, knocking her down, and seized the child. Baby M was placed in the custody of Mr. Stern, and the Whiteheads returned to New Jersey, where they attempted to regain custody. After a long and emotional court battle, Judge Harvey R. Sorkow ruled on March 31, 1987, that the surrogacy contract was valid, and that specific performance was justified in the best interests of the child. Immediately after reading his decision, he called the Sterns into his chambers so that Mr. Stern's wife, Dr. Elizabeth Stern, could legally adopt the child.

This outcome was unexpected and unprecedented. Most commentators had thought that a court would be unlikely to order a reluctant surrogate to give up an infant merely on the basis of a contract.[1] Indeed, if Ms. Whitehead had never surrendered the child to the Sterns, but had simply taken her home and kept her there, the outcome undoubtedly would have been different. It is also likely that Ms. Whitehead's failure to obey the initial custody order angered Judge Sorkow, and affected his decision.

The decision was appealed to the New Jersey Supreme Court, which issued its decision on February 3, 1988. Writing for a unanimous court, Chief Justice Wilentz reversed the lower court's ruling that the surrogacy contract was valid. The court held that a surrogacy contract that provides money for the surrogate mother, and that includes her irrevocable agreement to surrender her child at birth, is invalid and unenforceable. Since the contract was invalid, Ms. Whitehead did not relinquish, nor were there any other grounds for terminating, her parental rights. Therefore, the adoption of Baby M by Dr. Stern was improperly granted, and Ms. Whitehead remains the child's legal mother.

The court further held that the issue of custody is determined solely by the child's best interests, and it agreed with the lower court that it was in Melissa's best interests to remain with the Sterns. However, Ms. White-head, as Baby M's legal as well as natural mother, is entitled to have her own interest in visitation considered. The determination of what kind of visitation rights should be granted to her, and under what conditions, was remanded to the trial court.

The distressing details of this case have led many people to reject surrogacy altogether. Do we really want police officers wrenching infants from their mothers' arms, and prolonged custody battles when surrogates find they are unable to surrender their children, as agreed? Advocates of surrogacy say that to reject the practice wholesale, because of one unfortunate instance, is an example of a "hard case" making bad policy. Opponents reply that it is entirely reasonable to focus on the worst potential outcomes when deciding public policy. Everyone can agree on at least one thing: this particular case seems to have been mismanaged from start to finish, and could serve as a manual of how not to arrange a surrogate birth.

First, it is now clear that Mary Beth Whitehead was not a suitable candidate for surrogate motherhood. Her ambivalence about giving up the child was recognized early on, although this information was not passed on to the Sterns.[2] Second, she had contact with the baby after birth, which is usually avoided in "successful" cases. Typically, the adoptive mother is actively involved in the pregnancy, often serving as the pregnant woman's coach in labor. At birth, the baby is given to the adoptive, not the biological mother. The joy of the adoptive parents in holding their child serves both to promote their bonding and to lessen the pain of separation of the biological mother.

At Ms. Whitehead's request, no one at the hospital was aware of the surrogacy arrangement. She and her husband appeared as the proud parents of "Sara Elizabeth Whitehead," the name on her birth certificate. Ms. Whitehead held her baby, nursed her, and took her home from the hospital—just as she would have done in a normal pregnancy and birth. Not surprisingly, she thought of Sara as her child, and she fought with every weapon at her disposal, honorable and dishonorable, to prevent her being taken away. She can hardly be blamed for doing so.[3]

Why did Dr. Stern, who supposedly had a very good relation with Ms. Whitehead before the birth, not act as her labor coach? One possibility is that Ms. Whitehead, ambivalent about giving up her baby, did not want Dr. Stern involved. At her request, the Sterns' visits to the hospital to see the newborn baby were unobtrusive. It is also possible that Dr. Stern was ambivalent about having a child. The original idea of hiring a surrogate was not hers, but her husband's. It was Mr. Stern who felt a "compelling" need to have a child related to him by blood, having lost all his relatives to the Nazis.

Furthermore, Dr. Stern was not infertile, as was stated in the surrogacy agreement. Rather, in 1979 she was diagnosed by two eye specialists as suffering from optic neuritis, which meant that she "probably" had multiple sclerosis. (This was confirmed by all four experts who testified.) Normal conception was ruled out by the Sterns in late 1982, when a medical colleague told Dr. Stern that his wife, a victim of multiple sclerosis, had suffered a temporary paralysis during pregnancy. "We decided the risk wasn't worth it," Mr. Stern said.[4]

Ms. Whitehead's lawyer, Harold J. Cassidy, dismissed the suggestion that Dr. Stern's "mildest case" of multiple sclerosis determined the Sterns' decision to seek a surrogate. He noted that she was not even treated for multiple sclerosis until after the Baby M dispute had started. "It's almost as though it's an afterthought," he said.[5]

Judge Sorkow deemed the decision to avoid conception "medically reasonable and understandable." The Supreme Court did not go so far, noting that Dr. Stern's "anxiety appears to have exceeded the actual risk, which current medical authorities assess as minimal."[6] Nonetheless, the court acknowledged that her anxiety, including fears that pregnancy might precipitate blindness and paraplegia, was "quite real." Certainly, even a woman who wants a child very much may reasonably wish to avoid becoming blind and paralyzed as a result of pregnancy. Yet is it believable that a woman who really wanted a child would decide against pregnancy *solely* on the basis of *someone else's* medical experience? Would she not consult at least one specialist on her *own* medical condition before deciding it wasn't worth the risk? The conclusion that she was at best ambivalent about bearing a child seems irresistible.

This possibility conjures up many people's worst fears about surrogacy: that prosperous women, who do not want to interrupt their careers, will use poor and educationally disadvantaged women to bear their children. I will return shortly to the question of whether this is exploitive. The issue here is psychological: what kind of mother is Dr. Stern likely to be? If she is unwilling to undergo pregnancy, with its discomforts, inconveniences, and risks, will she be willing to make the considerable sacrifices that good parenting requires? Ms. Whitehead's ability to be a good mother was repeatedly questioned during the trial. She was portrayed as immature, untruthful, hysterical, overly identified with her children, and prone to smothering their independence. Even if all this is true—and I think that Ms. Whitehead's inadequacies were exaggerated—Dr. Stern may not be such a prize either. The choice for Baby M may have been between a highly strung, emotional, overinvolved mother, and a remote, detached, even cold one.[7]

The assessment of Ms. Whitehead's ability to be a good mother was biased by the middle-class prejudices of the judge and of the mental health officials who testified. Ms. Whitehead left school at fifteen, and is not conversant with the latest theories on child rearing: she made the egregious error of giving Sara teddy bears to play with, instead of the more "age-appropriate," expert-approved pans and spoons. She proved to be a total failure at patty-cake. If this is evidence of parental inadequacy, we're all in danger of losing our children.

The Supreme Court felt that Ms. Whitehead was "rather harshly judged" and acknowledged the possibility that the trial court was wrong in its initial award of custody. Nevertheless, it affirmed Judge Sorkow's decision to allow the Sterns to retain custody, as being in Melissa's best interests.

George Annas disagrees with the "best interests" approach. He points out that Judge Sorkow awarded temporary custody of Baby M to the Sterns in May 1986, without giving the Whiteheads notice or an opportunity to obtain legal representation. That was a serious wrong and injustice to the Whiteheads. To allow the Sterns to keep the child compounds the original unfairness: "justice requires that reasonable consideration be given to returning Baby M to the permanent custody of the Whiteheads."[8]

But a child is not a possession, to be returned to the rightful owner. It is not fairness to all parties that should determine a child's fate, but what is best for her. As Chief Justice Wilentz rightly stated, "The child's interests come first: we will not punish it for judicial errors, assuming any were made."[9]

Subsequent events have substantiated the claim that giving custody to the Sterns was in Melissa's best interests. After losing custody, Ms. Whitehead, whose husband had undergone a vasectomy, became pregnant by another man. She divorced her husband and married Dean R. Gould last November. These developments indicate that the Whiteheads were not able to offer a stable home, although the argument can be made that their marriage might have survived if not for the strains introduced by the court battle and the loss of Baby M. But even if Judge Sorkow had no reason to prefer the Sterns to the Whiteheads back in May 1986, he was still right to give the Sterns custody in March 1987. To take her away then, at nearly eighteen months of age, from the only parents she had ever known would have been disruptive, cruel, and unfair to her.

Annas' preference for a just solution is premised partly on his belief that there *is* no "best interest" solution to this "tragic custody case." I take it that he means that however custody is resolved, Baby M is the loser. Either way, she will be deprived of one parent. However, a best-interests solution is not a perfect solution. It is simply the solution that is on balance best for the child, given the realities of the situation. Applying this standard, Judge Sorkow was right to give the Sterns custody, and the Supreme Court was right to uphold the decision.

The best-interests argument is based on the assumption that Mr. Stern has at least a *prima facie* claim to Baby M. We certainly would not consider allowing a stranger who kidnapped a baby and managed to elude the police for a year to retain custody on the grounds that he was providing a good home to a child who had known no other parent. However, the Baby M case is not analogous. First, Mr. Stern is Baby M's biological father and, as such, has at least some claim to raise her, which no non-parental kidnapper has. Second, Mary Beth Whitehead *agreed* to give him their baby. Unlike the miller's daughter in *Rumpelstiltskin*, the fairy tale to which the Baby M case is sometimes compared, she was not forced into the agreement. Because both Mary Beth Whitehead and Mr. Stern have *prima facie* claims to Baby M, the decision as to who should raise her should be based on her present best interests. Therefore we must, regretfully, tolerate the injustice to Ms. Whitehead, and try to avoid such problems in the future.

It is unfortunate that the court did not decide the issue of visitation on the same basis as custody. By declaring Ms. Whitehead-Gould the legal mother, and maintaining that she is entitled to visitation, the court has prolonged the fight over Baby M. It is hard to see how this can be in her best interests. This is no ordinary divorce case, where the child has a relation with both parents that it is desirable to maintain. As Mr. Stern said at the start of the court hearing to determine visitation, "Melissa has a right to grow and be happy and not be torn between two parents."[10]

The court's decision was well-meaning but internally inconsistent. Out of concern for the best interests of the child, it granted the Sterns custody. At the same time, by holding Ms. Whitehead-Gould to be the legal mother, with visitation rights, it precluded precisely what is most in Melissa's interest, a resolution of the situation. Further, the decision leaves open the distressing possibility that a Baby M situation could happen again. Legislative efforts should be directed toward ensuring that this worst-case scenario never occurs.

SHOULD SURROGACY BE PROHIBITED?

On June 27, 1988, Michigan became the first state to outlaw commercial contracts for women to bear children for others.[11] Yet making a practice illegal does not necessarily make it go away: witness black-market adoption. The legitimate concerns that support a ban on surrogacy might be better served by careful regulation. However, some practices, such as slavery, are ethically unacceptable, regardless of how carefully regulated they are. Let us consider the arguments that surrogacy is intrinsically unacceptable.

Paternalistic Arguments

These arguments against surrogacy take the form of protecting a potential surrogate from a choice she may later regret. As an argument for banning surrogacy, as opposed to providing safeguards to ensure that contracts are freely and knowledgeably undertaken, this is a form of paternalism.

At one time, the characterization of a prohibition as paternalistic was a sufficient reason to reject it. The pendulum has swung back, and many people are willing to accept at least some paternalistic restrictions on freedom. Gerald Dworkin points out that even Mill made one exception to his otherwise absolute rejection of paternalism: he thought that no one should be allowed to sell himself into slavery, because to do so would be to destroy his future autonomy.

This provides a narrow principle to justify some paternalistic interventions. To preserve freedom in the long run, we give up the freedom to make certain choices, those that have results that are "far-reaching, potentially dangerous and irreversible."[12] An example would be a ban on the sale of crack. Virtually everyone who uses crack becomes addicted and, once addicted, a slave to its use. We reasonably and willingly give up our freedom to buy the drug, to protect our ability to make free decisions in the future.

Can a Dworkinian argument be made to rule out surrogacy agreements? Admittedly, the decision to give up a child is permanent, and may have disastrous effects on the surrogate mother. However, many decisions may have long-term, disastrous effects (e.g., postponing childbirth for a career, having an abortion, giving a child up for adoption). Clearly we do not want the state to make decisions for us in all these matters. Dworkin's argument is rightly restricted to paternalistic interferences that protect the individual's autonomy or ability to make decisions in the future. Surrogacy does not involve giving up one's autonomy, which distinguishes it from both the crack and selling-oneself-into-slavery examples. Respect for individual freedom requires us to permit people to make choices they may later regret.

Moral Objections

Four main moral objections to surrogacy were outlined in the Warnock Report.[13]

1) It is inconsistent with human dignity that a woman should use her uterus for financial profit.
2) To deliberately become pregnant with the intention of giving up the child distorts the relationship between mother and child.
3) Surrogacy is degrading because it amounts to child-selling.
4) Since there are some risks attached to pregnancy, no woman ought to be asked to undertake pregnancy for another in order to earn money.[14]

We must all agree that a practice that exploits people or violates human dignity is immoral. However, it is not clear that surrogacy is guilty on either count.

Exploitation

The mere fact that pregnancy is *risky* does not make surrogate agreements exploitive, and therefore morally wrong. People often do risky things for money; why should the line be drawn at undergoing pregnancy? The usual response is to compare surrogacy and kidney-selling. The selling of organs is prohibited because of the potential for coercion and exploitation. But why should kidney-selling be viewed as intrinsically coercive? A possible explanation is that no one would do it, unless driven by poverty. The choice is both forced and dangerous, and hence coercive.[15]

The situation is quite different in the case of the race-car driver or stunt-man. We do not think that they are *forced* to perform risky activities for money: they freely choose to do so. Unlike selling one's kidneys, these are activities that we can understand (intellectually, anyway) someone choosing to do. Movie stuntmen, for example, often enjoy their work, and derive satisfaction from doing it well. Of course they "do it for the money," in the sense that they would not do it without compensation; few people are willing to work "for free." The element of coercion is missing, however, because they enjoy the job, despite the risks, and could do something else if they chose.

The same is apparently true of most surrogates. "They choose the surrogate role primarily because the fee provides a better economic opportunity than alternative occupations, but also because they enjoy being pregnant and the respect and attention that it draws."[16] Some may derive a feeling of self-worth from an act they regard as highly altruistic: providing a couple with a child they could not otherwise have. If these motives are present, it is far from clear that the surrogate is being exploited. Indeed, it seems objectionally paternalistic to insist that she is.

Human Dignity

It may be argued that even if womb-leasing is not necessarily exploitive, it should still be rejected as inconsistent with human dignity. But why? As John Harris points out, hair, blood, and other tissue is often donated or sold; what is so special about the uterus?[17]

Human dignity is more plausibly invoked in the strongest argument against surrogacy, namely, that it is the sale of a child. Children are not property, nor can they be bought or sold.[18] It could be argued that surrogacy is wrong because it is analogous to slavery, and so is inconsistent with human dignity.

However, there are important differences between slavery and a surrogate agreement.[19] The child born of a surrogate is not treated cruelly or deprived of freedom or resold; none of the things that make slavery so awful are part of surrogacy. Still, it may be thought that simply putting a market value on a child is wrong. Human life has intrinsic value; it is literally priceless. Arrangements that ignore this violate our deepest notions of the value of human life. It is profoundly disturbing to hear in a television documentary on surrogacy the boyfriend of a surrogate say, quite candidly, "We're in it for the money."

Judge Sorkow accepted the premise that producing a child for money denigrates human dignity, but he denied that this happens in a surrogate agreement. Ms. Whitehead was not paid for the surrender of the child to the father: she was paid for her willingness to be impregnated and carry Mr. Stern's child to term. The child, once born, is his biological child. "He cannot purchase what is already his."[20]

This is misleading, and not merely because Baby M is as much Ms. Whitehead's child as Mr. Stern's. It is misleading because it glosses over the fact that the surrender of the child was part—indeed, the whole point— of the agreement. If the surrogate were paid merely for being willing to be impregnated and carrying the child to term, then she would fulfill the contract upon giving birth. She could take the money *and* the child. Mr. Stern did not agree to pay Ms. Whitehead merely to *have* his child, but to provide him with a child. The New Jersey Supreme Court held that this violated New Jersey's laws prohibiting the payment or acceptance of money in connection with adoption.

One way to remove the taint of baby-selling would be to limit payment to medical expenses associated with the birth or incurred by the surrogate during pregnancy (as is allowed in many jurisdictions, including New Jersey, in ordinary adoptions).[21] Surrogacy could be seen, not as baby-selling, but as a form of adoption. Nowhere did the Supreme Court find any legal prohibition against surrogacy when there is no payment, and when the surrogate has the right to change her mind and keep the child. However, this solution effectively prohibits surrogacy, since few women would become surrogates solely for self-fulfillment or reasons of altruism.

The question, then, is whether we can reconcile paying the surrogate, beyond her medical expenses, with the idea of surrogacy as prenatal adoption. We can do this by separating the terms of the agreement, which include surrendering the infant at birth to the biological father, from the justification for payment. The payment should be seen as compensation for the risks, sacrifice, and discomfort the surrogate undergoes during pregnancy. This means that if, through no fault on the part of the surrogate, the baby is stillborn, she should still be paid in full, since she has kept her part of the bargain. (By contrast, in the Stern-Whitehead agreement, Ms. Whitehead was to receive only $1,000 for a stillbirth).[22] If, on the other hand, the surrogate changes her mind and decides to keep the child, she would break the agreement, and would not be entitled to any fee or to compensation for expenses incurred during pregnancy.

The Right of Privacy

Most commentators who invoke the right of privacy do so in support of surrogacy.[23] However, George Annas makes the novel argument that the right to rear a child you have borne is also a privacy right, which cannot be prospectively waived. He says:

> [Judge Sorkow] grudgingly concedes that [Ms. Whitehead] could not prospectively give up her right to have an abortion during pregnancy. . . . This would be an intolerable restriction on her liberty and under *Roe v. Wade*, the state has no constitutional authority to enforce a

contract that prohibits her from terminating her pregnancy. But why isn't the same logic applicable to the right to rear a child you have given birth to? Her constitutional rights to rear the child she has given birth to are even stronger since they involve even more intimately, and over a lifetime, her privacy rights to reproduce and rear a child in a family setting.[24]

Absent a compelling state interest (such as protecting a child from unfit parents), it certainly would be an intolerable invasion of privacy for the state to take children from their parents. But Baby M has two parents, both of whom now want her. It is not clear why only people who can give birth (i.e., women) should enjoy the right to rear their children.

Moreover, we do allow women to give their children up for adoption after birth. The state enforces those agreements even if the natural mother, after the prescribed waiting period, changes her mind. Why should the right to rear a child be unwaivable before, but not after, birth? Why should the state have the constitutional authority to uphold postnatal, but not prenatal, adoption agreements? It is not clear why birth should affect the waivability of this right or have the constitutional significance that Annas attributes to it.

Nevertheless, there are sound moral and policy, if not constitutional, reasons to provide a postnatal waiting period in surrogate agreements. As the Baby M case makes painfully clear, the surrogate may underestimate the bond created by gestation and the emotional trauma caused by relinquishing the baby. Compassion requires that we acknowledge these findings, and not deprive a woman of the baby she has carried because, before conception, she underestimated the strength of her feelings for it. Providing a waiting period, as in ordinary postnatal adoptions, will help protect women from making irrevocable mistakes, without banning the practice.

Some may object that this gives too little protection to the prospective adoptive parents. They cannot be sure that the baby is theirs until the waiting period is over. While this is hard on them, a similar burden is placed on other adoptive parents. If the absence of a guarantee serves to discourage people from entering surrogacy agreements, that is not necessarily a bad thing, given all the risks inherent in such contracts. In addition, this requirement would make stricter screening and counseling of surrogates essential, a desirable side-effect.

Harm to Others

Paternalistic and moral objections to surrogacy do not seem to justify an outright ban. What about the effect on the offspring of such contracts? We do not yet have solid data on the effects of being a "surrogate child." Any claim that surrogacy creates psychological problems in the children is purely speculative. But what if we did discover that such children have deep feelings of worthlessness from learning that their natural mothers deliberately created them with the intention of giving them away? Might we ban surrogacy as posing an unacceptable risk of psychological harm to the resulting children?

Feelings of worthlessness are harmful. They can prevent people from living happy, fulfilling lives. However, a surrogate child, even one whose life is miserable because of these feelings, cannot claim to have been harmed by the surrogate agreement. Without the agreement, the child would never have existed. Unless she is willing to say that her life is not worth living because of these feelings, that she would be better off never having been born, she cannot claim to have been harmed by being born of a surrogate mother.[25]

Elsewhere I have argued that children can be *wronged* by being brought into existence, even if they are not, strictly speaking, *harmed*.[26] They are wronged if they are deprived of the minimally decent existence to which all citizens are entitled. We owe it to our children to see that they are not born with such serious impairments that their most basic interests will be doomed in advance. If being born to a surrogate is a handicap of this magnitude, comparable to being born blind or deaf or severely mentally retarded, then surrogacy can be seen as wronging the offspring. This would be a strong reason against permitting such contracts. However, it does not seem likely. Probably the problems arising from surrogacy will be like those faced by adopted children and children whose parents divorce. Such problems are not trivial, but neither are they so serious that the child's very existence can be seen as wrongful.

If surrogate children are neither harmed nor wronged by surrogacy, it may seem that the argument for banning surrogacy on grounds of its harmfulness to the offspring evaporates. After all, if the children themselves have no cause for complaint, how can anyone else claim to reject it on their behalf? Yet it seems extremely counter-intuitive to suggest that the risk of emotional damage to the children born of such arrangements is not even relevant to our deliberations. It seems quite reasonable and proper—even morally obligatory—for policy-makers to think about the possible detrimental effects of new reproductive technologies, and to reject those likely to create physically or emotionally damaged people. The explanation for this must involve the idea that it is wrong to bring people into the world in a harmful condition, even if they are not, strictly speaking, harmed by having been brought into existence.[27] Should evidence emerge that surrogacy produces children with serious psychological problems, that would be a strong reason for banning the practice.

There is some evidence on the effect of surrogacy on the other children of the surrogate mother. One woman reported that her daughter, now seventeen, who was eleven at the time of the surrogate birth, "is still having problems with what I did, and as a result she is still angry with me." She explains: "Nobody told me that a child could bond with a baby while you're still pregnant. I didn't realize then that all the times she listened to his heartbeat and felt his legs kick that she was becoming attached to him."[28]

A less sentimental explanation is possible. It seems likely that her daughter, seeing one child given away, was fearful that the same might be done to her. We can expect anxiety and resentment on the part of children whose mothers give away a brother or sister. The psychological harm to these children is clearly relevant to a determination of whether surrogacy is contrary to public policy. At the same time, it should be remembered that many things, including divorce, remarriage, and even moving to a new neighborhood, create anxiety and resentment in children. We should not use the effect on children as an excuse for banning a practice we find bizarre or offensive.

Conclusion

There are many reasons to be extremely cautious of surrogacy. I cannot imagine becoming a surrogate, nor would I advise anyone else to enter into a contract so fraught with peril. But the fact that a practice is risky, foolish, or even morally distasteful is not sufficient reason to outlaw it. It would be better for the state to regulate the practice, and minimize the potential for harm, without infringing on the liberty of citizens.

References

1. See, for example, "Surrogate Motherhood Agreements: Contemporary Legal Aspects of a Biblical Notion," *University of Richmond Law Review*, 16 (1982): 470; "Surrogate Mothers: The Legal Issues," *American Journal of Law & Medicine*, 7 (1981): 338, and Angela Holder, *Legal Issues in Pediatrics and Adolescent Medicine* (New Haven: Yale University Press, 1985), 8: "Where a surrogate mother decides that she does not want to give the baby up for adoption, as has already happened, *it is clear that no court will enforce a contract entered into before the child was born* in which she agreed to surrender her baby for adoption." Emphasis added.

2. Had the Sterns been informed of the psychologist's concerns as to Ms. White-head's suitability to be a surrogate, they might have ended the arrangement, costing the Infertility Center its fee. As Chief Justice Wilentz said, "It is apparent that the profit motive got the better of the Infertility Center." In the matter of Baby M, Supreme Court of New Jersey, A-39, at 45.

3. "[W]e think it is expecting something well beyond normal human capabilities to suggest that this mother should have parted with her newly born infant without a struggle. . . . We . . . cannot conceive of any other case where a perfectly fit mother was expected to surrender her newly born infant, perhaps forever, and was then told she was a bad mother because she did not." Id.: 79.

4. "Father Recalls Surrogate Was 'Perfect,' " *New York Times*, Jan. 6, 1987, B2.

5. Id.

6. In the matter of Baby M, supra note 2, at 8.

7. This possibility was suggested to me by Susan Vermazen.

8. George Annas, "Baby M: Babies (and Justice) for Sale," *Hastings Center Report*, 17, no. 3 (1987): 15.

9. In the matter of Baby M, supra note 2, at 75.

10. "Anger and Anguish at Baby M Visitation Hearing," *New York Times*, March 29, 1988, 17.

11. *New York Times*, June 28, 1988, A20.

12. Gerald Dworkin, "Paternalism," in R. A. Wasserstrom, ed., *Morality and the Law* (Belmont, Cal.: Wadsworth, 1971); reprinted in J. Feinberg and H. Gross, eds., *Philosophy of Law*, 3d ed. (Belmont, Cal.: Wadsworth, 1986), 265.

13. M. Warnock, chair, *Report of the Committee of Inquiry into Human Fertilisation and Embryology* (London: Her Majesty's Stationery Office, 1984).

14. As summarized in J. Harris, *The Value of Life* (London: Routledge & Kegan Paul, 1985), 142.

15. For an argument that kidney-selling need not be coercive, see B. A. Brody and H. T. Engelhardt, Jr., *Bioethics: Readings and Cases* (Englewood Cliffs, N.J.: Prentice-Hall, 1987), 331.

16. John Robertson, "Surrogate Mothers: Not So Novel after All," *Hastings Center Report*, 13, no. 5 (1983): 29; citing P. Parker, "Surrogate Mother's Motivations: Initial Findings," *American Journal of Psychiatry*, 140 (1983): 1.

17. Harris, supra note 14, at 144.

18. Several authors note that it is both illegal and contrary to public policy to buy or sell children, and therefore contracts that contemplate this are unenforceable. See B. Cohen, "Surrogate Mothers: Whose Baby Is It?," *American Journal of Law & Medicine*, 10 (1984): 253; "Surrogate Mother Agreements: Contemporary Legal Aspects of a Biblical Notion," *University of Richmond Law Review*, 16 (1982): 469.

19. Robertson makes a similar point, supra note 16, at 33.

20. In re Baby "M," 217 N.J. Super. 372, 525 A.2d 1157 (1987).

21. Cohen, supra note 18. See also Angela Holder, "Surrogate Motherhood: Babies for Fun and Profit," *Law, Medicine & Health Care*, 12 (1984): 115.

22. Annas, supra note 8, at 14.

23. See, for example, Robertson, supra note 16, at 32; and S. R. Gersz, "The Contract in Surrogate Motherhood: A Review of the Issues," *Law, Medicine & Health Care*, 12 (1984): 107.

24. Annas, supra note 8.

25. For discussion of these issues, see D. Parfit, "On Doing the Best for Our Children," in M. D. Bayles, ed., *Ethics and Population* (Cambridge, Mass.: Schenkman, 1976); M. D. Bayles, "Harm to the Unconceived," *Philosophy & Public Affairs*, 5 (1976): 292; J. Glover, *Causing Death and Saving Lives* (Harmondsworth, Eng.: Penguin, 1977), 67; John Robertson, "In Vitro Conception and Harm to the Unborn," *Hastings Center Report*, 8 (1978): 13; J. Feinberg, *Harm to Others* (Oxford: Oxford University Press, 1984), 95.

26. Bonnie Steinbock, "The Logical Case for 'Wrongful Life'," *Hastings Center Report*, 16, no. 2 (1986): 15.

27. For the distinction between being harmed and being in a harmful state, see Feinberg, supra note 25, at 99.

28. "Baby M Case Stirs Feelings of Surrogate Mothers," *New York Times*, March 2, 1987, B1.4

Is There Anything Wrong with Surrogate Motherhood?

An Ethical Analysis

Ruth Macklin

The Emotional Response

Is there anything ethically wrong with surrogate motherhood? Many people confess their inability to articulate their opposition in rational terms, yet they feel uneasy. The practice arouses negative emotions ranging from mild distaste to revulsion. Others say there is nothing wrong, in principle, with surrogate motherhood. It is a way of helping infertile women fulfill a fundamental human longing and, therefore, should be permitted and even facilitated. Many who are not fundamentally opposed to surrogacy nonetheless maintain that the practice ought to be regulated, in order to prevent abuses and to provide a mechanism for resolving conflicts that may develop in particular cases.

Surrogacy arrangements have been condemned by Roman Catholic spokesmen, in a legal brief by a conference of bishops in New Jersey,[1] and by the Vatican in a statement issued by the Pope in March 1987. Feminists have denounced the practice, using rhetoric rather than argument, with the slogan "woman as vessel." A group of women who agreed to bear children under surrogacy contracts has convened to speak out against such arrangements. A number of them, like Mary Beth Whitehead, the surrogate mother in the Baby M case, were seeking to get their babies back.[2]

Some critics charge that surrogacy exploits women, particularly those from lower economic classes, thus constituting a new form of "slavery."[3] Others contend that it dehumanizes babies, amounting to a new variety of "baby selling." The lawyer for Mary Beth Whitehead argued that surrogacy contracts are "against public policy" and ought to be outlawed, and called the idea of paying surrogate mothers to bear and surrender infants "repulsive and repugnant."[4]

Yet others disagree. Some, consistent with the feminist stance that women should be allowed to control their own bodies, insist that being a surrogate mother is just another reproductive choice, which ought to remain open to women. It is also pointed out that surrogacy fulfills an important biological and emotional need: couples in which the wife is infertile are often desperate to have a child with the father's genetic inheritance, and look to surrogacy as the only way to make this possible. And Noel P. Keane, the Detroit lawyer and founder of the Infertility Center in Manhattan, which arranged the contract between Mary Beth Whitehead and William Stern, Baby M's father, has argued that surrogacy permits "the furtherance of [a couple's] constitutionally protected right to procreation."[5]

The most striking feature of the controversy over surrogacy is the level of emotional response. Few people are neutral on the issue. Newspaper reports of the seven-week Baby M trial remarked on the "many basic emotions" touched by the legal proceedings.[6] An account of legislative hearings on a bill to regulate surrogacy in New York state described the proceedings as "an emotional State Senate committee hearing."[7] Many health professionals and academics confess to having strong feelings against surrogacy, but remain unable to come up with a rational position in defense of their view.

Not long ago, news accounts of a novel surrogacy arrangement stirred even deeper feelings. A forty-eight-year-old South African grandmother, Pat Anthony, served as a surrogate mother for her own daughter's biological infants. Ms. Anthony was implanted with four embryos resulting from ova produced by her daughter and fertilized in vitro with her son-in-law's sperm. On October 1, 1987, she give birth to triplets. Reactions to this story ranged from astonishment to repugnance. The trenchant comment of one biology professor was, "Yuk!"

Understanding Ethical Conflicts

Many ethical conflicts are soluble, while others are doomed never to be resolved. In the field of biomedical ethics, examples of both types of ethical conflicts exist.

An example of a basically resolvable ethical controversy is in vitro fertilization, the technique of fertilizing a female egg with a male sperm outside the human body. Although legal and regulatory details still need to be worked out, the ethical acceptability of in vitro fertilization is widely acknowledged. This is documented on an international level by fifteen extended committee statements, issued between 1979 and 1987, representing eight nations: Australia, the U.K., the U.S., Canada, the Federal Republic of Germany, France, the Netherlands, and Spain. The fifteen commissions stated the acceptability, in principle, of in vitro fertilization.[8]

However, some religious groups still oppose this mode of "artificial reproduction," as it is called. Most notably, the Vatican has made an official declaration (March 10, 1987) condemning this procedure and virtually any other departure from normal sexual intercourse between a husband and wife. Yet however bound Roman Catholics may be by such declarations, it does not follow that the practice under condemnation is morally wrong or even ethically controversial. A religion may impose duties and prohibitions on its believers that are morally neutral to others.

Other ethical conflicts are unlikely ever to be resolved. An example is the abortion controversy. Despite a rather clear public policy established in the United States fifteen years ago in *Roe v. Wade*, abortion remains a controversial issue in this country. Although opposition to abortion stems primarily from religious origins, a fundamental ethical question lies at the root of the controversy: the moral status of the fetus at various phases of development. Views on this topic range from the belief that a fertilized ovum is a person from the moment of conception and thus that it is immoral to destroy that life, to the belief that personhood begins at birth, or even later. No scientific evidence can possibly inform this debate, and no further facts can come to light that are likely to alter these various views about the "personhood" of the fetus.[9] The abortion controversy is probably an insoluble ethical conflict.

Is surrogate motherhood more like the issue of in vitro fertilization, or more like abortion? Is it simply a novel social situation, which requires us to establish safeguards against abuses and to resolve the question of who has rights to what in surrogacy arrangements? Or is it a practice that raises profound moral considerations that may forever resist resolution?

The statements of the fifteen extended committees on the new reproductive technologies illustrate the array of different surrogacy provisions found ethically acceptable.[10] Only three of the fifteen held that surrogate motherhood with payment of a fee is acceptable in principle (Ontario Law Reform Commission, 1985; American Fertility Society, 1986; and Dutch Health Council, 1984–86); all three required medical reasons for surrogate motherhood arrangements and specifically rejected surrogacy for reasons of convenience. A fourth committee (Council for Science and Society, U.K., 1984) held that it is acceptable in principle without payment of a fee. The Ethics Committee of the American Fertility Society called for surrogacy to be practiced only as a clinical experiment because not enough reliable data exist. According to this proposal, surrogate motherhood should be offered only as part of a research protocol approved by a local IRB or ethics committee. Also, clinics involved in surrogacy arrangements should publish data about the process and outcomes, to provide a firm basis for evaluating the practice.

In contrast to reactions stemming from gut feelings, a reasoned approach to the ethics of surrogacy can proceed by using either of two well-known ethical perspectives. The first perspective examines the good and bad consequences of an action or practice as a means of determining its moral rightness or wrongness, while the second tries to determine whether an act or practice is inherently or intrinsically wrong.

According to the first ethical perspective—consequentialism—if the good consequences outweigh the bad, the action or practice is ethically accept- able. If, on the other hand, there is a balance of bad consequences over good ones, then the action or practice is morally wrong. The best-known version of a consequentialist ethical theory is utilitarianism, but that is only one among several ways of articulating the details of this moral perspective.

Although a consequentialist mode of conducting an ethical analysis is basically sound, it is fraught with both theoretical and practical difficulties. Not only is it difficult to predict good and bad results; it is also hard to weigh consequences, even those that have already come about. Moreover, reasonable people frequently disagree over what should count as good and bad consequences, and how much weight should be assigned to each.

It is worth noting that hundreds of surrogacy arrangements have been successfully completed, with a distinct minority resulting in regrets by the surrogate mother and only a few leading to the sorts of devastating con- sequences exemplified by the Baby M case. If applying the utilitarian prin- ciple were simply a matter of subtracting the number of individuals who experienced bad consequences from the number of those who experienced good consequences, it would be an easy matter to determine the rightness or wrongness of surrogacy. But a proper application of the principle is methodologically much more complex. It requires assessing the magnitude of the good and bad consequences for every individual affected by the action or practice, a task that is fraught with problems of measurement and interpersonal comparisons.

The competing approach to ethics rejects as morally irrelevant the con- sequences of actions or practices. Sometimes known as formalism, this approach holds that certain actions are wrong because of the very type of action they are. It is the "form" the action takes that makes it right or wrong, not its consequences. Examples include killing innocent human beings, enslaving individuals or groups, the economic or social exploitation of persons or classes, and physical or mental torture. Debates erupt over just which human beings should be considered "innocent"; over whether some living entities, such as fetuses, should be considered human beings; and over just what should count as economic or social exploitation. But such debates do not detract from the respectability of formalism as a leading approach to ethics. A notable feature of this perspective is that it generates the morally important concept of rights.

ETHICAL ANALYSIS

In tackling the broader issue of surrogacy, the first and most fundamental ethical question is whether there is something intrinsically wrong with surrogacy arrangements. Couched in the language of ethical formalism, is this a practice whose very form makes it immoral? Does surrogate motherhood violate some basic ethical principle? Those who believe it does argue that surrogacy ought to be outlawed, not simply regulated. They contend that the practice of surrogacy is morally flawed, in principle, and that erecting safeguards cannot erase the fundamental ethical wrong of the practice. Within this category fall the objections of the Roman Catholic church and some feminist groups.

In a brief filed with the New Jersey Supreme Court prior to the appeal in the Baby M case, the New Jersey Catholic Conference, composed of the state's fourteen Roman Catholic bishops, argued that surrogate motherhood "promotes the exploitation of women and infertile couples and the dehumanization of babies." The bishops' brief focused largely (but not entirely) on the commercial aspects of surrogacy. "What is being paid for," they wrote, "is a living child."[11] But in trying to determine whether surrogacy is intrinsically immoral, it is necessary to separate the commercial aspects from the practice itself. In fact, just that separation is evident from developments in Britain. The Surrogacy Arrangements Act passed in 1985 bans commercial surrogacy and advertising of and for surrogacy services. But the act does not ban surrogacy itself.[12]

The Catholic bishops in New Jersey did not limit their criticism of surrogacy to its commercial aspects. Their brief also referred to the best interests of children born under such arrangements:

> In surrogacy, a child is conceived precisely in order to be abandoned to others and his or her best interests are the last factors to be considered. . . . There is great potential for psychological injury to the child when he realizes that he was born, not of a loving relationship, but from a cold, usually financial relationship.[13]

A similar position is argued by a feminist psychologist, who asserts that "no child wants to live in a womb for hire."[14]

When we begin to contemplate the possible consequences for the child born of surrogacy arrangements, and what is in the child's best interests, a new set of questions arises. Should the child be told, when old enough, the pertinent details about his or her conception and birth? Should the identity of the surrogate mother routinely be disclosed? What if the surrogate mother wants to be known to the child? What if she does not? What if she insists on visitation rights or other ongoing involvement with the child?

Such questions are identical to those that have been posed about adoption and about artificial insemination using the sperm of an anonymous donor. It is instructive that replies to these questions have changed over the years, and that even today there are no settled, universally accepted answers. In fact, some recent proposals mark a radical shift from earlier practices. Some people are now urging that the identity of birth mothers and fathers be disclosed to adoptive parents and, eventually, the child, and that the long-established practice of anonymous donor insemination be eliminated. These suggestions arise partly out of increasing efforts by many adopted children to discover the identity of their biological parents, and also from an assessment of the negative consequences for the children of secrecy surrounding the men who have anonymously donated their sperm for artificial insemination.

As important as these issues are, they are questions that pertain to the consequences of surrogate arrangements. They become pertinent only when the formalist approach to the morality of surrogacy has been rejected, or when it has been determined that the practice does not violate a prohibition against actions of an unacceptable type.

While some critics of surrogate motherhood base their opposition on the best interests of the children or on the motives of the surrogates, others oppose it as exploitative of women. This makes it appear that surrogacy is unethical because of the type of practice it is, namely, a form of exploitation. According to one writer: "When a woman provides womb service, the feminist issue surfaces. Women object to being baby factories or sex objects because it offends their human dignity."[15] And further: "This is going to end up as the final exploitation of women. It is always going to be poor women who have the babies and rich women who get them."[16]

These statements confuse two distinct issues: first, the exploitation of individual women, if that is indeed what really happens in surrogacy arrangements; and second, a form of class exploitation, since poorer women will be the ones serving as surrogates for the more well-to-do. My own view is that these would be sound, principled objections if it were clear that exploitation in some form actually occurs.

The feminist charge that the practice of surrogacy exploits women is paternalistic. It questions women's ability to know their own interests and to enter into a contractual arrangement knowingly and competently. There may well be a coercive aspect to commercial surrogacy, since money— especially a large enough sum—can serve as a coercive inducement to do something a person might not otherwise do voluntarily. But that speaks more to the exploitation of poorer classes of women, which I think is a genuine moral worry, than it does to the exploitation of women generally. Feminists who oppose surrogacy presume to speak for all women. But what they are really saying is that those who elect to enter surrogacy arrangements are incompetent to choose and stand in need of protection.

The charge of "exploitation" contradicts the moral stance that women have the ability and the right to control their own bodies. If that right grants women reproductive freedoms of other sorts, such as the right to abortion or to control the number and spacing of their children, why does it not similarly apply to the informed, voluntary choice to serve as a surrogate? Some feminists draw an analogy with prostitution, another practice believed to constitute exploitation of women. But the chief feminist complaint about prostitution pertains to its commercial aspect, the feature that transforms women's bodies into a commodity. Feminists who see nothing wrong with women engaging in sexual intercourse outside of marriage (in today's terms—as long as they practice safer sex) are inconsistent if they contend that noncommercial surrogacy arrangements are demeaning to women.

Still, it could be argued, to treat one's body as a mere means to the ends of others is degrading. It could be viewed as a violation of Kant's supreme moral principle, the categorical imperative, which prohibits treating persons merely as a means. But according to that interpretation, other acts and practices typically considered altruistic or even noble would similarly have to be viewed as degrading. A normal, healthy volunteer for biomedical or behavioral research is also acting as a "mere means" to the ends of others—of either the researchers, or future generations, or both. Monetary payments to research subjects would surely have to be outlawed, if it is exploitation to pay people for the use of their bodies or for services that use their bodies. And in the therapeutic context, requests for bone marrow donations would have to be considered suspect.

These analogies serve as a reminder that surrogate motherhood is a biomedical as well as a social practice, as it involves either artificial insemination or embryo transfer, then pregnancy and childbirth. It leads naturally to a consideration of informed consent.

Is Informed Consent Possible?

Although surrogacy arrangements are typically governed by a legal contract, the concept of informed consent is still applicable. Yet it has been argued that no one is capable of granting truly informed consent to be a surrogate mother. This argument contends that even if a woman has already borne children, she cannot know what it is like to have to give them up after birth. In fact, most surrogacy arrangements do require that women who offer to be surrogates already have children. This would seem to meet the objection that surrogate mothers cannot possibly know what it is like to go through pregnancy and childbirth. Yet according to those who say genuine informed consent to be a surrogate mother is impossible, it is the feature of having to give up the child that cannot be known in advance.

There is some merit to that argument. Yet as an argument against the very possibility of informed consent, it is too strong. If it holds for surrogate motherhood, it would seem to apply, as well, to a wide variety of other biomedical treatments and research maneuvers that people have never before experienced. The only time patients could give truly informed consent to treatment would be in those cases where they have already undergone the same or very similar treatment. If the standard for gaining informed consent had to be interpreted in that way, it would lose much of its ordinary meaning. As an ethical and legal concept pertaining to medical therapy and research, informed consent requires that the person understand the likely consequences. It is unrealistic to maintain that the only way to gain such understanding is to have had the actual experience, along with the accompanying feelings.

So, either the meaning of informed consent to become a surrogate mother is the same as that of informed consent to medical treatment, or it is different. If it should be understood in the usual sense, then women should be as capable of granting informed consent to carry a baby to term and then relinquish it as they are to grant consent for removal of a breast when they have breast cancer, or removal of their uterus if they develop a tumor, or for an operation to reduce or enlarge their breasts.

However, if a different, higher standard of informed consent is to be used, then the only women who could qualify would be those who had already undergone the experience of having had a baby and lost it. But that would surely be a bizarre requirement, and probably a cruel one, as well. Having experienced the loss of an infant, such women would be the only ones judged able to consent to enter a surrogacy agreement.

Additional Ethical Concerns

I believe it is not the element of understanding that poses the problem for the possibility of informed consent but, rather, the element of voluntariness when the arrangement is a commercial one and the surrogate is a person with limited financial assets. A fee of $10,000 paid to a woman of low income may well be an offer she cannot refuse. The remedy for this problem is to pay nothing at all, and to allow surrogacy arrangements only as purely altruistic acts on the part of the surrogate mother.

But is that fair? Is it reasonable? After all, the surrogate mother does have to undergo the inconvenience of pregnancy, with its possible discomforts, as well as take the time for prenatal visits to the obstetrician, and then undergo the risks and rigors of childbirth. Shouldn't she be paid for her time and inconvenience?

A physician colleague of mine has argued that she should. He said:

> If I wanted to hire a surrogate mother to bear my child, I'd want her to be adequately taken care of financially. I wouldn't want her to have to work at a grueling job. I'd want her to keep from exhausting herself, from being forced to go to work where she may be exposed to environmental hazards to the fetus. In short, I'd want her to be as comfortable and as free from stress as possible during the entire pregnancy.

I find this argument persuasive, but only to a point. For one thing, there is just so much that money can do to alleviate stress. And even if a woman is not exposed to the hazards of toxic fumes in a factory or to a video display terminal in an office, there is no way to eliminate entirely her exposure to potentially damaging substances, and surely no way to protect her from the emotional upset of daily life. It would take more evidence than is now available to conclude that monetary payments to surrogate mothers are likely to decrease the risks of harm to the fetus.

It is true, however, that contracts for surrogate arrangements impose obligations and restrictions on the woman during pregnancy. Most surrogacy contracts include prohibitions against smoking, drinking, and the use of prescription as well as recreational drugs. In the contract signed by Mary Beth Whitehead, the mother of Baby M, clause 15 required her "to adhere to all medical instructions given to her by the inseminating physician as well as her independent obstetrician." She had to agree "not to smoke cigarettes, drink alcoholic beverages, use illegal drugs, or take nonprescription medication or prescribed medications without written consent from her physician." She also had to agree to follow a prenatal medical examination schedule.[17]

These contractual provisions create a different sort of ethical problem: How can it be known whether the surrogate mother is adhering to the restrictions? How can such provisions be enforced? Should monitoring be permitted—for example, screening urine for drug use during pregnancy, installing cigarette smoke detectors in the home or in the car, doing random breathalizer tests for alcohol? These questions might seem far-fetched were it not for the fact that such tests are already in use in some places and for some purposes in our society, and have been recommended in many other settings. Would it be reasonable to require surrogate mothers to give up a substantial amount of privacy for the purpose of detecting violations of the surrogacy contract?

The discussion has now shifted to the provisions of surrogacy contracts, and away from the question with which we began: an ethical assessment of the practice of surrogacy itself. Yet a thorough evaluation of this new reproductive practice requires an examination of relevant public policy concerns.

Surrogacy and Public Policy

A factor that complicates the debate at the policy level is the contention that surrogate motherhood is a form of "baby selling." When the attorney for Mary Beth Whitehead asserted that a contract to be a surrogate mother for money is "against public policy," he was referring to his belief that the contract violated state adoption laws and public policies against the sale of babies.

Once again, this places the assessment of surrogacy in the context of a commercial arrangement. Although I have been urging that the commercial aspects be separated from the social arrangement of surrogacy for the purpose of ethical evaluation, the underlying conceptual question remains: Is this a form of baby-selling? Or should it be considered more like a fee for services rendered? People who express a strong emotional distaste for surrogate motherhood are quick to label it "baby selling." That term has such negative connotations, and the practice is so universally disapproved, that once surrogacy is categorized as a new variety of "baby selling," its rejection is sure to follow quickly. But fairness demands an objective examination of the issue. It is an old trick of argumentation to apply a concept that already carries negative connotations to a different situation, with the aim of persuading listeners that the new situation should, like the old one, be viewed in a negative light.

A Kentucky court, holding that surrogate contracts did not violate public policy, asked how it was possible for a natural father to be accused of buying his own child.[18] My own view on this question is that paying a woman to be a surrogate mother is more like "renting a womb" than it is like buying a baby. Monetary payment is for the woman's inconvenience and possible discomfort, including the risks of any complications of pregnancy. This interpretation can be supported by looking at the features of surrogacy contracts, features that impose certain duties and obligations on the surrogate mother during pregnancy. Also, one proposed law in the state of Michigan contains the provision that the surrogate agreement may not allow for a reduction of payment if the baby is stillborn or born alive but impaired.[19]

But an opposing interpretation is supported by some existing programs and proposed laws. In many surrogacy arrangements, the bulk of the payment is made after birth, and in some cases the surrogate mother does not receive full payment if she miscarries.[20] The law proposed in South Carolina would codify that approach by a provision that the woman will receive no compensation beyond her medical expenses if she miscarries before the fifth month of pregnancy, and will receive only 10 percent of the agreed-upon fee plus medical expenses if she miscarries during or after the fifth month.[21]

Despite my conclusion that contracts for surrogacy should not be considered a form of baby-selling, and therefore in violation of laws that prohibit that activity, I believe it is morally wrong to undertake commercial surrogacy transactions. There are two arguments in support of this view.

Two Arguments Against Commercial Surrogacy

The "Exploitation" Argument

The first argument goes back to an earlier point: there is a risk of richer women exploiting those who are poorer or less advantaged. The magnitude of this danger is probably exaggerated by the opponents of surrogate motherhood. Yet it is surely true that women who are poor, uneducated, or both have fewer options than those who are better off financially. They are more likely to be unemployed, receiving welfare payments, or forced to remain at home caring for their own young children. To offer money to a woman in these circumstances to bear the child of another woman is probably to offer her an undue inducement. It is an offer that may be difficult for a person of little financial means to refuse and would, in that case, be coercive.

Yet it would be hasty to conclude that any substantial amount of money offered to a person of little financial means, in return for services, is necessarily coercive. Payments to surrogates might be regulated so as to lessen the possibility of exploitation of the poor by the well-to-do. But what could serve as a proper basis for regulation? Although an offer of money almost always serves as an inducement to act in certain ways, it is difficult to determine when an incentive becomes an "undue" inducement.[22]

The attempt to distinguish between "due" and "undue" inducements is complicated by a number of considerations. First is the fact that different people attach different values to the same monetary sum. These differences may be due to the diminishing marginal utility of a unit of currency as one's income or wealth rises. Or they may stem from the varying importance people attach to money, even when they have roughly equal income or wealth.

A second complicating factor is the wide variation in people's willingness to undergo risks or discomforts. For some women, the discomfort of pregnancy and risks of childbirth are to be avoided at any cost, while others actually enjoy the experience, or at least do not consider the risks and discomforts especially burdensome.

Taken together, these differences in the degree to which people value money, along with variations in their willingness to undergo risks and discomforts, suggest that it is impossible to arrive at a single, objective criterion for separating "due" from "undue" inducements. What is merely an incentive for some would constitute a coercive offer for others. Practically speaking, it is unrealistic and would probably also be unfair to set a fixed sum of money as the "right amount" to pay surrogates.

Another possibility, however, is to relativize payments to the financial status of the surrogate. With this maneuver, the problems posed by the other alternatives—leaving the entire matter to market forces or seeking to devise a scheme of fixed payments—might be avoided. But a new difficulty would arise: to relativize acceptable monetary payments to each potential surrogate would result in providing different sums of money for essentially the same services. In effect, this would be giving unequal pay for "equal work." Leaving aside the further complication that some women labor much harder than others, nothing more need be said about the ethics of violating the precept of equal pay for equal work.

There is a lingering worry. The presumption that wealthier women who seek to employ surrogates are exploiting them could be viewed as paternalistic, since it seems to imply that poor women may not be able to assess their own interests. Why shouldn't they be permitted to commit themselves for nine months to the obligations of pregnancy and get paid for their efforts?

The answer to that question leads to considerations of justice. The particular concept of justice involved here is that of "distributive justice." Simply put, distributive justice requires that society's benefits and burdens be distributed fairly among different social classes and racial and ethnic groups. Since women who are less well off will almost always be the ones to serve as surrogates for wealthier or professional women, the distribution is not fair. This argument does not rebut the charge that it is paternalistic to prohibit women from being paid to be surrogates. Rather, it identifies considerations of justice as a higher value, one that may tolerate a certain amount of paternalism in public policy.

There is another objection to this argument, which points to considerations besides paternalism. Our capitalistic society already embodies many commercial arrangements in which a lower social class works for relatively low pay, providing services for a higher social class. Examples include domestic service, housekeeping and custodial work, and a wide range of other occupations. Since we already tolerate many such arrangements, this objection goes, why should it not be acceptable in surrogate motherhood?

It is arguable whether these social arrangements should be construed as a form of class exploitation, although this debate lies well beyond the scope of this article. But the already existing circumstances in which lower classes provide services for better-off members of society does not supply the basis for an argument that it is morally acceptable to create more such arrangements. The form of that philosophical argument is a variation of the attempt to derive an 'ought' from an 'is': "Because things are this way, it is morally permissible to continue in this way." If society is to achieve moral progress, that form of argument must be rejected.

Some feminists have provided a curious twist to the debate about commercial surrogacy. They argue that the standard $10,000 fee paid to a surrogate mother is too low, that it is exploitative precisely because it is not a fair wage for services rendered. As an hourly wage, they calculate, it comes to about $1.49 per hour. The idea of calculating a fair wage for surrogacy has all the marks of a reductio ad absurdum.

The "Commodification" Argument

The potential for better-off women to exploit those who are less well off is the first argument against commercial surrogacy arrangements. The second is a broader argument that applies to other biomedical concerns as well. Medical and other health services are a special sort of social good, one that should not be subject to the same market forces that govern the sale of pork bellies. The human body, its parts, and its reproductive products are not "mere meat."[23] The United States Congress wisely enacted a law prohibiting commercial arrangements for procuring and distributing organs for transplantation.[24] There is sufficient evidence of greed, corruption, and duplicity on the part of persons in financial markets, among defense contractors, local and federal officials, and others in the public and private sectors to make us wary of allowing commercial practices to invade and dominate the delivery of health care.

Medical services and other health-related activities should not be treated as commodities.[25] To do so is to feed the coffers of profiteers and enrich brokers and middlemen, people eager to reap personal gain from the misfortunes of others. Commercial arrangements drain monetary resources away from providing medical services and products directly to those in need.

The standard cost of a surrogacy arrangement is a case in point. When Noel P. Keane, the Detroit lawyer, appeared on the TV program "60 Minutes," he reported the breakdown of costs as follows: a one-time fee of $10,000 to the broker; $10,000 to the surrogate mother; and $5,000 for "other costs," for a total of $25,000.

CONCLUSION

From all of the considerations enumerated here, I conclude that it is not the practice of surrogate motherhood itself that is ethically wrong but, rather, its commercialization. This conclusion answers "no" to the question of whether there is something intrinsically unethical about surrogacy. It cannot be seen to violate any fundamental moral principle prohibiting certain types of action. But this conclusion does not yet answer the question of whether, on the whole, the bad consequences of allowing this practice outweigh the good ones. There is not enough evidence at this point for an empirically well-confirmed answer to that question.

But, it will be objected, if commercial surrogacy is prohibited, is that not likely to result in the disappearance of the practice? Who will come forward to serve as surrogate mothers—except for a few women who want to help their own sisters, or daughters, or even mothers, as the case may be?

My reply to this question is simple. The argument that there is nothing inherently unethical about surrogacy is not an argument that surrogacy is a good thing and that, therefore, it ought to be encouraged or promoted. It is simply an argument that noncommercial surrogacy is morally permissible and, therefore, should not be prohibited. If the practice disappears for lack of monetary incentive for women to act as surrogates, so be it. In the absence of evidence or arguments that surrogacy is such a desirable practice that its disappearance would constitute a harm or wrong to society, its loss should not be lamented.

Still, there is sufficient evidence from the Baby M case and that of other surrogate mothers who are seeking to get their babies back to suggest that even noncommercial surrogacy needs to be carefully regulated. Thought should be given to requiring the sort of provisions typical in adoption cases, which permit the birth mother to change her mind during a limited period after the baby is born. That would surely be preferable to lengthy trials, accompanied by the sensational publicity and humiliation that marked the Baby M case.

An ethical analysis of surrogate motherhood should proceed by seeking to determine the probable beneficial and harmful consequences. This requires an ongoing review of evidence as it becomes available. It brings to mind the recommendations of the Ethics Committee of the American Fertility Society noted earlier. Not only did the committee propose that surrogacy be practiced exclusively as a clinical experiment; it also recommended that clinics involved in surrogacy arrangements publish data about the process and outcomes. Some people might contend that it is too late to reverse social practices already set in motion, but that view is mistaken. Biomedical research involving human subjects was practiced for a long time before regulations and safeguards were introduced. It makes perfectly good sense to do the same for novel reproductive arrangements, in order to provide a scientific basis on which they can be evaluated for the purpose of fashioning public policy.

The argument that surrogacy is a morally flawed activity because of exploitation, dehumanization, or the base motives of the participants does not stand up to critical analysis. The moral flaws are tied to the commercial features of surrogacy, not to the arrangement itself. Although there is nothing ethically wrong, in principle, with surrogate motherhood, if it becomes evident that surrogacy arrangements result in more overall harm than benefits, we shall have to conclude that the practice is morally wrong.

REFERENCES

1. Joseph Sullivan, "Bishops File Brief Against Surrogate Motherhood," *New York Times,* July 19, 1987, 28.

2. Keith Schneider, "Mothers Urge Ban on Surrogacy as Form of 'Slavery,' " *New York Times,* Sept. 1, 1987.

3. Id.

4. Quoted in "Who's Who in the Fight for Baby M," *New York Times,* April 1, 1987, sec. B2.

5. Quoted in Schneider, supra note 2.

6. Robert Hanley, "Seven-Week Trial Touched Many Basic Emotions," *New York Times,* April 1, 1987, sec. B2.

7. James Feron, "Testimony Is Given on Surrogate Bill," *New York Times*, April 11, 1987.

8. LeRoy Walters, "Ethics and New Reproductive Technologies: An International Review of Committee Statements," *Hastings Center Report*, 17 (June 1987, Special Supplement): 3–9.

9. Ruth Macklin, "Personhood in the Bioethics Literature," *Milbank Memorial Fund Quarterly*, 61 (1983): 35–37.

10. Walters, supra note 8.

11. Sullivan, supra note 1, at 28.

12. Diana Brahams, "The Hasty British Ban on Commercial Surrogacy," *Hastings Center Report*, 17 (Feb. 1987): 16–19.

13. Sullivan, supra note 1, at 28.

14. Sidney Callahan, "No Child Wants to Live in a Womb for Hire," *National Catholic Reporter*, Oct. 11, 1985.

15. Id.

16. Sidney Callahan, as quoted in Iver Peterson, "Baby M Trial Splits Ranks of Feminists," *New York Times*, Feb. 24, 1987, sec. B1.

17. George Annas, "Baby M: Babies (and Justice) for Sale," *Hastings Center Report*, 17 (June 1987): 13–15, at 14.

18. Commonwealth of Kentucky v. Surrogate Parenting Associates, Inc. (Oct. 26, 1983), Kentucky Circuit Court, Franklin County.

19. Lori Andrews, "The Aftermath of Baby M: Proposed State Laws on Surrogate Motherhood," *Hastings Center Report*, 17 (Oct./Nov. 1987): 31–40, at 35.

20. Id.

21. Id.

22. See Ruth Macklin, " 'Due' and 'Undue' Inducements: On Paying Money to Research Subjects," *IRB: A Review of Human Subjects Research*, 3 (May 1981): 1–6. The arguments in this section are excerpted from the article.

23. See Leon Kass, " 'Making Babies' Revisited," *The Public Interest*, 54 (Winter 1979): 32–60.

24. National Organ Transplant Act of 1984, 42 U.S.C. Para. 274(e) (1982).

25. See, gen., Margaret Radin, "Market Inalienability," *Harvard Law Review*, 100 (June 1987): 1849–1937.

THE ETHICS OF
SURROGATE MOTHERHOOD
Biology, Freedom, and Moral Obligation

Lisa Sowle Cahill

Proponents of the new reproductive arrangements tend to speak in terms of "reproductive freedom," "the right to be a parent," "contractual obligation," and infertility "therapy," while opponents speak of "the natural bond of motherhood," "the gift of a child," "the integrity of the family," and "playing God with the reproductive process." Underlying the rhetorical slogans are deep differences about the values that should guide evaluation of the disputed practices and policies. The proponents of surrogacy contracts place a high value on freedom and autonomy, and consequently on legally binding agreements to embark on birth projects that will alleviate for some the physiological blight of infertility. The opponents of surrogacy and other forms of nontraditional reproduction, on the other hand, defend the physical and genetic foundations not only of parenthood but also of marriage and family. The right to self-determination, they hold, should not extend beyond the personal relationships derived from the basic biological realities of marriage cemented sexually and "natural" parenthood.

The first position is "liberal" in the sense that it affirms the value of the individual, understood primarily in terms of his or her freedom, autonomy, self-determination, and privacy. The liberal political and philosophical outlook is very much at home in the Western tradition of constitutional democracy, and lies at the root of our legislative and judicial protection of individual civil and political rights. A legal scholar and liberal feminist, Lori B. Andrews, exemplifies this outlook in her assertion that parenthood does

The present essay was originally commissioned for publication in the journal *Law, Medicine, and Health Care*, to whose editors it was submitted in July 1987. It was then anticipated that it would be published before the decision of the New Jersey Supreme Court in the case of "Baby M." Hence the essay refers only to the New Jersey Superior Court decision of Judge Harvey R. Sorkow (March 1987). However, the basic ethical approach outlined in the essay is intended to apply to surrogacy in general. The decision of the New Jersey Supreme Court (February 1988) is much more consistent with this approach, insofar as it refuses to uphold the surrogacy contract, recognizes the parental rights of both Mary Beth Whitehead and William Stern, and gives a central place to the best interests of the child.

not depend on biology and would well be dissociated from it in order to enlarge options for family formation. "The new reproductive technologies," she writes, "by so clearly separating gestational from genetic parenthood and biological from rearing parenthood, open up the possibility for creating nontraditional family forms other than two-parent families."[1] In order to protect the child, however, "it is important *to choose* a primary family for the infant before his or her birth. One approach would be to have a policy that always holds that the intended parents are the legal parents."[2] In other words, it is choice and intention that determine parenthood, and the social and legal task is to ensure that such choices will be secure.

Yet to affirm the moral and legal legitimacy of surrogacy contracts is to take the position that there is little morally important connection either between marriage and genetic reproductive cooperation, or between one's genetic reproductive contribution and the social role of parent. To affirm surrogacy is to deny that moral obligations can be contingent upon physical relationships, and to affirm that the only morally binding relationships are the ones to which persons freely consent.

Unfortunately, many opponents of reproductive technologies take it as self-evident that these biological realities determine the morally proper family relationships, but fail to consider whether it is ever appropriate for human intelligence and freedom to intervene in the exceptional cases where normal biological function fails. Many proponents of the same technologies take it for granted that freedom means autonomy and implies a right to self-determination, but fail to demonstrate how freedom can function responsibly to protect all the parties and biologically based relationships involved.

I hope to persuade that biological relationships can and should exercise some constraints upon freedom to choose (or not choose) the parental relation, although I still affirm, within limits, free and intelligent reproductive choice. The toughest philosophical and policy question is the precise placement of these limits. I cannot hope to resolve policy questions about surrogate motherhood in any detail, but I think it is possible at least to offer considerations against the encouragement of surrogate motherhood.

THE MORAL ISSUES

My analysis will focus on the moral ramifications of surrogate motherhood undertaken by means of artificial insemination, especially on the moral status of decisions (1) to conceive a child one does not intend to raise, or to induce another to do so; and (2) to enter into a reproductive relationship with an individual with whom one has no significant and enduring interpersonal relationship, especially when one is already married to someone else.[3]

Conception without Intent to Raise

The fact that the surrogate mother conceives the child without intending to raise it makes surrogacy significantly different from traditional adoption. Adoption is usually a measure taken after the facts of conception, pregnancy, and birth; conception is not undertaken with adoption in mind. While the decision to offer a baby for adoption is usually morally admirable in itself, for both the birth parents and the adoptive parents, the commendability of adoption says nothing about the moral acceptability of the circumstances in which conception occurred. Indeed, one can safely say that most birth parents look on the circumstances leading to the adoption with regret, if not anguish and anger. Adoption generally brings good out of an undeniably unfortunate set of events. That does not mean it is morally commendable to create, intentionally and with a great deal of forethought, a reproductive scenario in which the genetic child of one person (or persons) is yielded to the care of another person (or persons), who may or may not also be genetically related to the child.

Is it morally appropriate to contract for the production of a child, or to undertake to produce a child for someone else, whether out of altruism or for profit? Our moral repugnance against child-selling, to take the extreme case, arises from the common perception that persons should not be treated merely as means to the ends of others. Of course, most parents who want a child and conceive one do so because they see the child as a potential "benefit" to themselves. In some cultures and economic circumstances, this can even include economic benefit. However, the long-term parent-child association, in which an interpersonal relation is established and that in at least the early years requires the parents to make considerable personal sacrifices, serves as a safeguard against, if not an absolute barrier to, purely self-interested motives for child-bearing. The fulfillment parents receive through their children also leads them to act protectively toward them, and teaches them to value and respect their children as persons of intrinsic worth. Buying or selling a child implies that the child is of value to the parent only instrumentally.

Reproductive Arrangements Between Non-Spouses

If conception occurs outside the marriage(s) of one (or both) of the biological parent(s), the nature of the marital trust is called into question. Indeed, the "surrogate" is "substituting" not for the *mother*—she is a real mother, even if she intentionally limits her role to its biological aspects—but for the *wife* of her child's biological father, making a biological contribution usually made by the wife. The relationships of parenthood and spousehood clearly can be established independently of one another. But is it morally acceptable to separate the biological from the interpersonal aspects of the basic human relationships of spouse and parent? After-the-fact contract disputes highlight unresolved questions about whether what the surrogate contract promises to accomplish can be accomplished and sustained successfully in reality.

The Moral Status of the Surrogacy Contract

What is intended in a surrogacy contract? In the type of contract that has prevailed to date, what is intended is both the acts we have been discussing: the mother's voluntary and complete dissociation from her fetus and child, and the formation of a reproductive alliance outside of the marital relationship. Such an intention is exemplified in the agreement between William Stern and the Whiteheads. Mary Beth Whitehead agreed to be inseminated with William Stern's sperm and to bear their child; her husband, Richard, agreed to give up any legal right to be considered the father; and both Whiteheads agreed that the child would upon birth be given to the biological father to be adopted by his wife and raised by the Sterns.

In this and other surrogacy arrangements, the surrogate retains obligations to the fetus during pregnancy. These are based, however, not on her own independent relation to the fetus but on her relation to the father and the prospective adoptive mother, who may prescribe the surrogate's behavior during pregnancy, including obstetrical care, abstinence from possibly harmful substances, genetic testing, and even whether or not to abort. The surrogate ostensibly agrees that the child is not "hers" but the biological father's and the adoptive-mother-to-be's, and perceives her responsibility to the child only as an aspect of her contractual relation to the couple and the pregnancy she undertakes on their behalf. Such a contract presupposes that a woman has no intrinsic moral responsibility to and for a child she conceives and no rights to a relationship with him or her.

A dispute subsequent to the birth of the child, in which the surrogate claims a bond to the child based on their biological relationship, challenges this crucial premise. Such a dispute occurred between William Stern and Mary Beth Whitehead, with Ms. Whitehead refusing to yield the child permanently to the custody of Mr. Stern and his wife, and eventually absconding with the child to another state. Although she returned to face court adjudication of the matter, she has continued to resist the decision that favored the Sterns and allowed her only visitation rights. Her major claim is that as the baby's natural mother, she has a right to custody at least equal to that of the father, her prior contractual agreement notwithstanding.

THE JUDGMENT IN "BABY M"

Present but unintegrated in Judge Harvey Sorkow's opinion in the Baby M case[4] are legal formulations of the two competing points of view we have been discussing. The idea that moral bonds can be freely undertaken or abandoned emerges in the language defending reproductive self-determination contractually undertaken and legally protected. The idea that *prima facie* moral bonds are linked to biological parenthood emerges in the judge's defense of William Stern's fatherhood and in his recourse to the child's "best interests" as an excuse to override the maternal claim of Mary Beth Whitehead.

These contradictory and unresolved elements result in a philosophically unstable series of arguments. Thus while upholding the legality of the surrogacy contract, Judge Sorkow nonetheless keeps invoking the child's best interests as a reason for enforcing that contract. And while defending the right to reproductive self-determination he cannot abandon the concepts of biological motherhood and fatherhood. I will examine and respond to each of these conflicts in turn.

Contract vs. Best Interests

Judge Sorkow opens his deliberations by defining the "best interests" of Baby M as the "primary issue." However, he recognizes the subsidiary importance of

> the need to determine if a unique arrangement between a man and woman, unmarried to each other, creates a contract. If so, is the contract enforceable; and if so, by what criteria, means and manner. If not, what are the rights and duties of the parties with regard to custody, visitation and support.[5]

He subsequently describes the "Surrogate Parenting Agreement" signed not only by William Stern and Mary Beth Whitehead but also by Richard Whitehead, who otherwise would be presumed legally to be the child's father. In essence Ms. Whitehead agreed, for $10,000, "to attempt conception by artificial insemination, upon conception to carry the child to term, deliver the child and surrender the child to Mr. Stern renouncing at that time all of her parental rights and acknowledging that doing so is in the child's best interest."[6]

Some interpret this $10,000 as a payment for Ms. Whitehead's gestational services, not for the child herself. But this interpretation is weakened by the fact that in the process of providing these services, Ms. Whitehead also contributed half of the genes that became constitutive of the baby. Ms. Whitehead cannot be said to have sold "her" child to Mr. Stern, who is after all the father; but it might be said that she sold her "half" of the child, a notion that one can scarcely articulate without suggesting that the child is property.

Judge Sorkow asserts repeatedly that the dispute is to be concluded on the best interest of the child alone. "The sole legal concepts that control are *parens patriae* and best interest of the child."[7] "It is with her welfare that this court concerns [itself]."[8] He insists that the parents cannot enact a contract that can be enforced against the welfare of the child: "An agreement between parents is inevitably subservient to the considerations of best interests of the child. The welfare of a child cannot be subscribed by an agreement of the parents. . . . It must follow that 'best interests' are paramount to the contract and this court must answer a best interests inquiry if it is to specifically perform the surrogate parenting agreement."[9]

Yet Judge Sorkow is unwilling to abandon considerations of contractual validity. He asserts: "[T]his court concludes and holds that the surrogate parenting agreement is a valid and enforceable contract pursuant to the Laws of New Jersey. . . . This court further finds that Mrs. Whitehead had breached her contract," by failing to surrender Baby M and to "renounce her parental rights."[10] Thus, he adds, "The surrogate parenting agreement of February 6, 1985, will be specifically enforced."[11] Best interests thus seems both to override any prior attempt at a contract and to be the criterion by which the contract is to be implemented. But why is contractual remedy via "specific performance" even an issue if the child will be turned over to the Sterns in her own best interests, not because her parents had made, prior to her birth, a decision concerning her fate?

All other things being equal, it is surely in the interests of a child both to be raised within its biological family and to be nurtured by persons who are willing and able to nurture it lovingly and capably. The "best interests" standard has the potential to reconcile considerations both of intentional commitment and of socially recognized biological relation, by focusing on the need of a child for both and on the necessity to balance these needs within the parameters of the options practically available in specific cases. However, in Judge Sorkow's interpretation of "best interests," the interrelational aspects of parenthood not only take precedence over the biological, as they properly should, but function as virtually the sole criterion of best interests, as they should not. As a consequence, Mary Beth Whitehead's stake in her child is almost completely overridden in favor of the Sterns' preferable psychosocial status. In effect this sets aside, without adequate warrant, the customary and morally valid criteria that govern custody assignment in other disputes between biological parents, especially in divorce cases. A divorced parent is not deprived of custody simply because his or her ex-spouse offers a better environment. Each parent retains a *prima facie* right to share custody, unless he or she is demonstrably incompetent.

Reproductive Freedom vs. Biological Motherhood and Fatherhood

Perhaps one reason that Judge Sorkow continues to retain an interest in the contract even after he has set it aside in favor of the child's best interests is that he puts a high priority on a right of free self-determination, extending to the right to conceive a child and form a family. He recognizes "the social and psychological importance" of persons having children who are "genetically theirs" and the powerful desire "to reproduce blood lines."[12] Under the rubric of a "right to privacy," affirmed in relation to reproductive matters by *Roe v. Wade,* Judge Sorkow claims that

> if one has a right to procreate coitally, then one has the right to reproduce non-coitally. If it is the reproduction that is protected, then the means of reproduction are also to be protected. The value and interests underlying the creation of family are the same by whatever means obtained. This court holds that the protected means extends to the use of surrogates. The contract cannot fall because of the use of a third party.[13]

Striking here is the emphasis on one's "interests" in forming a family and the uncritical extension of approval to the means necessary in realizing that interest, to include measures that are at the least morally dissimilar. The "interests" in question seem primarily to be those of Mr. Stern, who is the only member of his family to have survived the Holocaust, and whose wife was considered at the time of the contract to be at risk of severe physical debilitation if she were to embark on a pregnancy. However, as George Annas comments, "The 'right to procreate' is determinative in this case only if we assume it is exclusively a male right, and not one that Mary Beth Whitehead herself retains." Why is her "genetic and gestational" contribution counted as significantly less important than his sperm?[14]

Perhaps more fundamentally, the physiological conditions affecting one's exercise of the "right to reproduce" are considered significantly less important than the choice to exercise it. Mary Beth Whitehead is cut out of the picture not only because she is of lower socioeconomic standing but also because the parental status of each partner is defined by their contractual agreement, not by their biological contribution. Each parent may have a fundamental right to reproduce, but each parent also has a right to sign that right away.

The freedom of persons to make binding commitments as part of their right to self-determination, and their responsibility to abide by what they have chosen, is a central theme in the liberal defense of autonomy and of its legal protection. Lori Andrews defends surrogacy contracts from a liberal feminist perspective that takes the decision-making prerogative as the *sine qua non* of egalitarian moral agency. She rejects the idea that women's biological tie to their children compels them into a parental relationship. Her "personal opinion" is that "it would be a step backward for women to embrace any policy argument based on a presumed incapacity of women to make decisions. That, after all, was the rationale for so many legal principles oppressing women for so long, such as the rationale behind the laws not allowing women to hold property."[15]

Compare to the liberal position of Andrews the rather similar "socialist" feminist position of Barbara Katz Rothman, who argues against surrogacy, seeing "the fetus as a part of a woman's body." Thus she has absolute control over it; the father does not. This control cannot be contracted away. Yet a libertarian element seems to creep in via Rothman's assertion that what she values most are "the interpersonal relations people establish." The woman may *choose* to establish (or not establish, as in abortion) a maternal relationship to her unborn offspring. "The relationship that a woman has established by the time she births her baby has more weight, in my value system, than claims of genetic ties, of contracts signed, or of down payments made."[16]

Andrews and Rothman are certainly right that public policy should hold women equal to men in responsibility and rights. If the freedom to make a choice and stick by it is the standard of moral responsibility and legal rights, then it is a standard that women as well as men can meet and to which they must be held. But is this standard in fact sufficient to define the moral and legal responsibilities of parents? I would argue that, for both women and men, parenthood is a relation whose existence cannot be made entirely contingent on choice, as both Andrews and Rothman indicate it can.

Judge Sorkow offers some recognition of a biological parent-child tie in his opinion. Against the claim of Ms. Whitehead, he asserts: "Mr. Stern agreed to pay Mrs. Whitehead $10,000.00 for conceiving and bearing his child,"[17] and "At birth, the father does not purchase the child. It is his own biological genetically related child. He cannot purchase what is already his."[18] Yet the infant is at least equally the "biological genetically related child" of Mary Beth Whitehead. She was in fact paid not only to undergo a pregnancy but also to sign away her parental interest in and responsibility for her biological offspring. Even in the case of post-natal adoption, where birth parents are understood to have severed their ties to the child permanently, the statement of absolute relinquishment is in a sense a legal fiction, put in place prudently to protect the "best interests" of the child and of the yielding parents as well. The immense interest of adopted children in discovering their biological "roots," and the frequent reciprocation by birth parents, however, testify to the fact that natural kinship bonds remain, whatever the intentions of individuals to step outside them. Adoptive parents create real parental bonds, but these bonds may remain in an ambiguous moral (even if not legal) relationship to the natural bonds of the biological parents with the child. Along with her advocacy of the non-traditional family, Andrews cautions that "[t]here is considerable evidence from the adoption context that no matter where legal parenthood resides, many adopted children feel a need for information about (and potential contact with) their biological parents."[19]

Feminists object that the notion of a natural biological bond between parents and children seems to enshrine traditional, patriarchal kinship and family structures, and to confine women to a patriarchally defined maternal role. But the moral significance of kinship is a separate question from that of the moral acceptability of the patriarchal institutionalization of sexuality, parenthood, and kinship. Since the most intimate human physical relationships have been institutionalized in ways detrimental to women, it is appropriate to exercise extreme caution in attaching enduring moral significance to those relationships. However, caution need not become the equivalent of a moratorium. The task is to determine what moral value sex, conception, pregnancy, and biological parenthood may have within a perspective that views the moral agency of men and women equally.

Surrogate motherhood contracts also involve the spouses of the two biological parents, highlighting the tension between their marital commitments and their reproductive contract. A Western monogamous marriage carries with it at least an implicit promise to procreate with one's spouse, if at all. An assumption in the Sterns' marriage was the eventual accomplishment of mutual biological and social parenthood. The very fact that William Stern sought *as a remedial measure* a woman not his spouse to bear his child testifies to the initial commitment of the Sterns to conceive a child together, if feasible. That Richard Whitehead had to sign away his legal entitlement to paternity testifies to the legal and social presupposition that the husband of a married woman is the natural father of her children. The adoption of Baby M by Elizabeth Stern has in view precisely the creation of a relation between her and the baby analogous to that of a biological mother who is the wife of her child's father. In fact, both couples tend to refer to Baby M as "our" child. The day after Ms. Whitehead originally relinquished the three-day-old child to the Sterns, for instance, her husband advised her to go "get our baby."[20]

STANDARDS FOR RESOLVING SURROGATE CONFLICTS

The deciding factor in surrogate arrangements—granting that they are going to take place with or without legal protection and ethical justification—should be the best interests of the child. An important but secondary and modifying consideration should be the rights and duties of parents in regard to their biological offspring.

Best Interests

The life and thus the welfare of a child have two dimensions: the psychosocial and the physical. The first consideration of a "best interests" criterion, then, is to ensure as far as possible the child's physical and psychological nurturance. Would-be raisers of the child can, accordingly, be evaluated on the basis of their potential physical and psychological contributions. How should these two dimensions of infant need and of parental contribution be weighed and compared? The psychological, intentional, affective, and cognitive aspects of personhood are more important morally than the material and physical, because the former most define humanity as distinctive from other life forms and are indispensable to what we think of as a virtuous and happy life. Generally, if made to choose, we would give priority to a loving home over a wealthy home, to an atmosphere of trust and cooperation over financial security. The most important standard of "best interests" in a child custody case, as expert witnesses testified regarding Baby M, is a firm and reliable determination on the part of a parent to provide permanent care and love to the child, and the emotional and psychological ability of the adult to carry through with that commitment.[21] This is not to say that the physical and material preconditions of psychospiritual flourishing are dispensable or insignificant. A second standard is ability to support the basic physical needs of the child and, when possible, to provide relative comfort as well as minimal necessities.

The Rights and Duties of Biological Parents

Parents' interests are distinct from and secondary to the child's interests, but the two are integrally related in that biological relations typically ground interpersonal relations among family members.

Obviously, parental and familial love for a child does not absolutely require a biological foundation, but a biological relation will undergird and enhance the interpersonal one, exceptional cases notwithstanding. For instance, the U.S. social welfare system goes to some lengths to keep families together, or to separate them only temporarily, rather than forcing indigent parents to put their children up for adoption by others who undoubtedly could support them better and who often are desperate to adopt. A birth mother's consent to relinquish her child for adoption is given significant legal protection. Willing and able relatives should be candidates of first choice in seeking placement for a child whose biological parents are unable to rear him or her. In custody assignments following divorce, the presumption is that each biological parent has a right and even duty to maintain contact with the child, barring inability or a reasonable determination of the parent's harmful effects on the child. A biological parent is not excluded from custody merely because the other parent—much less an unrelated person—can offer a superior environment, nor because it is better for children in general to be raised in an intact home, nor because prior to the child's birth—or even after—there had been some contrary understanding about the arrangement of parental responsibility. Yes, it would be better ideally for Baby M to be nurtured within a single family and in a two-parent home; yes, the Sterns are financially and socially better placed; yes, Mary Beth Whitehead has shown erratic, impulsive, and even irrational behavior. But unless it can be demonstrated that she is an unfit and positively harmful mother, the basic biological relation that she retains to her child entitles her to at least some of the rights and responsibilities of social parenthood.

Neither the rights of Mary Beth Whitehead as biological mother nor those of William Stern as biological father straightforwardly dictate the best interests of their child. But their rights may converge with her interests, insofar as the child's own biological identity and "kinship" community are part of her existence as a human being, and potentially part of her self-understanding. Sometimes it is morally commendable to set aside these physical substrata of identity and relatedness, when to give them explicit social recognition causes disproportionate damage to the child or its natural family, or interferes with the child's psychosocial welfare. This is the case in adoption, or in the denial of custody or visiting rights to destructive parents. However, generally speaking, it serves the welfare of both parent and child to be able to build an interpersonal relation on their biological one.

Yet the kinship bond between children and their biological families has been far from equitably protected in the Stern-Whitehead case. Mr. Stern's fatherhood was given more explicit and positive recognition than Ms. Whitehead's motherhood; Ms. Whitehead's claim as biological mother was given little if any recognition in establishing the best interests of the child herself; and the viability of surrogate contracts was not as such denied, resulting in tacit legitimation of the idea that kinship relations of parents and children are morally significant only when individual parents decide they are.

The extent and limit of *each* competing parent's access to the child must be determined in the light of best interests fully and adequately defined, so as to incorporate psychological nurturance and growth, material welfare, and the affirmation of kinship bonds, especially the biological parent-child bond. As George Annas persuasively argues, Judge Sorkow portrayed the "facts" of Mary Beth Whitehead's situation and capabilities in egregiously biased language.[22] This is not to say that more serious consideration would lead to a reversal of his decision. However, a proposal such as joint custody cannot so easily be dismissed. In the first place it is far from clear that, as the judge asserted, two people with virtually no previous relationship would be less capable of sharing custody than a couple whose marriage broke down after many years of gradually accumulating bitterness and acrimony, nor that the former would more readily attempt to manipulate the child in their continuing mutual siege.

To place on the viability of surrogacy arrangements the weight of "best interests" (interpreted to include an interest in socially validated kinship), qualified by a recognition of the rights and responsibilities of biological parents, would serve to discourage surrogacy without explicit legal prohibition. I concur with Charles Krauthammer that in regard to surrogate contracts "the proper role of the state," or at least its most feasible present role, is "tolerant discouragement: no overt interference with private arrangements, but a refusal by the state to enforce the contract, particularly the part that compels a surrogate gestator to give up her child."[23] By referring disputes to the best-interests standard primarily, the court would effectively undercut the sustainability of pre-conception agreements to bear children in order to give them up. Parties to such agreements would have to rely on mutual trust alone, which would limit surrogate arrangements largely to situations characterized by a close relationship between the parties to the agreement and by a motive of altruistic concern, as for a friend or sister, thus deterring the commercialization of birth.

Real problems no doubt remain with such an approach, particularly the likelihood of leading surrogacy clients to seek out women so economically desperate that they would be unlikely to forfeit the surrogacy payment, and whose very impoverishment makes them unlikely to win a custody fight. The alternatives, however, are either to outlaw surrogacy entirely or to make surrogate contracts irreversibly binding. The former would require a close supervision of reproductive activities that would be both difficult to accomplish and offensive to the moral and political sensitivities of many Americans. The latter enshrines the radically libertarian view that in the matter of parenthood, biology can be separated from morality by fiat, an extreme view not consistent with our full experience of personhood and of human relationships and not in the end espoused thoroughly even by the defenders of surrogacy.

CONCLUSIONS

Surrogate motherhood should not be outlawed, but neither should it be given the legal protection that would encourage it as a social practice. If disputed cases are decided on the best interests of the child, with weight given to the importance of maternal and paternal kinship to the child, then not only will the welfare of the children so born be protected but surrogate contracts will also be deprived of the security on which their wide-spread success depends.

Surrogate arrangements are morally objectionable because they insist on free choice about human relations to an extent that constitutes a virtual denial of important material and physical aspects both of the relations of spousehood and parenthood, and of moral obligation in general. Individuals cannot choose in all cases whether they have a certain moral obligation. The mutual obligations of biological family members—children, parents, siblings—are a paradigmatic case of obligations that one cannot simply decide do not exist. In addition, surrogacy seems a practice almost guaranteed to encourage financially and economically well-disposed couples to take advantage of poorer women, and to induce those women not only to undergo pregnancy for pay but also to agree to give up children to whom they have a real if incomplete parental relationship.

REFERENCES

1. Lori B. Andrews, "Feminist Perspectives on Reproductive Technologies," unpublished conference paper. Available from the author: Lori B. Andrews, American Bar Foundation, 750 Lake Shore Drive, Chicago, IL 60611.

2. Id.: 40 (emphasis added).

3. A prior question, which I consider less morally problematic, is the morality of interfering technologically in the human reproductive process in order to enable conception through an action other than sexual intercourse. Although strong statements have been made against such interference, I do not find the moral arguments against them to be strong, nor are such interventions legally questionable in the United States. For the negative arguments, see the Vatican's *Instruction on Respect for Human Life in Its Origin and on the Dignity of Procreation: Replies to Certain Questions of the Day*, dated Feb. 22, 1987, and issued on March 10 with the signature of Cardinal Joseph Ratzinger, Prefect of the Congregation for the Doctrine of the Faith. The full text was published in the *New York Times, March* 11, 1987. For critical discussion of these arguments, see Lisa Sowle Cahill and R. A. McCormick, "The Vatican Document on Bioethics: Two Responses," *America*, 156, no. 12 (March 28, 1987): 245–48; and C. Krauthammer, "The Ethics of Human Manufacture," *Conscience*, 3, no. 3(May/June 1987): 8–12 (originally published in *The New Republic*, 1987).

4. In re Baby "M," 217 N.J. Super. 313, 525 A.2d 1128 (1987).

5. Id. at 323, 525 A.2d at 1132.

6. Id. at 373–74, 525 A.2d at 1158.

7. Id. at 375, 525 A.2d at 1159.

8. Id. at 328, A.2d at 1135.

9. Id. at 391, A.2d at 1167.

10. Id. at 388–89, A.2d at 1166.

11. Id. at 408, A.2d at 1175.

12. Id. at 331, A.2d at 1136.

13. Id. at 386, A.2d at 1164.

14. George J. Annas, "Baby M: Babies (and Justice) for Sale," *Hastings Center Report*, 17, no. 3 (June 1987): 13–14.

15. Andrews, supra note 1, at 14.

16. B. K. Rothman, "Surrogacy: A question of values," *Conscience*, 8, no. 3 (May/June 1987): 2–3.

17. In re Baby "M," 217 N.J. Super. 374, 525 A.2d at 1158.

18. Id. at 372, 525 A.2d at 1157.

19. Andrews, supra note 1, at 33.

20. In re Baby "M," 217 N.J. Super. 348, 525 A.2d at 1144.

21. See especially the nine criteria offered by Dr. L. Salk, in id. at 362–63, 525 A.2d at 1151–52.

22. Annas, supra note 14.

23. Krauthammer, supra note 3, at 12.

WOMEN'S AUTONOMY

Surrogate Motherhood
The Challenge for Feminists

Lori B. Andrews

Surrogate motherhood presents an enormous challenge for feminists. During the course of the *Baby M* trial, the New Jersey chapter of the National Organization of Women met and could not reach consensus on the issue. "The feelings ranged the gamut," the head of the chapter, Linda Bowker, told the *New York Times*. "We did feel that it should not be made illegal, because we don't want to turn women into criminals. But other than that, what you may feel about the Baby M case may not be what you feel about another.

"We do believe that women ought to control their own bodies, and we don't want to play big brother or big sister and tell them what to do," Ms. Bowker continued. "But on the other hand, we don't want to see the day when women are turned into breeding machines."[1]

Other feminist groups have likewise been split on the issue, but a vocal group of feminists came to the support of Mary Beth Whitehead with demonstrations[2] and an amicus brief[3]; they are now seeking laws that would ban surrogate motherhood altogether. However, the rationales that they and others are using to justify this governmental intrusion into reproductive choice may come back to haunt feminists in other areas of procreative policy and family law.

As science fiction has taught us, the types of technologies available shape the nature of a society. Equally important as the technologies—and having much farther-reaching implications—are the policies that a society devises and implements to deal with technology. In Margaret Atwood's *A Handmaid's Tale*, a book often cited as showing the dangers of the technology of surrogacy, it was actually policy changes—the criminalization of abortion and the banning of women from the paid labor force—that created the preconditions for a dehumanizing and harmful version of surrogacy.

THE FEMINIST LEGACY

In the past two decades, feminist policy arguments have refashioned legal policies on reproduction and the family. A cornerstone of this development has been the idea that women have a right to reproductive choice—to be able to contracept, abort, or get pregnant. They have the right to control their bodies during pregnancy, such as by refusing Cesarean sections. They have a right to create non-traditional family structures such as lesbian households or single-parent families facilitated by artificial insemination by donor. According to feminist arguments, these rights should not be overridden by possible symbolic harms or speculative risks to potential children.

Another hallmark of feminism has been that biology should not be destiny. The equal treatment of the sexes requires that decisions about men and women be made on other than biological grounds. Women police officers can be as good as men, despite their lesser strength on average. Women's larger role in bearing children does not mean they should have the larger responsibility in rearing children. And biological fathers, as well as nonbiological mothers or fathers, can be as good parents as biological mothers.

The legal doctrine upon which feminists have pinned much of their policy has been the constitutional protection of autonomy in decisions to bear and rear one's biological children.[4] Once this protection of the biologically related family was acknowledged, feminists and others could argue for the protection of non-traditional, non-biological families on the grounds that they provide many of the same emotional, physical, and financial benefits that biological families do.[5]

In many ways, the very existence of surrogacy is a predictable outgrowth of the feminist movement. Feminist gains allowed women to pursue educational and career opportunities once reserved for men, such as Betsy Stern's position as a doctor and medical school professor. But this also meant that more women were postponing childbearing, and suffering the natural decline in fertility that occurs with age. Women who exercised their right to contraception, such as by using the Dalkon Shield, sometimes found that their fertility was permanently compromised. Some women found that the chance for a child had slipped by them entirely and decided to turn to a surrogate mother.

Feminism also made it more likely for other women to feel comfortable being surrogates. Feminism taught that not all women relate to all pregnancies in the same way. A woman could choose not to be a rearing mother at all. She could choose to lead a child-free life by not getting pregnant. If she got pregnant, she could choose to abort. Reproduction was a condition of her body over which she, and no one else, should have control. For some women, those developments added up to the freedom to be a surrogate.

In the surrogacy context, feminist principles have provided the basis for a broadly held position that contracts and legislation should not restrict the surrogate's control over her body during pregnancy (such as by a requirement that the surrogate undergo amniocentesis or abort a fetus with a genetic defect). The argument against enforcing such contractual provisions resounds with the notion of gender equality, since it is in keeping with common law principles that protect the bodily integrity of both men and women, as well as with basic contract principles rejecting specific performance of personal-services provisions.[6] It is also in keeping with constitutional principles giving the pregnant woman, rather than the male progenitor, the right to make abortion decisions. In this area, feminist lobbying tactics have met with considerable success. Although early bills on surrogacy contained provisions that would have constrained surrogates' behavior during pregnancy, most bills regulating surrogacy that have been proposed in recent years specifically state that the surrogate shall have control over medical decisions during the pregnancy.[7] Even the trial court decision in the Baby M case, which enforced the surrogacy contract's termination of parental rights, voided the section that took from the surrogate the right to abort.[8]

Now a growing feminist contingent is moving beyond the issue of bodily control during pregnancy and is seeking to ban surrogacy altogether. But the rationales for such a ban are often the very rationales that feminists have fought against in the contexts of abortion, contraception, non-traditional families, and employment. The adoption of these rationales as the reasons to regulate surrogacy could severely undercut the gains previously made in these other areas. These rationales fall into three general categories: the symbolic harm to society of allowing paid surrogacy, the potential risks to the woman of allowing paid surrogacy, and the potential risks to the potential child of allowing paid surrogacy.

THE SYMBOLIC HARM TO SOCIETY

For some feminists, the argument against surrogacy is a simple one: it demeans us all as a society to sell babies. And put that way, the argument is persuasive, at least on its face. But as a justification for policy, the argument is reminiscent of the argument that feminists roundly reject in the abortion context: that it demeans us as a society to kill babies.

Both arguments, equally heartfelt, need closer scrutiny if they are to serve as a basis for policy. In the abortion context, pro-choice people criticize the terms, saying we are not talking about "babies" when the abortion is done on an embryo or fetus still within the woman's womb. In the surrogacy context, a similar assault can be made on the term "sale." The baby is not being transferred for money to a stranger who can then treat the child like a commodity, doing anything he or she wants with the child. The money is being paid to enable a man to procreate his biological child; this hardly seems to fit the characterization of a sale. Am I buying a child when I pay a physician to be my surrogate fallopian tubes through in vitro fertilization (when, without her aid, I would remain childless)? Am I buying a child when I pay a physician to perform a needed Cesarean section, without which my child would never be born alive?

At most, in the surrogacy context, I am buying not a child but the pre-conception termination of the mother's parental rights. For decades, the pre-conception sale of a father's parental rights has been allowed with artificial insemination by donor. This practice, currently facilitated by statutes in at least thirty states, has received strong feminist support. In fact, when, on occasion, such sperm donors have later felt a bond to the child and wanted to be considered legal fathers, feminist groups have litigated to hold them to their pre-conception contract.[9]

Rather than focusing on the symbolic aspects of a sale, the policy discussion should instead analyze the advisability of pre-conception terminations for both women and men. For example, biological parenting may be so important to both the parent and the child that either parent should be able to assert these rights after birth (or even later in the child's life). This would provide sperm donors in artificial insemination with a chance to have a relationship with the child.

Symbolic arguments and pejorative language seem to make up the bulk of the policy arguments and media commentary against surrogacy. Surrogate motherhood has been described by its opponents not only as the buying and selling of children but as reproductive prostitution,[10] reproductive slavery,[11] the renting of a womb,[12] incubatory servitude,[13] the factory method of childbearing,[14] and cutting up women into genitalia.[15] The women who are surrogates are labeled paid breeders,[16] biological entrepreneurs,[17] breeder women,[18] reproductive meat,[19] interchangeable parts in the birth machinery,[20] manufacturing plants,[21] human incubators,[22] incubators for men's sperm,[23] a commodity in the reproductive marketplace,[24] and prostitutes.[25] Their husbands are seen, alternatively, as pimps[26] or cuckolds.[27] The children conceived pursuant to a surrogacy agreement have been called chattel[28] or merchandise to be expected in perfect condition.[29]

Feminists opposing surrogacy have also relied heavily on a visual element in the debate over Baby M. They have been understandably upset at the vision of a baby being wrenched from its nursing mother or being slipped out a back window in a flight from governmental authorities. But relying on the visceral and visual, a long-standing tactic of the right-to-life groups, is not the way to make policy. Conceding the value of symbolic arguments for the procreative choice of surrogacy makes it hard to reject them for other procreative choices.

One of the greatest feminist contributions to policy debates on reproduction and the family has been the rejection of arguments relying on tradition and symbolism and an insistence on an understanding of the nature and effects of an actual practice in determining how it should be regulated. For example, the idea that it is necessary for children to grow up in two-parent, heterosexual families has been contested by empirical evidence that such traditional structures are not necessary for children to flourish.[30] This type of analysis should not be overlooked in favor of symbolism in discussions of surrogacy.

THE POTENTIAL HARM TO WOMEN

A second line of argument opposes surrogacy because of the potential psychological and physical risks that it presents for women. Many aspects of this argument, however, seem ill founded and potentially demeaning to women. They focus on protecting women against their own decisions because those decisions might later cause them regret, be unduly influenced by others, or be forced by financial motivations.

Reproductive choices are tough choices, and any decision about reproduction—such as abortion, sterilization, sperm donation, or surrogacy—might later be regretted. The potential for later regrets, however, is usually not thought to be a valid reason to ban the right to choose the procedure in the first place.

With surrogacy, the potential for regret is thought by some to be enormously high. This is because it is argued (in biology-is-destiny terms) that it is unnatural for a mother to give up a child. It is assumed that because birth mothers in traditional adoption situations often regret relinquishing their children, surrogate mothers will feel the same way. But surrogate mothers are making their decisions about relinquishment under much different circumstances. The biological mother in the traditional adoption situation is already pregnant as part of a personal relationship of her own. In many, many instances, she would like to keep the child but cannot because the relationship is not supportive or she cannot afford to raise the child. She generally feels that the relinquishment was forced upon her (for example, by her parents, a counselor, or her lover).[31]

The biological mother in the surrogacy situation seeks out the opportunity to carry a child that would not exist were it not for the couple's desire to create a child as a part of their relationship. She makes her decision in advance of pregnancy for internal, not externally enforced reasons. While 75 percent of the biological mothers who give a child up for adoption later change their minds,[32] only around 1 percent of the surrogates have similar changes of heart.

Entering into a surrogacy arrangement does present potential psychological risks to women. But arguing for a ban on surrogacy seems to concede that the *government*, rather than the individual woman, should determine what risks a woman should be allowed to face. This conflicts with the general legal policy allowing competent individuals to engage in potentially risky behavior so long as they have given their voluntary, informed consent.

Perhaps recognizing the dangers of giving the government widespread powers to "protect" women, some feminists do acknowledge the validity of a general consent to assume risks. They argue, however, that the consent model is not appropriate to surrogacy since the surrogate's consent is neither informed nor voluntary.

It strikes me as odd to assume that the surrogate's consent is not informed. The surrogacy contracts contain lengthy riders detailing the myriad risks of pregnancy, so potential surrogates are much better informed on that topic than are most women who get pregnant in a more traditional fashion. In addition, with volumes of publicity given to the plight of Mary Beth Whitehead, all potential surrogates are now aware of the possibility that they may later regret their decisions. So, at that level, the decision is informed.

Yet a strong element of the feminist argument against surrogacy is that women cannot give an informed consent until they have had the experience of giving birth. Robert Arenstein, an attorney for Mary Beth Whitehead, argued in congressional testimony that a "pre-birth or at-birth termination, is a termination without informed consent. I use the words informed consent to mean full understanding of the personal psychological consequences at the time of surrender of the child."[33] The feminist amicus brief in *Baby M* made a similar argument.[34]

The New Jersey Supreme Court picked up this characterization of informed consent, writing that "quite clearly any decision prior to the baby's birth is, in the most important sense, uninformed."[35] But such an approach is at odds with the legal doctrine of informed consent. Nowhere is it expected that one must have the experience first before one can make an informed judgment about whether to agree to the experience. Such a requirement would preclude people from ever giving informed consent to sterilizations, abortions, sex change operations, heart surgery, and so forth. The legal doctrine of informed consent presupposes that people will predict in advance of the experience whether a particular course will be beneficial to them.

A variation of the informed consent argument is that while most competent adults can make such predictions, hormonal changes during pregnancy may cause a woman to change her mind. Virtually a whole amicus brief in the *Baby M* appeal was devoted to arguing that a woman's hormonal changes during pregnancy make it impossible for her to predict in advance the consequences of her relinquishment.[36] Along those lines, adoption worker Elaine Rosenfeld argues that

> [t]he consent that the birth mother gives prior to conception is not the consent of . . . a woman who has gone through the chemical, biological,

endocrinological changes that have taken place during pregnancy and birth, and no matter how well prepared or well intentioned she is in her decision prior to conception, it is impossible for her to predict how she will feel after she gives birth.[37]

In contrast, psychologist Joan Einwohner, who works with a surrogate mother program, points out that

> women are fully capable of entering into agreements in this area and of fulfilling the obligations of a contract. Women's hormonal changes have been utilized too frequently over the centuries to enable male dominated society to make decisions for them. The Victorian era allowed women no legal rights to enter into contracts. The Victorian era relegated them to the status of dependent children. Victorian ideas are being given renewed life in the conviction of some people that women are so overwhelmed by their feelings at the time of birth that they must be protected from themselves.[38]

Surrogate Carol Pavek is similarly uncomfortable with hormonal arguments. She posits that if she is allowed the excuse of hormones to change her mind (thus harming the expectant couple and subjecting the child to the trauma of litigation), what's to stop men from using their hormones as an excuse for rape or other harms? In any case, feminists should be wary of a hormone-based argument, just as they have been wary of the hormone-related criminal defense of premenstrual syndrome.

The consent given by surrogates is also challenged as not being voluntary. Feminist Gena Corea, for example, in writing about another reproduction arrangement, in vitro fertilization, asks, "What is the real meaning of a woman's 'consent' . . . in a society in which men as a social group control not just the choices open to women but also women's *motivation* to choose?"[39]

Such an argument is a dangerous one for feminists to make. It would seem to be a step backward for women to argue that they are incapable of making decisions. That, after all, was the rationale for so many legal principles oppressing women for so long, such as the rationale behind the laws not allowing women to hold property. Clearly, any person's choices are motivated by a range of influences—economic, social, religious.

At a recent conference of law professors, it was suggested that surrogacy was wrong because women's boyfriends might talk them into being surrogates and because women might be surrogates for financial reasons. But women's boyfriends might talk them into having abortions or women might have abortions for financial reasons; nevertheless, feminists do not consider those to be adequate reasons to ban abortions. The fact that a woman's decision could be influenced by the individual men in her life or by male-dominated society does not by itself provide an adequate reason to ban surrogacy.

Various feminists have made the argument that the financial inducement to a surrogate vitiates the voluntariness of her consent. Many feminists have said that women are exploited by surrogacy.[40] They point out that in our society's social and economic conditions, some women—such as those on welfare or in dire financial need—will turn to surrogacy out of necessity, rather than true choice. In my view, this is a harsh reality that must be guarded against by vigilant efforts to assure that women have equal access to the labor market and that there are sufficient social services so that poor women with children do not feel they must enter into a surrogacy arrangement in order to obtain money to provide care for their existing children.

However, the vast majority of women who have been surrogates do not allege that they have been tricked into surrogacy, nor have they done it because they needed to obtain a basic of life such as food or health care. Mary Beth Whitehead wanted to pay for her children's education. Kim Cotton wanted money to redecorate her house.[41] Another surrogate wanted money to buy a car. These do not seem to be cases of economic exploitation; there is no consensus, for example, that private education, interior decoration, and an automobile are basic needs, nor that society has an obligation to provide those items. Moreover, some surrogate mother programs specifically reject women who are below a certain income level to avoid the possibility of exploitation.

There is a sexist undertone to an argument that Mary Beth Whitehead was exploited by the paid surrogacy agreement into which she entered to get money for her children's education. If Mary Beth's husband, Rick, had taken a second job to pay for the children's education (or even to pay for their mortgage), he would not have been viewed as exploited. He would have been lauded as a responsible parent.

It undercuts the legitimacy of women's role in the workforce to assume that they are being exploited if they plan to use their money for serious purchases. It seems to harken back to a notion that women work (and should work) only for pin money (a stereotype that is the basis for justifying the firing of women in times of economic crisis). It is also disturbing that in most instances, when society suggests that a certain activity should be done for altruism, rather than money, it is generally a woman's activity.

Some people suggest that since there is a ban on payment for organs, there should be a ban on payment to a surrogate.[42] But the payment for organs is different from the payment to a surrogate, when viewed from either the side of the couple or the side of the surrogate. As the New Jersey Supreme Court has stated, surrogacy (unlike organ donation) implicates a fundamental constitutional right—the right to privacy in making procreative decisions.[43] The court erroneously assumed that the constitutional right did not extend to commercial applications. This is in conflict with the holdings of other right-to-privacy cases regarding reproductive decisions. In *Carey v. Population Services*, for example, it was acknowledged that constitutional protection of the use of contraceptives extended to their commercial availability.[44] The Court noted that "in practice, a prohibition against all sales, since more easily and less offensively enforced, might have an even more devastating effect on the freedom to choose contraception" than a ban on their use.[45]

Certainly, feminists would feel their right to an abortion was vitiated if a law were passed prohibiting payment to doctors performing abortions; such a law would erect a major barrier to access to the procedure. Similarly, a ban on payment to surrogates would inhibit the exercise of the right to produce a child with a surrogate. For such reasons, it could easily be argued that the couple's right to pay a surrogate is constitutionally protected (unlike the right to pay a kidney donor).

From the surrogate's standpoint, the situation is different as well. An organ is not meant to be removed from the body; it endangers the life of the donor to live without the organ. In contrast, babies are conceived to leave the body and the life of the surrogate is not endangered by living without the child.[46]

At various legislative hearings, women's groups have virtually begged that women be protected against themselves, against their own decisions. Adria Hillman testified against a New York surrogacy bill on behalf of the New York State Coalition on Women's Legislative Issues. One would think that a women's group would criticize the bill as unduly intruding into women's decisions—it requires a double-check by a court on a contract made by a woman (the surrogate mother) to assure that she gave voluntary, informed consent and does not require oversight of contracts made by men. But the testimony was just the opposite. The bill was criticized as empowering the court to assess whether a surrogacy agreement protects the health and welfare of the potential child, without specifying that the judge should look into the agreement's potential effect on the natural mother.[47] What next? Will women have to go before a court when they are considering having an affair—to have a judge discern whether they will be psychologically harmed by, or later regret, the relationship?

Washington Post writer Jane Leavy has written:

> I have read volumes in defense of Mary Beth, her courage in taking on a lonely battle against the upper classes, the exploited wife of a sanitation man versus the wife of a biochemist, a woman with a 9th grade education versus a pediatrician. It all strikes me as a bit patronizing. Since when do we assume that a 29-year-old mother is incapable of making an adult decision and accepting the consequences of it?[48]

Surrogate mother Donna Regan similarly testified in New York that her will was not overborne in the surrogacy context: "No one came to ask me to be a surrogate mother. I went to them and asked them to allow me to be a surrogate mother.[49]

"I find it extremely insulting that there are people saying that, as a woman, I cannot make an informed choice about a pregnancy that I carry," she continued, pointing out that she, like everyone, "makes other difficult choices in her life."[50]

POTENTIAL HARM TO POTENTIAL CHILDREN

The third line of argument opposes surrogacy because of the potential harm it represents to potential children. Feminists have had a long-standing concern for the welfare of children. But much feminist policy in the area has been based on the idea that mothers (and family) are more appropriate decision-makers about the best interests of children than the government. Feminists have also fought against using traditions, stereotypes, and societal tolerance or intolerance as a driving force for determining what is in a child's best interest. In that respect, it is understandable that feminists rallied to the aid of Mary Beth Whitehead in order to expose and oppose the faulty grounds on which custody was being determined.[51]

However, the opposition to stereotypes being used to determine custody in a best-interests analysis is not a valid argument against surrogacy itself (which is premised not on stereotypes about the child's best interest being used to determine custody, but on a preconception agreement being used to determine custody). And when the larger issue of the advisability of surrogacy itself comes up, feminists risk falling into the trap of using arguments about potential harm to the child that have as faulty a basis as those they oppose in other areas of family law.

For example, one line of argument against surrogacy is that it is like adoption and adoption harms children. However, such an argument is not sufficiently borne out in fact. There is evidence that adopted children do as well as non-adopted children in terms of adjustment and achievement.[52] A family of two biological parents is not necessary to assure the child's well-being.

Surrogacy has also been analogized to baby-selling. Baby-selling is prohibited in our society, in part because children need a secure family life and should not have to worry that they will be sold and wrenched from their existing family. Surrogacy is distinguishable from baby-selling since the resulting child is never in a state of insecurity. From the moment of birth, he or she is under the care of the biological father and his wife, who cannot sell the child. There is thus no psychological stress to that child or to *any other existing child* that he or she may someday be sold. Moreover, no matter how much money is paid through the surrogacy arrangement, the child, upon birth, cannot be treated like a commodity—a car or a television set. Laws against child abuse and neglect come into play.

Paying a biological mother to give her child up for traditional adoption is criticized since the child may go to an "undeserving" stranger, whose mere ability to pay does not signify sufficient merit for rearing a child. In paid surrogacy, by contrast, the child is turned over to the biological father. This biological bond has traditionally been considered to be a sufficient indicator of parental merit.

Another argument about potential harm to the resulting children is that parents will expect more of a surrogate child because of the $10,000 they have spent on her creation. But many couples spend more than that on infertility treatments without evidence that they expect more of the child. A Cesarean section costs twice as much as natural childbirth, yet the parents don't expect twice as much of the children. Certainly, the $10,000 is a modest amount compared to what parents will spend on their child over her lifespan.

Surrogacy has also been opposed because of its potential effect on the surrogate's other children. Traditionally, except in cases of clear abuse, parents have been held to be the best decision-makers about their children's best interests. Applying this to surrogacy, the surrogate (and not society) would be the best judge of whether or not her participation in a surrogacy program will harm her children. Not only are parents thought best able to judge their child's needs, but parents can profoundly influence the effects of surrogacy on the child. Children take their cues about things from the people around them. There is no reason to believe that the other children of the surrogate will necessarily feel threatened by their mother's contractual pregnancy. If the children are told from the beginning that this is the contracting couple's child—not a part of their own family—they will realize that they themselves are not in danger of being relinquished.

Surrogate Donna Regan told her child that "the reason we did this was because they [the contracting couple] wanted a child to love as much as we love him." Regan contrasted her case to the Whitehead case: "In the Mary Beth Whitehead case, the child did not see this as something her mother was doing for someone else, so, of course, the attitude that she got from that was that something was being taken away rather than something being given."[53]

It seems ironic for feminists to embrace the argument that certain activities might inherently lead their children to fear abandonment, and that consequently such activities should be banned. Feminists have fought hard to gain access for women to amniocentesis and late-stage abortions of fetuses with a genetic defect[54]—even in light of similarly anecdotal evidence that when the woman aborts, her *other* children will feel that, they too, might be "sent to heaven" by their mother.[55] Indeed, it could be argued that therapeutic abortion is more devastating to the remaining children than is surrogacy. After all, the brother or sister who is aborted was intended to be part of the family; moreover, he or she is dead, not just living with other people. I personally do not feel that the potential effect of either therapeutic abortion or surrogacy on the pregnant woman's other children is a sufficient reason to ban the procedures, particularly in light of the fact that parents can mediate how their children perceive and handle the experiences.

The reactions of outsiders to surrogacy may, however, be beyond the control of parents and may upset the children. But is this a sufficient reason to ban surrogacy? William Pierce seems to think so. He says that the children of surrogates "are being made fun of. Their lives are going to be ruined."[56] It would seem odd to let societal intolerance guide what relationships are permissible. Along those lines, a judge in a lesbian custody case replied to the argument that children could be harmed by stigma by stating:

> It is just as reasonable to expect that they will emerge better equipped to search out their own standards of right and wrong, better able to perceive that the majority is not always correct in its moral judgments, and better able to understand the importance of conforming their beliefs to the requirements of reasons and tested knowledge, not the constraints of currently popular sentiment or prejudice.[57]

FEMINISM REVISITED

Feminists are taking great pride that they have mobilized public debate against surrogacy. But the precedent they are setting in their alliance with politicians like Henry Hyde and groups like the Catholic church is one whose policy is "protect women, even against their own decisions" and "protect children at all costs" (presumably, in latter applications, even against the needs and desires of women). This is certainly the thrust of the New Jersey Supreme Court decision against surrogacy, which cites as support for its holding the notorious *In re A. C.* case. In that case a woman's decision to refuse a Cesarean section was overridden based on an unsubstantiated possibility of benefit to her future child.[58]

In fact, the tenor of the New Jersey Supreme Court decision is reminiscent of earlier decisions "protecting" women that have been roundly criticized by feminists. The U.S. Supreme Court in 1872 felt it was necessary to prevent Myra Bradwell and all other women from practicing law—in order to protect women and their children. And when courts upheld sexist employment laws that kept women out of employment that men were allowed to take, they used language that might have come right out of the New Jersey Supreme Court's decision in the Baby M case. A woman's

> physical structure and a proper discharge of her maternal functions—having in view not merely her health, but the well-being of the race—justify legislation to protect her from the greed as well as the passion of

man. The limitations which this statute place upon her contractual powers, upon her right to agree with her employer as to the time she shall
labor, are not imposed solely for her benefit, but also largely for the benefit
of all.[59]

The New Jersey Supreme Court rightly pointed out that not everything
should be for sale in our society. But the examples given by the court, such
as occupational safety and health laws prohibiting workers from voluntarily
accepting money to work in an unsafe job, apply to both men and women.
In addition, an unsafe job presents risks that we would not want people
to undertake, whether or not they received pay. In contrast, a policy against
paid surrogacy prevents women from taking risks (pregnancy and relinquishment) that they are allowed to take for free. It applies disparately—
men are still allowed to relinquish their parental rights in advance of conception and to receive money for their role in providing the missing male
factor for procreation.

Some feminists are comfortable with advocating disparate treatment on
the grounds that gestation is such a unique experience that it has no male
counterpart at law and so deserves a unique legal status.[60] The special
nature of gestation, according to this argument, gives rise to special rights—
such as the right for the surrogate to change her mind and assert her legal
parenthood after the child is born.

The other side of the gestational coin, which has not been sufficiently
addressed by these feminists, is that with special rights come special responsibilities. If gestation can be viewed as unique in surrogacy, then it
can be viewed as unique in other areas. Pregnant women could be held to
have responsibilities that other members of society do not have—such as
the responsibility to have a Cesarean section against their wishes in order
to protect the health of a child (since only pregnant women are in the
unique position of being able to influence the health of the child).

Some feminists have criticized surrogacy as turning participating women,
albeit with their consent, into reproductive vessels. I see the danger of the
anti-surrogacy arguments as potentially turning *all* women into reproductive vessels, without their consent, by providing government oversight for
women's decisions and creating a disparate legal category for gestation.
Moreover, by breathing life into arguments that feminists have put to rest
in other contexts, the current rationales opposing surrogacy could undermine a larger feminist agenda.

REFERENCES

1. Iver Peterson, "Baby M Custody Trial Splits Ranks of Feminists over Issue
of Exploitation," *New York Times*, Feb. 24, 1987 (quoting Linda Bowker).

2. Bob Port, "Feminists Come to the Aid of Whitehead's Case," *St. Petersburg Times*, Feb. 23, 1987, 1A.

3. Brief filed on behalf of Amici Curiae, the Foundation on Economic Trends et al., In the matter of Baby M, New Jersey Supreme Court, Docket No. FM-25314–86E (hereafter cited as "Brief"). (The feminists joining in the brief included Betty Friedan, Gloria Steinem, Gena Corea, Barbara Katz Rothman, Lois Gould, Michelle Harrison, Kathleen Lahey, Phyllis Chesler, and Letty Cottin Pogrebin.)

4. See, e.g., Roe v. Wade, 410 U.S. 113 (1973); Griswold v. Connecticut, 381 U.S. 479 (1965); Meyer v. Nebraska, 262 U.S. 390 (1923); Pierce v. Society of Sisters, 268 U.S. 510 (1928).

5. See, e.g., Karst, "The Freedom of Intimate Association," *Yale Law Journal*, 89 (1980): 624.

6. Prior to conception and during pregnancy, the surrogate mother contract is a personal service contract. However, after the child's birth, no further services on the part of the surrogate are needed. Thus, enforcing a provision providing for the father's custody of the child is not the enforcement of a personal services contract. It is like the enforcement of a court order on custody or the application of a paternity statute.

7. Lori Andrews, "The Aftermath of Baby M: Proposed State Laws on Surrogate Motherhood," *Hastings Center Report*, 17 (Oct./Nov. 1987): 31–40, at 37.

8. In re Baby M, 217 N.J. Super. 313, 525 A.2d 1128, 1159 (1987).

9. Jhordan C. v. Mary K., 179 Cal. App. 3d 386, 224 Cal. Rptr. 530 (1986).

10. *Surrogate Parenthood and New Reproductive Technologies, A Joint Public Hearing, before the N.Y. State Assembly, N.Y. State Senate, Judiciary Committees* (Oct. 16, 1986) (statement of Bob Arenstein at 103–4, 125); *In The Matter of a Hearing on Surrogate Parenting before the N.Y. Standing Committee on Child Care* (May 8, 1987) (statement of Adria Hillman at 174, statement of Mary Ann Dibari at 212 ["the prostitution of motherhood"]).

11. *Surrogacy Arrangements Act of 1987: Hearing on H. R. 2433, before the Subcomm. on Transportation, Tourism, and Hazardous Materials*, 100th Cong., 1st Sess. (Oct. 15, 1987) (statement of Gena Corea at 3, 5); Robert Gould, N.Y. Testimony (May 8, 1987), supra note 10, at 233 (slavery).

12. Arthur Morrell, U.S. Testimony (Oct. 15, 1987), supra note 11, at 1.

13. William Pierce, U.S. Testimony (Oct. 15, 1987), supra note 11, at 2, citing Harvard Law Professor Lawrence Tribe.

14. Brief, supra note 3, at 19.

15. Port, supra note 2, at 7A, quoting Phyllis Chesler.

16. Gena Corea, U.S. Testimony (Oct. 15, 1987), supra note 11, at 3; Hillman, N.Y. Testimony (May 8, 1987), supra note 10, at 174.

17. Ellen Goodman, "Checking the Baby M Contract," *Boston Globe*, March 24, 1987, 15.

18. Gena Corea, U.S. Testimony (Oct. 15, 1987), supra note 11, at 5; Hillman, N.Y. Testimony (May 8, 1987) supra note 10, at 174.

19. Gena Corea, U.S. Testimony (Oct. 15, 1987), supra note 11, at 5.

20. Id.

21. Id.: 2.

22. Elizabeth Kane, U.S. Testimony (Oct. 15, 1987), supra note 11, at 1.

23. Kay Longcope, "Standing up for Mary Beth," *Boston Globe*, March 5, 1987, 81, 83 (quoting Janice Raymond).

24. Brief, supra note 3, at 14.

25. Robert Gould, N.Y. Testimony (May 8, 1987), supra note 10, at 232.

26. Judianne Densen-Gerber, N.Y. Testimony (May 8, 1987), supra note 10, at 253; Robert Gould, N.Y. Testimony (May 8, 1987), supra note 10, at 232.

27. Robert Gould, N.Y. Testimony (May 8, 1987), supra note 10, at 232.

28. Henry Hyde, U.S. Testimony (Oct. 15, 1987), supra note 11, at 1 ("Commercial surrogacy arrangements, by rendering children into chattel, are in my opinion, immoral."); DiBari, N.Y. Testimony (May 8, 1987), supra note 10, at 212.

29. John Ray, U.S. Testimony (Oct. 15, 1987), supra note 11, at 7.

30. See, e.g., Maureen McGuire and Nancy J. Alexander, "Artificial Insemination of Single Women," *Fertility and Sterility*, 43 (Feb. 1985): 182–84; Raschke and Raschke, "Family Conflict and Children's Self-Concept: A Comparison of Intact and Single Parent Families," *Journal of Marriage and the Family*, 41 (1979): 367; Weiss, "Growing up a Little Faster," *Journal of Social Issues*, 35 (1979): 97.

31. See, e.g., Rynearson, "Relinquishment and Its Maternal Complications: A Preliminary Study," *American Journal of Psychiatry*, 139 (1982): 338; Deykin, Campbell, Patti, "The Postadoption Experience of Surrendering Parents," *American Journal of Orthopsychiatry*, 54 (1984): 271.

32. Betsy Aigen, N.Y. Testimony (May 8, 1987), supra note 10, at 18.

33. Robert Arenstein, U.S. Testimony (Oct. 15, 1987), supra note 11, at 9.

34. Brief, supra note 3, at 30–31.

35. In re Baby M, 109 N.J. 396; 537 A.2d 1227, 1248 (1988).

36. See Brief filed on behalf of Amicus Curiae the Gruter Institute, In the Matter of Baby M, New Jersey Supreme Court, Docket No. FM-25314–86E.

37. *Hearing in re Surrogate Parenting: Hearing on S. B. 1429, before Senators Goodhue, Dunne, Misters Balboni, Abramson, and Amgott* (April 10, 1987) (statement of Elaine Rosenfeld at 187). A similar argument made by Adria Hillman, N.Y. Testimony (May 8, 1987), supra note 10, at 175.

38. Joan Einwohner, N.Y. Testimony (April 10, 1987), supra note 37, at 110–11.

39. Gena Corea, *The Mother Machine* (New York: Harper & Row, 1985), 3.

40. Brief, supra note 3, at 10, 13; Judy Breidbart, N.Y. Testimony (May 8, 1987), supra note 10, at 168.

41. K. Cotton and D. Winn, *Baby Cotton: For Love and Money* (1985).

42. Karen Peters, N.Y. Testimony (May 8, 1987), supra note 10, at 121.

43. In re Baby M, 109 N.J. 396; 537 A.2d 1227, 1253 (1988).

44. Carey v. Population Services Int'l., 431 U.S. 678 (1977).

45. Carey v. Population Services, Int'l., 431 U.S. 678, 688 (1976) (citation omitted).

46. Betsy Aigen, N.Y. Testimony (May 8, 1987), supra note 10, at 11–12.

47. Adria Hillman, N.Y. Testimony (May 8, 1987), supra note 10, at 177–78.

48. Jane Leavy, "It Doesn't Take Labor Pains to Make a Real Mom," *Washington Post*, April 4, 1987.

49. Donna Regan, N.Y. Testimony (May 8, 1987), supra note 10, at 157.

50. Id.

51. Michelle Harrison, "Social Construction of Mary Beth Whitehead," *Gender and Society*, 1 (Sept. 1987): 300–311.

52. Teasdale and Owens, "Influence of Paternal Social Class on Intelligence Level in Male Adoptees and Non-Adoptees," *British Journal of Educational Psychology*, 56 (1986): 3.

53. Donna Regan, N.Y. Testimony (May 8 1987), supra note 10, at 156.

54. See, e.g., the briefs filed by feminist organizations in Thornburgh v. American College of Obstetricians, 476 U.S. 747 (1986).

55. See, e.g., J. Fletcher, *Coping with Genetic Disorders: A Guide for Counseling* (San Francisco: Harper & Row, 1982).

56. William Pierce, N.Y. Testimony (May 8, 1987), supra note 10, at 86. It should be pointed out that kids hassle other kids for a wide range of reasons. A child might equally be made fun of for being the recipient of a kidney transplant or being the child of a garbage man.

57. M. P. v. S. P., 169 N.J. Super. 425, 438, 404 A.2d 1256, 1263 (Super. Ct. App. Div. 1979).

58. In re Baby M, 109 N.J. 396; 537 A.2d 1227, 1254 n. 13 (1988), citing In re A. C., 533 A.2d 611 (D.C. App. 1987).

59. Muller v. Oregon, 208 U.S. 412, 422 (1907).

60. See Brief, supra note 3, at 11.

An Essay on Surrogacy and Feminist Thought

Joan Mahoney

Surrogacy is not an easy issue for feminists.[1] On one hand, it raises concerns about exploitation; one is faced with images of poor women being enlisted to produce babies for wealthy men and their wives, either because of fertility problems or because pregnancy is simply too inconvenient for those women who can afford to hire someone to do it for them. On the other hand, there is the specter of the state passing laws, once again, that tell women what they can and cannot do with their bodies. If we believe, as many of us do, that the state has no right to prohibit a woman from selling the sexual use of her body, doesn't she also have the right to sell the reproductive use? And if many of us, doctors, lawyers, law professors, have been willing to employ other women, less privileged women, to take care of our children after they are born, what is so different in moving the date back a bit and hiring them to carry our children *before* birth as well?

Assuming that surrogacy is not legally prohibited, does that mean that surrogacy contracts must be enforced? If we find something abhorrent in the idea of babies being taken from their mothers' arms because, after all, a contract is a contract,[2] we might argue that the contracts can be legal but unenforceable. But then we are accused of being patronizing, paternalistic. Can we protect women who enter into these contracts and then change their minds from losing their babies only at the cost of having women described as irrational, emotional, not to be trusted?

If surrogacy is permitted but not enforced and the agreement breaks down, the bottom line question, of course, is: Who gets the baby? It is not an easy question to answer in the context of divorce, when the baby is probably not a newborn, when there is a family history and tradition and one can determine which parent has been primary caretaker or the "psychological parent." But when the baby is just born and the father has never lived with the mother, has perhaps never even *met* the mother of the baby, how do we decide who gets the baby? If it is the mother—because she is the one who has been relating to the child for nine months, she has done all the caring for it, at risk to her health and even risk to her life—are we not perpetuating the stereotype of women as nurturers? And, if so, is that such a bad stereotype?

Those are a few of the questions that arise and the dilemmas that face a feminist trying to come to terms with surrogacy. This essay is an attempt to lay out some of the issues raised by surrogacy and some of the answers feminist jurisprudence might suggest to them, including those areas in which theories of feminist jurisprudence are likely to produce different answers. Although surrogacy agreements have probably existed informally for any number of years (at least since Hagar bore Ishmael for Isaac), and commercial surrogacy has gone on in this country since 1976,[3] it has only recently attracted significant attention, perhaps because of the Baby M case[4] and all its attendant publicity.

PROHIBITION OF SURROGACY CONTRACTS

The threshold question regarding surrogacy is: Should such agreements be permitted or not? If, as many feminists believe, surrogacy exploits women—particularly women with limited education and earning ability (based on the going rate of $10,000, and given that pregnancy lasts twenty-four hours per day for roughly nine months, the rate of pay is just over $1.54 per hour)—would it be in their interests to have the agreements prohibited by the state?

If prohibition by the state means the imposition of criminal penalties on those who enter into the agreements, it would be hard to muster a feminist argument in support of such legislation. The purpose of protecting women from exploitation is not likely to be furthered by jailing them for participating in an exploitive relationship. It makes as much sense as it does to put prostitutes in jail.

On the other hand, if the prohibition simply meant that surrogacy contracts would be void as against public policy, or that adoptions by the father's spouse would not be permitted if it was shown that money, other than to reimburse the gestational mother for her costs, had changed hands,[5] the legislation would be less offensive on its face. Such laws do, however, raise interesting issues. They certainly appear to restrict women in ways that men are not. Men, after all, are free to donate sperm or, to be more precise, to sell sperm, while women would be prohibited by the application of these laws from selling their full reproductive capability, although they would presumably remain free to sell their genetic material just as men do.

One could also argue that laws restricting commercial surrogacy contracts discriminate against men rather than women. Women with infertile husbands may pay sperm banks for sperm and then be artificially inseminated; men with infertile wives are prohibited from paying fertile women to carry their children for them. Under the doctrine generally applied by the Supreme Court in sex discrimination cases, it is irrelevant whether it is men or women who are suffering from the discrimination. So long as a statute is distinguishing on the basis of sex without a sufficient showing by the state of a rationale for the distinction, it will be struck down.[6]

If such statutes were framed as prohibiting babyselling rather than as protecting women, and if they applied to prevent both men and women from entering into surrogacy contracts, they would be less likely to be viewed as discriminatory. The argument that surrogacy is a form of baby-selling derives both from constitutional concerns,[7] and from the parallel to adoption. Some authors have argued that surrogacy is unlike adoption in that the contract is written before the child is conceived; the pregnant woman is not agreeing to give up her child while under the stress of an unwanted pregnancy.[8] Using that logic, it should also be legal for a couple in which, for example, both parties are infertile, to contract with a woman to become pregnant by an anonymous sperm donor on the assumption that the couple would adopt the resulting baby. This would certainly appear to violate state prohibitions on payment for adoptions. The only difference in the surrogacy context is that the baby the woman is carrying is genetically related to one of the prospective parents. Either of these situations would seem to result in the "commodification" of babies.[9]

Even if laws prohibiting surrogacy were seen as gender-neutral, and therefore not discriminatory, it could be argued that they violate both the woman's right to control her reproductive capabilities[10] and the man's right to procreate.[11] It has been held that reproductive rights are not absolute and that there are state interests sufficient to limit them.[12] A state interest in preventing the sale of babies might be held to be sufficiently strong to overcome the interests of the parents. Furthermore, it is arguable that reproductive freedom does not necessarily encompass the right to *sell* one's reproductive capabilities. One is free to donate organs but generally not free to sell them,[13] and the adoption laws mentioned above would clearly prohibit a woman from choosing to carry an unwanted baby to term and then receiving a substantial payment for the child once it is born.

In a recent article, Sylvia Law develops an approach to feminist jurisprudence that supports sex-based equality while taking into account biological differences.[14] Prof. Law rejects the assimilationist view—that sex, like race and eye color, does not describe a difference that ought to have any legal significance.[15] She also rejects the respect-for-difference theory—that there are a variety of social and psychological as well as physical differences between men and women that ought to be recognized in a positive way in the law. She views this approach as overbroad and perhaps tending to perpetuate socially created differences.[16] Instead, Prof. Law would take into account only biological and immutable characteristics, or those that will be immutable until we create some form of reproduction that does not require a uterus. As to laws governing reproductive biology, she would ask whether the state can meet the burden of showing either that the law "has no significant impact in perpetuating the oppression of women or culturally imposed sex role constraints on individual freedom" or that it is "the best means for meeting a compelling state purpose."[17]

If we see laws banning surrogacy as a control on reproductive biology, the question would be: Do such laws perpetuate the oppression of women? An attempt to ban surrogacy would be based primarily on the protection of children and secondarily on avoiding the exploitation of women by encouraging society to view them as manufacturers of children. Such a prohibition could hardly be seen as perpetuating the oppression of women, except insofar as it denies women the choice to sell, but not give away, their reproductive capabilities.

ENFORCEABILITY OF SURROGACY CONTRACTS

If a state does choose to allow surrogacy contracts, it would have to decide whether to make the contracts enforceable against a woman who changed her mind. Surrogacy contracts usually contain very detailed provisions regarding the health of the gestational mother and her activities and medical care during pregnancy.[18] If the woman decides, for example, not to have amniocentesis, could the father require her to undergo the procedure? Could he require her to have an abortion, if the baby has a genetic defect? If she decides not to continue the pregnancy, can she be prohibited from having an abortion?

It seems fairly clear, based on the line of cases starting with *Roe*,[19] that an order requiring a woman to have or not have an abortion, based on a contract entered into before the pregnancy began, would not be enforceable. If a husband cannot force a woman to continue a pregnancy against her will,[20] it is most unlikely that a court would allow the contractual father to do so. It is not necessary to delve into feminist theory at any depth to arrive at the conclusion that feminists are unlikely to support the enforcement of contracts that deprive women of control over their own bodies.

Some people might argue that the refusal to enforce the contract is paternalistic and prohibits women from choosing to enter into enforceable contracts. This idea will be discussed at some length below regarding the promise to terminate parental rights. In the area of abortion and bodily integrity, I find that line of reasoning particularly unpersuasive. Imagine, for example, that a famous doctor advertised for male volunteers to be subjects in her study (a study she was sure would win her the Nobel Prize). The men were to stay in bed for several months eating only the foods prescribed by the doctor, after which she was to perform open-heart surgery. If a man signed up for the study, stayed in bed, ate the foods, and then, at the last minute, announced that he could not possibly have the surgery, no court in the country would order him to go through with it, contract or no contract. Would a court make him pay back the value of the food he had eaten or the room he had occupied? If his attorney argued that to do so would violate his constitutional right to bodily integrity by, in essence, forcing him to go through with the operation or pay damages, perhaps the court would agree that such a contract was simply unenforceable.

The argument, then, is that no one has the power to sell his or her right to bodily integrity, that the choice of having an abortion or not is not commodifiable.[21] In that case, the decision to allow a woman to rescind the contract prior to the birth of the child without being liable for specific performance or damages is not patronizing, nor is it a way of preferring women. Rather, it is a sex-neutral measure based on fundamental values of our society.

In a sense, the questions raised about abortion and bodily integrity are easy to resolve from a feminist perspective. Other than the argument that the refusal of the state to enforce the promise is patronizing, there is almost no case that can be made for the enforceability of such agreements. The prospect of women being forced to undergo medical procedures against their will is truly horrifying, especially when conflicts arise between the health of the woman and the baby. If the state were to find these provisions enforceable, would the father be able to require the gestational mother to have a Cesarean section if the doctor advised it? Could he require her to continue the pregnancy if her health were threatened—by a sudden increase in her blood pressure, for example? It is strange to envision a situation where the father of a child would have more power because of a contract than does a non-contractual father whose baby is being carried by his wife.

The more difficult question has to do with the enforceability of the promise to give up the child to the father and his wife, if he has one, and to terminate parental rights so that the father's wife may adopt the baby. Some people contend that the refusal of the state to enforce such agreements, whether by a statute declaring them void as against public policy or by a judicial refusal to order specific enforcement, is paternalistic and patronizing.[22] Their position is that women are being denied the right to enter into contracts in order to protect them from making contracts they might later regret.

Some feminists object to any legislation that provides special benefits for women.[23] Wendy Williams, for example, takes what is referred to as the "equal treatment" position, that women should reject laws that appear to be for their benefit as well as those that apparently discriminate. She argues that the same doctrinal approach that permits pregnancy to be treated *worse* than other disabilities is the same one that will allow the state constitutional freedom to create special *benefits* for pregnant women. . . . If we can't have it both ways, we need to think carefully about which way we want to have it.[24]

The question, then, for the equal treatment feminists is whether the refusal of the state to specifically enforce surrogacy contracts is the kind of special treatment to which they should object. The answer may depend on whether the refusal was based on the assumption that *women* ought not to be bound by such agreements or on the better rationale that *no one* ought to be permitted to waive constitutional rights in the future. For example, I could go down to the local police station today and inform the staff that if I am ever arrested, they need not give me my Miranda warnings. Nonetheless, I could, in fact, withdraw that consent at any time I chose, even if I had accepted money for the waiver of my rights.[25] If the argument is simply that advance waiver of rights ought not to be permitted, the application of such a rule in the surrogacy context does not violate the principle of equal treatment.

Men, however, are routinely expected to waive any parental rights to a resulting child at the time that they donate sperm.[26] If men can waive parental rights before a child is conceived and women cannot, isn't that establishing a gender-based distinction after all? The answer, I think, is that women can also waive their parental rights in advance when they donate genetic material. It makes perfect sense (and establishes a nice analogy to the sperm donation situation) to allow, and even require, egg donors, at the time that the eggs are "harvested," to waive their rights and obligations as to any children created from their eggs. Gestating, however, is different from donating eggs or sperm. The *activity* itself is not over until the baby is born, whereas the activity of donating genetic material is completed before the baby is conceived. Sperm or egg donors do not waive their rights in advance, but at the time that they perform the acts necessary for the donation, while the gestational mother does not *begin* performing her share of the required process until conception.

The primary alternative approach to feminist jurisprudence takes the opposite position in the special treatment/equal treatment debate. It would look not to whether a particular rule or practice treated women differently from men, but at what effect both the rule and the practice would have on the status of women.[27] Catharine MacKinnon, for example, states that what she calls the "inequality" approach "understands the sexes to be not simply socially differentiated but socially *unequal*. In this broader view, all practices which subordinate women to men are prohibited."[28] Ruth Colker has called this principle the "anti-subordination" approach.[29]

The problem with the anti-subordination approach is in determining which practices encourage and which discourage the subordination of women.[30] It is not always easy. On one hand, since it can be argued that surrogacy exploits women, the anti-subordination approach should support its ban. On the other hand, it can also be argued that a law prohibiting women from doing what they wish with their bodies is also demeaning, and therefore, although surrogacy ought not to be encouraged, it ought not to be prohibited either. Similarly, the enforcement of contracts may be seen as empowering women, in that it allows them to determine their own fate, or as maintaining the hierarchy, in that women are being encouraged to use their bodies to produce children for men.

The view that the refusal to enforce surrogacy contracts is restricting the rights of women to contract compares the laws to those the Supreme Court upheld in *Muller v. Oregon*,[31] which restricted the hours women could work. *Muller* upheld protective legislation for women at a time when protective legislation for men was being struck down.[32] Since the passage of the Fair Labor Standards Act,[33] it has been perfectly clear that the government, federal or state, has the right to pass laws that protect workers from exploitive relationships. The arguments that a prohibition on surrogacy would restrict women's rights to contract sound more like the reasoning of the Court in *Lochner*, upholding the right of bakers to contract to work as many hours as they please. No one currently has the legal right to work for less than the minimum wage, unless the position is exempt from coverage, and no one has a right to contract away protection provided by occupational safety legislation. Only women can bear children, so a refusal to enforce surrogacy contracts protects only women from making bad agreements. But such a provision would be only one of many that restrict the freedom of employees to contract for their own exploitation.

Whether or not the state may ban surrogacy, regulating the lawyers and agencies that set up surrogacy arrangements would not appear to violate the rights of the individuals involved and, in fact, might actually increase their knowledge of and ability to exercise their rights. For example, a requirement that each party to the contract have separate counsel, rather than being represented by the same person (or rather, as is often the case, having an attorney who represents the father and none for the mother), does not perpetuate the oppression of women but may help to diminish it. Such a regulation is also quite obviously even-handed, since it would treat men and women entering the arrangements the same way, and would therefore comport with the equality model as well. Even an absolute prohibition on agencies that arrange surrogacy contracts would not seem to violate the rights of the parties, so long as, for example, couples seeking surrogates could advertise or women seeking to act as surrogates could do the same. Presumably, any regulation that was framed in a way that implied an inability of women to act for themselves would be offensive to most feminists, but any even-handed regulation for the protection of both parties—or of all the parties, if you include the mates of the biological parents and the baby itself—would be acceptable.

The Determination of Custody

Even if a state bans commercial surrogacy, there will still be informal agreements, and even if commercial surrogacy is allowed but not enforced, there will still be disputes over what to do with the child if the agreement breaks down. An enormous number of questions arise in the custody context. If, for example, the state has a joint custody presumption, would that apply to a surrogacy case? How does one determine the "best interests" of a newborn baby, if that is the standard chosen? Do parental concerns play any role at all in the custody determination? May the surrogacy contract be introduced to demonstrate that the surrogate did not initially want the baby? Or that she is a bad person who breaks her promises? Or to show the father's intent to become a parent? These are very different purposes, and thus different considerations underlie their resolution.

There are other questions regarding custody that are unique to surrogacy. Who is to take the baby if no one wants it? Would either parent be liable for child support if the adoption does not go through and one or the other gets the baby in a custody fight? Should the non-custodial parent get visitation? And does the "step-parent" (the mate of the biological parent who ends up with custody) have any right to the child? For example, what will happen to Baby M if the Sterns get divorced, or if Mr. Stern should die before she reaches adulthood? Normally, a biological parent is presumed to have preference over one related by marriage. Would that be the case here?

What about the situations where the child has both a gestational and a genetic mother? Does it matter if the latter is a donor, in the same sense as an anonymous donor of artificially inseminated sperm, or whether she is the wife of the biological father and has the same intent to raise the child? In the latter case, if the gestational mother chooses not to honor the contract, there are three people who are arguably the child's parents and two who are both the mother. Surely, if a genetic *father* has a claim to the child, so does a genetic mother, but what about a gestational mother who is not a genetic parent? Even where the gestational mother is also the genetic mother, it is not simply the contribution of her egg that creates her interest, because if that were the case, she could waive her rights to the child before birth, just as a sperm donor does. But if we admit that there is something special about gestation, are we saying that there *is* a difference between men and women that the law cannot ignore? That there are ways in which men and women are not and never can be equal?

To begin with the question of custody itself, there are three possible ways to resolve these conflicts. One is to assume that the father should get the baby, not because of the contract but because he wanted it the most from the beginning, having created this agreement for the sole purpose of obtaining a child, while the mother had entered the agreement to produce a child for someone else, only deciding after she became pregnant that she wanted the child. A second possibility is to give the child to the mother, engaging in something like the tender years presumption.[34] The assumption is that women form a bond with the child during gestation and childbirth that a father cannot form.[35] Finally, there is the possibility of leaving the decision up to the courts as in any other custody case, with the determination to be made based on the best interests of the child.

There is actually a fourth possibility. It is to argue that it is impossible to decide what the best interests of a newborn baby are, or that the decision in the surrogacy context is simply too difficult, and that therefore the court should engage in a rebuttable presumption that one parent or the other should get the baby, with a court battle ensuing only where one parent can make a colorable claim that the other is unfit.

The problem with this solution is that one then has to decide *which* of the parents should get the advantage of the rebuttable presumption, leading back to one of the first three possibilities above. That is, whether one decides that the mother should get the baby because newborns are better off with their mothers or because one parent or the other should, as a general rule, get the child and for whatever reason it should be the mother, the results are the same. Similarly, if the decision is made to give the baby to the father to avoid a custody battle or because he should get the benefit of his bargain, he still has the advantage at the time that the agreement breaks down. It is therefore necessary to consider whether the preference for either parent is consistent with feminist theory or whether, unpleasant as the prospect appears, the decision must be left to the courts in each case. And, if the latter, are there underlying considerations that the courts should keep in mind?

It seems clear that if preference is given to the father in any custody fight following a breakdown in a surrogacy agreement, the policy against the enforcement of such agreements is illusory. In other words, it is meaningless to tell a woman that she will not be bound by any promise made to give up her child before birth if in fact the father, unless he is unfit, will get the baby and the agreement will be enforced indirectly.

On the other hand, if the baby is given to the mother, whether because of a straight maternal preference or as a way of avoiding a custody fight, the choice becomes a gender-based distinction. Only women can carry and bear children. In the surrogacy context, the father has done all that he can to facilitate his becoming a father, at least in a situation where he is not married to or living with the mother and cannot provide care and support (other than financial) during the pregnancy.

One would expect that feminists who adhere to the equality model would be forced to reject this proposal, consistent with their position on the *CalFed* case[36] that women should be treated equally, rather than either discriminated for or against because of their ability to, among other things, bear children.[37] The argument against *Geduldig v. Aiello*[38] and *General Electric Co. v. Gilbert*[39] is not that women should get an advantage where men do not, but that women ought not to be discriminated against, or the disabilities suffered by women ought not to be discriminated against, where those suffered by men are covered. The purpose of the equal treatment approach is to "get the law out of the business of reinforcing traditional, sex-based family roles."[40] A maternal preference in surrogacy cases is based on a traditional conception of male and female roles within the family and would pretty clearly result in the perpetuation of those roles.

If one approaches the custody question from the anti-subordination perspective rather than the equality model, a rule of maternal preference in custody cases is less clearly objectionable. Certainly the anti-subordination principle does not rule out discrimination against men, since they are not a historically discriminated-against group.[41] This, then, is the point at which the difference between the two models of feminist jurisprudence becomes significant in the surrogacy context. The anti-subordination feminists would not ask whether the rule treats men and women equally but "whether the policy or practice in question integrally contributes to the maintenance of an underclass or a deprived position because of gender status."[42]

An argument could certainly be made that giving custody to women in surrogacy cases does nothing to advance the cause of women's rights and may, in fact, retard it. It is possible that some feminists who adhere to the anti-subordination model would reject a maternal custody preference on the grounds that it continues the stereotype of women as nurturers, while others would argue that it is reasonable and fair to give a preference based on women's unique capacity to bear children and thus form a bond even before the birth.

If the issue of custody *is* to be left up to the courts, some effort must be made to structure a way to make the determination. Until the eighteenth century, fathers had an absolute right to the custody of their legitimate minor children.[43] Children, like wives, were treated as chattels that belonged to the husband. Although there were cases before the middle of the eighteenth century in which the father was denied custody, those were extraordinary occurrences.[44] The tender years doctrine, in which custody of young children is presumed to go to the mother, was enacted by statute in Britain in 1839 and by either statute or caselaw in the United States during the nineteenth century.[45]

The tender-years doctrine served as a presumption that children would be better off with their mothers, but it could be rebutted by sufficient showing of maternal unfitness. In any event, it served as a way of defining the best interests of the child. In recent years, there has been a move away from the presumption of maternal custody towards a gender-neutral best interests test.[46] Some states provide a list of factors to be taken into account in determining best interests,[47] while others look to see which parent has been the primary caretaker or psychological parent.[48] Obviously the latter test is inapposite when the custody of a newborn is being determined, unless we count gestation as caregiving—in which case we are back to a maternal preference.

If custody battles arising out of surrogacy contracts were to be treated no differently from those between other natural parents, a determination would still have to be made whether to treat the fathers like ex-husbands or like unwed fathers.[49] If the fathers in surrogacy cases were treated like other unwed fathers, they would apparently stand very little chance of obtaining custody, or even of preventing the termination of their parental rights.

In *Stanley v. Illinois*,[50] the Supreme Court rejected the action of Illinois in terminating Stanley's right to his children. He had lived with the childrens' mother for eighteen years prior to her death, although they were not married. Following her death the children were declared wards of the state and Stanley was denied a hearing on his fitness as a parent. The Court held that the denial deprived Stanley of both due process and equal protection. In *Quilloin v. Walcott*,[51] however, an unmarried father who had not attempted to legitimate the child was denied any opportunity to prevent the adoption of the child by the mother's husband. The next year, in *Caban v. Mohammed*,[52] the rights of the unwed father were again upheld, as against a New York law that permitted adoption without his consent, although in this case, like *Stanley*, the father had lived with the mother for several years.

Relying on *Stanley* and *Caban*, the father in *Lehr v. Robertson*[53] argued that he had an absolute right to notice and the opportunity to be heard before his daughter was adopted. Although he had lived with the child's mother before the child was born and had visited her in the hospital, the parents had not lived together after the birth and Lehr had not paid support. As the dissent, by Justice White, points out, the mother had concealed her whereabouts from Lehr after she left the hospital, and he had continuously tried to find them until the time the adoption petition was filed.[54] The majority rejected Lehr's due process argument, stating:

> The significance of the biological connection is that it offers the natural father an opportunity that no other male possesses to develop a relationship with his offspring. If he grasps that opportunity and accepts some measure of responsibility for the child's future, he may enjoy the blessings of the parent-child relationship and make uniquely valuable contributions to the child's development. If he fails to do so, the Federal Constitution

will not automatically compel a State to listen to his opinion of where the child's best interests lie.[55]

In this case, Lehr claimed that he had done everything he could to make contact with his child and establish a parental relationship. The majority seems to be saying, therefore, that the extent of protection available to fathers depends on the access to the child allowed by the mother. If that is the case in surrogacy as well, the mother could effectively prevent the father from ever obtaining custody simply by not allowing him to approach the baby after its birth and by not accepting support for the child.

The unwed-father line of cases seems to offer women a power they have not had before: if they choose to raise a child by themselves or with the help of a partner who is not the child's father, they can exclude the child's father from any role at all. Perhaps it is foolish to look the proverbial gift horse in its proverbial mouth, but that offer of power makes me, and I assume other feminists, very nervous. If mothering is more important than fathering (or parenting), then maybe it is too important to society to justify the provision of day care centers, or to allow parental leaves so that fathers can have the option of staying home with small children (and mothers can have the option of going back to work). It seems to me that in *Lehr* the Court is perpetuating the stereotype of women as nurturers that has so often been used to justify the subordination of women. If in this instance the stereotype gives women power instead of diminishing it, that doesn't make the stereotype any less offensive or dangerous.

The image of the police snatching Mary Beth Whitehead's baby from her arms[56] is not a pleasant one. Neither, however, is the image of all the women left to rear their children alone because raising babies is, after all, women's work. As Wendy Williams puts it, we can't have it both ways.[57] We had better think very hard about whether we want to pay the price that a preference in custody, even if limited to the surrogacy context, would cost.

CONCLUSION

It seems clear that feminist thought raises more questions than it answers about surrogacy agreements. This essay has attempted to pose some of the questions and present ways in which feminists might provide answers to them. I have tried to go through each of the stages in the creation and enforcement of a surrogacy contract to look at the relationship between the parties, and between the parties and the state, at each. While I feel that feminists are likely to agree on the resolution of certain issues, such as the enforceability of promises to forgo abortion, others are more problematic, and I have tried to show the way different schools of feminist jurisprudence might approach their resolution. The whole idea of women producing babies for money makes me profoundly uneasy, although I am afraid my uneasiness will not make the whole situation go away. Feminists must give the matter some thought, whether or not thinking about it makes us uneasy and whether or not we are dismayed by the absence of easy answers. Surrogacy will be permitted or prohibited depending on what state courts and legislatures decide to do about it, and the time to make our voices heard is while the process of decision-making is going on.

REFERENCES

Many of the ideas that went into this essay were thought out while I was serving on an American Civil Liberties Union committee drafting policy on the surrogacy issue. I would like to thank the other members of the committee—Larry Gostin, Wendy Williams, Susan Wolf, and Leslie Harris—for their helpful contributions.

1. See, e.g., Hubbard, "A Birthmother Is a Birthmother Is a . . . ," *Sojourner: The Women's Forum*, 71 (Sept. 1987); Pollitt, "The Strange Case of Baby M," *The Nation* (May 23, 1987); Levine, "Motherhood Is Powerless," *Village Voice* (April 14, 1987): 15.

2. In the Matter of Baby M, 217 N.J. Super. 313 (1987), rev'd in part,—A.2d—, 1988 WL 6251 (N.J.).

3. N. Keane and D. Breo, *The Surrogate Mother* (1981), 33.

4. In the Matter of Baby M,—A.2d—, 1988 WL 6251 (N.J.), overruling in part 217 N.J. Super. 313 (1987).

5. See, e.g., Ky. Rev. Stat. §199.590(2) (Baldwin 1982); Mich. Comp. Laws Ann. §710.69 (Supp. 1974).

6. See, e.g., Mississippi University for Women v. Hogan, 458 U.S. 718 (1982) (striking down a state statute that excluded men from enrolling in a state-supported nursing school); Orr v. Orr, 440 U.S. 268 (1979) (holding unconstitutional a state law that imposed alimony obligations on men but not women); and Craig v. Boren, 429 U.S. 190 (1976) (striking down a state law that set a lower drinking age for females than males). But see, Rostker v. Goldberg, 453 U.S. 57 (1981) (upholding the military registration of males but not females) and Michael M. v. Superior Court, 450 U.S. 464 (1981) (upholding California's statutory rape law, which made it a crime for men to have sexual intercourse with an underage woman but did not impose a similar penalty on women).

7. Both the Thirteenth Amendment prohibition on slavery and, by implication, on the sale of persons as chattels, and the Fourteenth Amendment protection of liberty are implicated by these concerns.

8. See, e.g., Coleman, "Surrogate Motherhood: Analysis of the Problems and Suggestions for Solutions," *Tennessee Law Review*, 50 (1982): 71, 109–10; Black, "Legal Problems of Surrogate Motherhood," *New England Law Review*, 16 (1981): 373, 381–83.

9. See Radin, "Market-Inalienability," *Harvard Law Review*, 100: 1849, 1925–30.

10. See, Akron v. Akron Center for Reproductive Health, 462 U.S. 416 (1983) (striking down restrictions on availability of abortion); Roe v. Wade, 410 U.S. 113 (1973) (holding that women have a privacy right that encompasses the abortion decision); Griswold v. Connecticut, 381 U.S. 479 (1965) (striking down state laws criminalizing the use of contraceptives).

11. See, Skinner v. Oklahoma, 316 U.S. 535 (1942) (holding invalid a state law providing for compulsory sterilization of criminals).

12. See, Planned Parenthood Association of Kansas City v. Ashcroft, 462 U.S. 476 (1983) (upholding requirement of a second physician in post-viability abortions and a pathologist's report for all abortions, while striking down a requirement that all abortions after twelve weeks be performed in a hospital); Roe v. Wade, 410 U.S. 113 (1973) (holding that the right to abortion was not unqualified and the state's interest increased in each trimester of the pregnancy).

13. California permits the sale of organs but prohibits brokering. Cal. Penal Code §367f(e) (West 1986).

14. Law, "Rethinking Sex and the Constitution," *University of Pennsylvania Law Review*, 132 (1984): 955.

15. Id.: 963–66.

16. Id.: 966–68. As will be discussed below, Catharine MacKinnon's approach to feminist jurisprudence comes closest to what Prof. Law calls the respect-for-difference theory.

17. Id.: 1016–17.

18. See, e.g., the contract in the Baby M case, In the Matter of Baby M,—A.2d—, 1988 WL 6251 (N.J.) Appendix A.

19. See, e.g., Akron v. Akron Center for Reproductive Health, 462 U.S. 416 (1983); Roe v. Wade, 410 U.S. 113 (1973).

20. Planned Parenthood of Missouri v. Danforth, 428 U.S. 52 (1976) (striking down state statute requirement for spousal consent).

21. Radin, supra note 9, at 1934.

22. See "Rumpelstiltskin Revisited: The Inalienable Rights of Surrogate Mothers," *Harvard Law Review*, 99 (1986): 1936, 1942–46.

23. See, e.g., Williams, "Equality's Riddle: Pregnancy and the Equal Treatment/Special Treatment Debate," *N.Y.U. Review of Law and Social Change*, 13 (1984–85): 325 (hereinafter cited as Williams, "Equality's Riddle"); Williams, "The Equality Crisis: Some Reflections on Culture, Courts and Feminism," *Women's Rights Law Reporter*, 7 (1982): 175 (hereinafter cited as Williams, "The Equality Crisis"); Taub, Book Review, *Columbia Law Review*, 80 (1980): 1686.

24. Williams, "The Equality Crisis," supra note 23, at 196.

25. See "Rumpelstiltskin Revisited," supra note 22, for a discussion of alienability and waivability of rights.

26. See, e.g., Cal. Civil Code §7005(b) (West 1987).

27. See, e.g., Colker, "Anti-Subordination Above All: Sex, Race and Equal Protection," *N.Y.U. Law Review*, 61 (1986): 1003; Scales, "The Emergence of Feminist Jurisprudence: An Essay," *Yale Law Journal*, 95 (1986): 1373; C. MacKinnon, *Sexual Harassment of Working Women: A Case of Sex Discrimination* (1979).

28. C. MacKinnon, supra note 27, at 4.

29. Colker, supra note 27.

30. The test in fact reminds me of the only question my grandmother ever asked about world events. Whether people were talking about the election of the president of the United States, the results of the World Series, or the recognition of a new country by the United Nations, my grandmother wanted to know, "Will it be good for the Jews?"

31. 208 U.S. 412 (1908).

32. See, e.g., Lochner v. N.Y., 198 U.S. 45 (1905).

33. 29 USC 201–19 amnd. 1977.

34. See Klaff, "The Tender Years Doctrine: A Defense," *California Law Review*, 70 (1982): 335.

35. Hubbard, supra note 1.

36. California Fed. Savings & Loan v. Guerra, 107 S.Ct. 683 (1987).

37. See Williams, "Equality's Riddle," supra note 23.

38. 417 U.S. 484 (1974) (holding that the equal protection clause does not require employers to provide disability coverage for pregnancy when they choose to cover other disabilities).

39. 429 U.S. 125 (1976) (holding that Title VII does not prohibit the exclusion of pregnancy coverage from employee disability plans).

40. Williams, "Equality's Riddle," supra note 23, at 352.

41. See Colker, supra note 27, at 1007–8: "From an anti-subordination perspective, both facially differentiating and facially neutral policies are invidious only if they perpetuate racial or sexual hierarchy."

42. C. MacKinnon, supra note 27, at 117.

43. Klaff, supra note 34, at 337.

44. Id.: 337–39.

45. Id.: 340–41.

46. Id.: 336.

47. Mich. Stat. Ann. §25.312(3) (Callaghan 1987).

48. See, e.g., Garska v. McCoy, 278 S.E.2d 357 (W.Va., 1981).

49. See, e.g., Surrogate Parenting Assocs. v. Kentucky *ex rel* Armstrong, 707 S.W.2d 209, 213 (Ky. 1986), stating that if a surrogate mother decided to keep her child, "[s]he would be in the same position vis-a-vis the child and the biological father as any other mother with a child born out of wedlock."

50. 405 U.S. 645 (1972).

51. 434 U.S. 246 (1978).

52. 441 U.S. 380 (1979).

53. 463 U.S. 248 (1983).

54. 463 U.S. 248, 269 (1983).

55. 463 U.S. 248, 262 (1983).

56. In the Matter of Baby M,—A.2d—, 1988 WL 6251, at 9 (N.J.).

57. Williams, "The Equality Crisis," supra note 23.

PUBLIC HEALTH

Surrogacy and the Health Care Professional

Baby M and Beyond

Karen H. Rothenberg

Introduction

William and Elizabeth Stern wanted to have a child of their own, but believed it too dangerous when they learned that Elizabeth might have multiple sclerosis, a disease that in some cases renders pregnancy a serious health risk. As the sole member of his family to survive the Holocaust, Mr. Stern wanted to continue his bloodline. Initially, the Sterns considered adoption, but they became discouraged by the long delay and by potential problems arising from their age and differing religions. The Sterns then contacted a surrogacy agency, the Infertility Center of New York (ICNY).

Mary Beth Whitehead, a married woman with two children of her own, responded to an advertisement for ICNY to contract as a surrogate mother. She stated that she wanted to give another couple the "gift of life,"[1] and she wanted the $10,000 contractual fee to help her family. Mrs. Whitehead had been a potential surrogate mother with another couple, but after a number of unsuccessful inseminations, that effort was abandoned.

In February of 1985, Mr. Stern and Mr. and Mrs. Whitehead executed a surrogate parenting agreement. After several artificial inseminations, Mrs. Whitehead became pregnant. On March 6, 1986, a baby girl was born. Immediately after the baby's birth, Mrs. Whitehead realized she could not relinquish the baby. So began the legal battle over Baby M.

Mr. and Mrs. Stern brought suit seeking to compel Mrs. Whitehead's surrender of Baby M, to restrain any interference with their custody, and to terminate Mrs. Whitehead's parental rights to allow adoption of the child by Mrs. Stern. The trial court[2] held the surrogate contract valid, ordered Mrs. Whitehead's parental rights be terminated, granted sole custody of the child to Mr. Stern, and authorized adoption by Mrs. Stern. Mrs. Whitehead appealed.

On February 3, 1988, the New Jersey Supreme Court reversed the trial court.[3] The Court held that the surrogate contract conflicted with state laws concerning baby-selling, adoption, and termination of parental rights. The Court voided Mrs. Stern's adoption proceeding and reinstated Mrs. Whitehead's status as the child's legal mother, but upheld the trial court's order to award custody to Mr. Stern, based on the child's best interests. The issue of visitation was remanded to the trial court for factual reconsideration.[4]

The Baby M case[5] has forced us to take sides in the public debate over surrogate motherhood. Public reaction has been swift, and at least five states have passed legislation restricting the use of surrogacy contracts. Meanwhile, "[l]awyers, doctors and other brokers report a rush of recent applications from infertile couples anxious to beat possible legislative cut-offs."[6] More state legislation is predicted. Inevitably, the surrogacy process will continue to raise questions for the health care provider.

This paper will first analyze the Baby M decision. The second section will briefly outline public reaction and legislative action to ban or regulate surrogacy. The third section will highlight the professional response to surrogacy. The final section will analyze in detail the issues health care professionals face throughout the surrogacy process.

THE DECISION

In its unanimous opinion, the New Jersey Supreme Court refused to enforce the surrogacy contract that provided money to a surrogate mother to be artificially inseminated with the semen of another woman's husband, to conceive a child, to carry it to term, and to irrevocably agree to relinquish her parental rights and surrender her child to the natural father and his wife, regardless of the best interests of the child. The Court believed that its "declaration that this surrogacy contract is unenforceable and illegal is sufficient to deter similar agreements."[7]

The Court based its ruling on its interpretation of New Jersey adoption law and public policy. It was particularly offended by the payment of money in exchange for bearing and relinquishing a baby: "There are, in a civilized society, some things that money cannot buy."[8] Payment of money to the surrogate was "illegal, perhaps *criminal*, and degrading to women."[9]

The Baby M case was a dispute about a contract and the custody of Baby M, not about criminal liability. Yet the Court stated, albeit in dictum, that the surrogate arrangement was "perhaps criminal" under New Jersey law.[10] The Court found "no offense" to present laws where a woman without payment serves as a surrogate, provided she is not subject to a binding agreement to surrender her child.[11]

New Jersey law prohibits the use of money in connection with adoptions. Violation of this "baby selling" law is a high misdemeanor, a third-degree crime carrying a three- to five-year prison term.[12] Excepted are fees of an approved agency and payment or reimbursement for medical, hospital, or related expenses incurred in connection with the birth of the child. Although the Baby M contract provided that the fees paid were for services and expenses, the Court concluded that the parties knew it was nothing other than a private placement adoption for money. The contract provided for "the sale of a child, or at the very least, the sale of a mother's right to her child, the only mitigating factor being that one of the purchasers is the father."[13]

The Court concluded that the evils that prompted the prohibition against the payment of money in connection with adoption are present in the surrogacy arrangement. In both cases, "the essential evil is the same, taking advantage of the woman's circumstances (the unwanted pregnancy or the need for money) in order to take away the child. . . . "[14] In the Court's view, it was the middleman—the surrogate broker—motivated by the desire for profit, who promoted the sale.[15] The profit motive—and not the best interests of the parties—"predominates, permeates, and ultimately governs the transaction."[16]

The Court completed its ninety-five–page opinion with a prediction— and perhaps a hope for the future: "Legislative consideration of surrogacy may also provide the opportunity to begin to focus on the overall implications of the new reproductive biotechnology. . . . The problem can be addressed only when society decides what its values and objectives are in this troubling, yet promising, area."[17] Thus, the Court did not preclude the legislature from altering the statutory scheme to permit surrogacy contracts, within constitutional limits—limits which the Court did not define and which are not easily definable.

Public Reaction and Legislative Action[18]

Immediate legislative reaction to the Court's decision was targeted at banning commercial surrogacy. At least five state bills passed making it unlawful[19] to compensate the surrogate and third-party surrogate brokers.[20] Florida, Indiana, Kentucky, Michigan, and Nebraska passed legislation during the 1988 session making surrogate parenthood contracts void and unenforceable if compensation is involved.[21]

The determination of these states to discourage and ban surrogacy is apparent in their enforcement provisions. Penalties for brokering a surrogacy contract for compensation have been assessed under the baby-selling statutes, and range from a minimum $500 fine and/or a six-month imprisonment in Kentucky, to a maximum $50,000 fine and up to five years of imprisonment in Michigan.[22] Penalties for engaging in a surrogacy contract have been established as both misdemeanors and felonies, with penalties of $10,000 fines and at least a one-year imprisonment.[23]

Only the Florida statute specifically identifies physicians as potential brokers or agents who are prohibited from collecting a finder's fee.[24] Kentucky states that no person, agency, institution, or intermediary shall act as a facilitator,[25] while Michigan inclusively states that "a person" shall not act as an agent in the formation of a surrogate parentage contract for compensation.[26]

The constitutionality of the recently enacted Michigan Surrogate Parenting Act[27] was upheld by a circuit court in Wayne County, Michigan after a challenge by the American Civil Liberties Union on behalf of couples who received children through surrogacy.[28] The state argued that it would enforce the law only if the contract required the mother to give up the baby.[29] This narrow interpretation judicially accorded to the new law (permitting contracts if the surrogate did not have to decide until after birth whether she wants to terminate parental rights) allowed both sides to claim victory.[30] An order will issue shortly detailing what will be permitted in surrogate arrangements. Professional opinion is divided on whether this judgment will contribute to the demise of surrogacy contracts.[31]

In the meantime, without clearer legislation nationwide, the hint of immorality and potential criminality should at least cause those persons participating in a surrogacy contract to analyze their roles throughout the process. Since the Court's decision last February, surrogate parenting agencies have come under heightened scrutiny for criminal investigation.[32] The National Coalition Against Surrogacy, a group of 17 surrogate mothers now opposed to the practice, recently wrote to the attorneys general in 12 states where surrogate brokers operate, demanding the closure of agencies.[33]

Approximately half of the states have laws prohibiting baby-selling.[34] The Baby M Court never mentioned the role of the health professional in the context of baby-selling prohibitions. Yet the taint of immorality and possible criminality permeates the Court's analysis. If baby-selling laws are interpreted to cover the surrogacy arrangement, it may be interpreted broadly enough to subject health care professionals to criminal liability for their participation.[35] Unless the health care professional also serves as a broker, makes referrals, or owns a surrogacy agency, it is highly unlikely that there will be fair notice under most existing state laws to be criminally liable.[36] Yet the charge of "aiding and abetting" a crime would not be out of the question.

A more realistic fear for the health care professional may be the impact of the surrogacy process having been characterized as immoral, illegal, and "perhaps criminal." For couples desperate to have a child, for women desperate for money,[37] and for brokers desperate to get rich, the risks may still be worth taking. Criminalization of surrogacy may simply drive the business underground.[38]

In the meantime, what is to be the professional's role in the surrogacy process? Subsequent to the initial flurry of bills to ban surrogacy outright, some state proposals focused on regulating the surrogacy process.[39] Various trends emerged in the bills introduced in 1988 which could lead to an increasing role for the health care professional. For example, in some bills physicians and other providers would be required to file affidavits verifying that infertility testing, genetic testing, and counseling were completed prior to insemination of the surrogate. Some legislation would require that a physician perform and monitor insemination and insure that the surrogate has an active role in medical decision-making.[40]

THE PROFESSIONAL RESPONSE TO SURROGACY

Nineteen Amici briefs, expressing various interests and views on surrogacy, were filed with the New Jersey Supreme Court in the Baby M case.[41] Yet not one brief was filed on behalf of health professional associations. One can only speculate that such groups either did not view the Baby M case as a relevant health care case of nationwide importance or had not officially considered their positions on surrogacy. Not one of the major mental health associations, such as the American Psychological Association and the American Psychiatric Association, had officially considered the issue. In fact, very little attention has been given to surrogacy in any of the scientific journals. Either the Baby M decision will increase demand for evidence on the effects of surrogacy, or it will dry up interest. Or perhaps the issue will continue to be too controversial for health professional groups struggling for consensus.

Yet, as early as 1983, The Judicial Council of the American Medical Association (AMA), and the Executive Board of the American College of Obstetrics and Gynecology (ACOG) issued policy statements on surrogacy.[42] As late as Sept. 1987, the AMA reiterated its opposition to surrogacy in a statement to the Drafting Committee on the "Status of Children of the New Biology" of the National Conference of Commissioners on Uniform State Laws: "surrogate parent contracts do not represent a satisfactory reproductive alternative for those who wish to become parents."[43] The AMA opposed state legislation to sanction such arrangements.

Although ACOG is reevaluating its position, its present ethical guidelines do not condemn the practice but express "significant reservations about this approach to parenthood."[44] Of particular concern is its difficulty in differentiating between payments for the service of carrying the child and payment for the child itself—a practice that is clearly "illegal and morally objectionable."[45] ACOG also warns against accepting money for recruiting or referring potential surrogates or investing in surrogacy businesses. The physician "should not participate in a surrogate program where the financial arrangements are likely to exploit any of the parties."[46] Yet in the end, the decision about whether to participate in a surrogacy arrangement is left up to the physician. Physicians should contemplate the ethical obligations inherent either in contracting with a surrogacy agency as a staff physician or in serving as an independently contracting consultant. At the very least, they should consider the potential subrogation liability should an agency be sued.[47] A decision to participate in a surrogacy arrangement should be made only after the physician has weighed all the "legal, psychological, societal, medical and ethical aspects."[48]

In 1986 the Ethics Committee of the American Fertility Society issued its report on "Ethical Considerations of the New Reproductive Technologies."[49] The Committee concluded that, if surrogate motherhood is pursued, it should be as a "clinical experiment."[50] Unfortunately, this experiment will not answer the current concerns about the enforceability of the surrogate contract and the custody of the child. In fact, a few members of the Committee questioned whether, given the small number of couples involved, it was likely that significant research would be performed. Others would not endorse a procedure that was so highly controversial and whose risk/benefit ratio did not justify support.[51]

In spite of the fact that these groups did not play an active role in the Baby M appeal, surrogacy will continue to raise a number of unanswered questions for the health care professional. Future regulation may also increase the role of the surrogacy agreement.[52]

THE SURROGACY PROCESS AND THE HEALTH PROFESSIONAL[53]

Pre-Insemination: Evaluation, Counseling, and "Informed Consent"

New Jersey law mandates extensive counseling prior to the termination of parental rights, and the Baby M Court found that the surrogacy contract did not provide adequate "counseling, independent or otherwise, of the natural mother, no evaluation, no warning."[54] This lack of counseling and evaluation reinforced the Court's determination to void the surrogacy agreement.

Apparently the only psychological evaluation performed on Mrs. Whitehead was almost two years prior to her agreement with Mr. Stern. According to the trial court, Mrs. Whitehead received a "psychological evaluation to determine her suitability as a potential surrogate candidate" at the Infertility Center of New York (ICNY).[55] Although the "examiner" thought it important to explore her ability to relinquish the child in more depth, she was recommended as an appropriate candidate.[56] "It was this fact of prior evaluation that the Sterns relied on."[57] According to the trial court, Mrs. Whitehead also testified that she received two counseling sessions at ICNY, a point ignored by the New Jersey Supreme Court.

The Supreme Court raised a number of concerns about the role of evaluation and counseling. It questioned whether the evaluation served anyone but ICNY.[58] Nothing in the record stated that the evaluation was for the surrogate's benefit. Rather Mrs. Whitehead testified that all she was told was that "she had passed."[59] The Sterns never asked to see the evaluation. They assumed that ICNY had made an evaluation and "had concluded that there was no danger that the surrogate would change her mind."[60]

The Court stressed the fact that a psychologist warned that Mrs. Whitehead demonstrated certain traits that "might make surrender of the child difficult and that there should be further inquiry."[61] The Court speculated that to inquire further could have jeopardized the deal, believing that the "profit motive got the better" of ICNY.[62]

The Court ignored the provision in the contract that specifically stated that a *"psychiatric"* evaluation, which Mr. Stern was to pay for, was to be arranged for both Mr. and Mrs. Whitehead, and that the Whiteheads were to sign a release permitting dissemination of the evaluation report to ICNY or the Sterns.[63] Did this evaluation ever take place as provided in the contract? If so, what were the results? Is this the evaluation the Supreme Court was describing? Or did the Sterns in fact waive this contract requirement for a current psychiatric evaluation and rely on the evaluation done almost two years earlier by a clinical psychologist under contract with ICNY?

The facts are not clear from the record. It is clear, however, that the Court envisioned a process of both evaluation and counseling, one entailing not only a more in-depth evaluation of whether Mrs. Whitehead would change her mind, but also extensive counseling in which she would have been warned about the impact of relinquishing her child.

Should the mental health professional be in a position to guarantee that the mother will not change her mind or that her consent is voluntary?[64] Would the Court agree that such an assessment was impossible until after birth?[65] How would the professional make such assessments?

A recent demographic survey revealed some characteristics of prospective surrogates.[66] Generally, the women were white and in their mid- to late twenties. Half as many of the surrogates were married as were single. Virtually all had been pregnant, and approximately two out of ten had lost a child through miscarriage or abortion. Surprisingly, 12 percent of the women were adopted. Less than 10 percent had given up one of their own children through adoption. As regards education, over half had some high school background, and about a third had some college study. Financially, half of the households had incomes ranging between $15,000 and $30,000, 30 percent between $30,000 and $50,000, 13 percent less than $15,000, and 5 percent over $50,000.[67] To some extent, these statistics reflect the selection requirements imposed by agencies mandating minimum age, education, income, and life experiences.[68]

What traits, in fact, is the professional or agency to look for when choosing surrogates—stability, monetary motivation, detachment, sensitivity?[69] Will the surrogate with a detached personality have the easiest time relinquishing, but also be most unconcerned and medically noncompliant during the pregnancy? Perhaps the most sensitive personality will feel a sense of duty to the infertile couple and find it easiest to relinquish a child. What was it about Mrs. Whitehead's personality that caused doubt? Do psychologists on contract with a surrogacy agency ever recommend that a candidate not be approved? If the initial evaluation appears to raise questions, does one stop there, or should the mental health professional reevaluate following counseling? Should counseling include surrogate "support groups" in which the surrogate candidate can minimize feelings of doubt? And how often should an evaluation take place? For example, would the Baby M Court require evaluation and counseling each month prior to insemination?

The Court speculated that if either the Sterns or Mrs. Whitehead had been told the details of the evaluation, the agreement might never have been signed.[70] The evaluation, if shared, might have warned both parties and put them on notice. It has been suggested that the psychiatrist's duty to warn potential victims of a patient's anticipated harmful acts (the *Tarasoff* rule)[71] might conceivably be extrapolated to surrogacy. It is unclear whether such a duty to warn could be extended to potential victims of a contractual breach, i. e., the natural father.[72]

In any case, the Court pointed out that both parties suffered severe emotional distress, something that might have been avoided with proper evaluation, full disclosure, and counseling.[73] Yet the contract between Mr. Stern and ICNY made quite clear that ICNY would "not guarantee or warrant" that the surrogate would comply . . . including, but not limited to her "refusal to surrender custody of the child upon birth."[74] Mr. Stern also specifically released ICNY from any liability[75] "related to or arising from any agreement or understanding between himself and a 'surrogate mother' located through the services of ICNY."[76]

The Court questioned whether a surrogate could ever grant "informed consent" to the terms of the surrogate contract, even with sufficient evaluation and counseling. Traditionally, informed consent requires the patient to be told of the risks and benefits of treatment options. For the trial court, informed consent was defined as a "concept used in the trial of medical malpractice cases."[77] The trial court rejected the argument by Mrs. Whitehead that, not having "felt the emotion of birth and sensed the child, she could not give informed consent at the time she signed the contract."[78] To accept this expanded concept of informed consent would put "all contracts in limbo."[79]

To the contrary, the Supreme Court's concern was not so much with informed consent to a medical procedure (the insemination procedure is a simple, non-material risk) but rather with the consent—at the time of signing the contract—to relinquish the baby. The Court embraced a broad definition of informed consent, somewhat foreign to contract law. A standard contract requires only that both parties be competent at the time the agreement is made. In fact, the contract stated that both parties "freely and voluntarily" signed the agreement.[80]

Perhaps the Court deemed it "impossible" or "impracticable" for a natural mother to consent to relinquish her child until a reasonable time after birth. Without any scientific evidence cited, the Court took judicial notice that the "natural mother is irrevocably committed before she knows the strength of her bond with her child."[81] In the "most important sense" her decision is "uninformed."[82]

As a practical matter, what should the consent process include? Is a health care professional qualified to disclose medical, psychological, legal, and financial risks and benefits to the surrogate contract? How certain is any of this information? Medical risks associated with insemination and pregnancy are presently to be disclosed. But what about the long-term psychological risks to the parties, their families, and the child? Furthermore, the uncertainty of the legal and financial issues clouds consent even more. At best, "informed consent" will require a *warning* to all potential parties about all foreseeable risks.

Some states may attempt to regulate surrogacy by delineating standards for screening, evaluation, counseling, and informed consent prior to the signing of a contract. For example, recent proposals require the surrogate and natural father to submit to physical and genetic screening. The surrogate may also be required to undergo psychological evaluation to determine whether any medical disability would prevent her from abiding by the terms of the contract. A few proposals require that a psychologist, psychiatrist, or licensed marriage counselor certify that "the consequences and responsibilities of surrogate parenthood" were explained to the natural father and his wife, that "the surrogate had the capacity to consent," and that "the potential psychological consequence of her consent" had been discussed.[83] A proposal in Connecticut, for example, prohibits insemination unless the "physician is professionally satisfied with the mental and physical suitability of the surrogate and the natural father."[84]

Such requirements might have the effect of putting the health care professional in the position of "guarantor" of the surrogacy process. Professionals will have to guarantee or warrant that the mother will remain compliant and will not change her mind, that the medical and genetic makeup of both natural parents proves acceptable, that the psychological evaluation assures no problems, and that the parties have been warned of all risks.

Such attempts at regulation may re-characterize surrogacy as a medically controlled reproductive choice rather than a commercial enterprise. More involvement of health care professionals will legitimize the surrogacy process. Is this a role that health care professionals want to accept? Quality control under these contracts may improve, but who will monitor compliance? Ultimately, such a role may increase exposure to professional liability suits.

Insemination

In the typical surrogacy arrangement, the surrogate candidate is artificially inseminated with the semen of another woman's husband. This process does not require any complex reproductive technology, and the expertise of the physician is not essential. In fact, artificial insemination can be done at home with a turkey baster. State laws regulate artificial insemination to varying degrees.[85] In a few states it is in fact a criminal offense for anyone other than a licensed physician to perform artificial insemination.[86]

The Baby M contract specifically provided that the surrogate would be "artificially inseminated with the semen of the natural father by a *physician*."[87] Although contracts may vary as to the role of screening and evaluation at the pre-conception stage, it is clear that the physician takes a role in initiating conception. Prior to each attempt, the sperm donor and the surrogate should be screened for sexually transmitted diseases.[88] As in the Baby M case, it may be necessary to attempt insemination several times before conception occurs.

The health care professional's involvement is necessary for the surrogacy contract to proceed (assuming rejection of the at-home turkey-baster method or sexual intercourse). At this stage, the inseminating physician appears to have a physician-patient relationship with the surrogate and the natural father, as well as a business relationship with the surrogacy agency.[89] While the majority of statutes governing artificial insemination by donors specify the participation of a physician to guarantee legitimization of the offspring,[90] quality control is also a rationale for physician participation in surrogacy insemination. The standard of care for evaluating the physician's role in this process is uncertain.[91]

Prenatal Care

Once insemination is successful and conception occurs, the contract may provide for a continuing role for the inseminating physician. How does the surrogacy contract shape medical decision-making, and how does it affect the health care professional? Typical contractual provisions create limitations on the surrogate's behavior and control during pregnancy.[92] Such provisions raise constitutional issues regarding an individual's right to privacy, personal autonomy, and bodily integrity.[93]

The Baby M contract set out a number of specific terms related to prenatal care. First, Mrs. Whitehead would agree not to abort unless "in the professional medical opinion of the *inseminating physician*" it was necessary for her "physical health" or unless the child had been found to be "physiologically abnormal."[94] Furthermore, "upon the request" of the inseminating physician, she would agree to "undergo amniocentesis or similar tests to detect genetic and congenital defects."[95]

These provisions place all the decision-making authority with the inseminating physician.[96] What relationship does this physician have with the surrogate? What role does her independent obstetrician have in her care? To what extent does the inseminating physician know of her physical health, and what about her emotional health? Does the inseminating physician take orders from the surrogate agency and/or those who pay his fee? Will the profit motive "get the best of him" under these circumstances? In spite of the contract, it was Mrs. Stern, a physician herself, who insisted that Mrs. Whitehead undergo amniocentesis. The actual role of any other physician is unknown from the record.[97]

The Baby M contract provided that the surrogate would receive no compensation if she miscarried prior to the fifth month.[98] What if an ordered amniocentesis brought about a miscarriage? Who would have the cause of action against which physician? And in the event the baby was stillborn subsequent to the fourth month, the surrogate would receive only $1,000.[99] Would the surrogate and the natural father have a cause of action against the physician for negligence if they could prove the physician caused the stillbirth? Could the surrogate sue for the $9,000 she would have lost and for her expenses? Could the father sue for all his expenses? Obviously, if the contract is unenforceable, the contract remedy would not be available, but what about a negligence case? Could all parties establish a duty of the professional to provide a perfect, final "product?"

The Baby M contract did provide that if prenatal testing revealed any defects, the surrogate would abort the fetus "upon demand" of Mr. Stern or forfeit the money.[100] Even the trial court determined that this provision was clearly void and unenforceable.[101] Relying on *Roe v. Wade*,[102] it found "[t]hat only the woman has the constitutionally protected right to determine the manner in which her body and person shall be used."[103]

In another contract provision ignored by both courts, the surrogate would agree "to adhere to all medical instructions given to her by the inseminating physician as well as her independent obstetrician."[104] But what if there was a conflict between the physicians? Was she the patient of both physicians?[105] Did she have a relationship only with her independent physician? And if so, why should the inseminating physician have a role in her prenatal care?—Because the contract said so. And which physician's instructions was she to consider?

The contract further set out that the surrogate was not to "smoke cigarettes, drink alcoholic beverages, use illegal drugs, or take nonprescription medications or prescribed medications without written consent from her physician."[106] And which physician is this? What if she tells her "independent" physician she has been drinking or smoking a cigarette in violation of the contract? And what if she misses an appointment scheduled according to the contract? Is her physician to write these facts in the chart because they are medically relevant? Or should the physician not put such facts in her record because they violate the contract? The physician's interest is in protecting the welfare of the patient and the fetus.[107] Is the physician required to report this information to anyone? Even if she agreed by contract, should the physician report compliance or lack thereof to anyone else? Should a copy of the contract and its terms be placed in the surrogate's medical record? What if she gives the contract to the physician or the surrogate agency sends it? Should the physician ignore it and act as if it did not exist?[108]

Since her "independent obstetrician" is not part of the business deal, maybe the surrogate will not tell this physician about the contract. Does she have a reason to "deceive" the physician? Her physician might be better off not knowing about the terms of the contract and its "rules" on medical decision-making. It certainly would be less complicated. Yet this information may be relevant to her prenatal care. What if she begins to experience increasingly high blood pressure? Perhaps it is being caused by the ambivalence she feels about giving up the child—or maybe she fears that if she refuses to give up the child she will be sued. And what about the stress that her husband may feel about her pregnancy? Maybe her children are pressuring her not to give up the baby. Shouldn't the physician have this information? The physician may believe that the stress of the arrangement is causing psychological and perhaps physical harm to the mother and the fetus. With this information, what should the physician do? Should counseling be ordered to reduce her feelings of stress and bonding, or should counseling be directed toward validating her "natural" feelings about not wanting to relinquish the child—the possible position of the Baby M Court?

What may be in the surrogate's best interests medically may be to her disadvantage financially if she refuses to relinquish the baby. Is this a risk the surrogate assumes? Should the natural father pay all the expenses as foreseeable under the arrangement, whether or not the surrogate decides to keep the baby? The Baby M contract provided that the natural father should pay all expenses "not covered or allowed by her present health and major medical insurance, including all extraordinary medical expenses and all reasonable expenses for treatment of any emotional or mental conditions or problems related to said pregnancy. . . . "[109] What are deemed "reasonable" expenses for "emotional problems?" Who makes this determination? If counseling results in failure to relinquish the child, is the surrogate financially liable? If the natural father pays, does he have a role in directing the medical and psychological care provided? In the end, it may be the physician who ultimately determines the "success" of the surrogacy deal for all the parties. The health care professional will be forced to balance patient care needs with financial, legal, and ethical uncertainties.

The Birth

At the birth of Baby M, no one on the hospital staff appeared to know that the baby was the "product" of a surrogate contract. The Court described the following scene: "Not wishing anyone at the hospital to be aware of the surrogacy arrangement, Mr. and Mrs. Whitehead appeared to all the proud parents of a healthy female child. . . . In accordance with Mrs. Whitehead's request, the Sterns visited the hospital unobtrusively to see the newborn child."[110] Contrary to a specific provision in the contract,[111] Mrs. Whitehead named the child Sara Elizabeth Whitehead on the birth certificate and Mr. Whitehead was named as the father.[112] In short, the hospital staff had been deceived.

But what if the facts are different? What if hospital staff is advised of the arrangement and the mother appears uncertain about relinquishing the baby? Should the physician or nurse give the baby to the mother to hold or nurse? Such action, part of standard practice, might encourage even more bonding or attachment—something not agreed to in the contract. In fact, some proposed surrogate contracts provide that the surrogate not breast-feed following the birth. And who would take the baby home at the time of discharge? Without a court order or formal proof of relinquishment for adoption, most hospitals would release a child only to the natural mother. Hospital policy and fear of liability would not allow otherwise.

Furthermore, what if the baby had not been born healthy? Which parent would be granting or denying consent for immediate medical care? If Baby M had needed medical care, the hospital staff would have sought consent from Mr. and Mrs. Whitehead. What if there had been a conflict about medical care? Or what if a baby is deformed and no one wants to take responsibility for its care? The physician could be forced—as he was in a 1983 case—to get a court order to treat the medical problems of a child born with microcephaly.[113] The disappointment of the less-than-perfect child is hard for any parent to accept. It is also one of the most difficult problems for the physician to work out with parents. In fact, hospital ethics committees have been formed to assist the medical staff and family to make complex ethical and medical decisions about treatment for the severely defective newborn. To further complicate matters, the physician and hospital staff must figure out which possible parent speaks on behalf of the best interests of the child.

A few legislative proposals regulate decision-making at the time of birth. Some give authority to the natural mother through birth and immediately thereafter,[114] while others shift authority at the time of viability to the natural father and his wife.[115] For the physician and the hospital staff, it seems safest to place these decisions with the natural mother, assuming she is acting in the best interests of the child. But what if the natural mother then relinquishes the less-than-perfect baby to the natural father pursuant to the contract? It is conceivable than he will not want the "damaged goods" either, and the child will be abandoned by all parties.[116] In a recent case reported in the *New England Journal of Medicine*, a surrogate mother passed HIV infection to the fetus, and neither the surrogate nor the natural father wanted custody of the infant.[117]

Even if a natural father is granted custody, he may not have had a role in making decisions about medical care for the infant at birth. The physician may not have known of the surrogacy arrangement. Faced with significant medical and related expenses for his defective child, the father, detached from the medical decision-making process, may look for a "deep pocket" to sue. Both the health care professional and the hospital will face increasing liability risks from all parties.

CONCLUSION

Baby M was not a case about health care professionals. Yet examination of the surrogacy contract reveals the importance of the health care professional as a player in the process. From the initial evaluation through the birth, the health care professional faces a number of complex legal and ethical questions. Many of these questions have no answers. As state legislatures continue to address surrogacy, health care professionals will be expected to assume an increasing role as a "guarantor" in the process. This is a role that the health care professional should not accept without a clear recognition of the inevitable conflicts.

REFERENCES

1. 109 N.J. 396, 413; 537 A.2d 1227, 1236 (Sup. Ct. 1988).
2. 217 N.J. Super. 313, 525 A.2d 1128 (1988).
3. *Matter Of Baby M*, 109 N.J. 396, 537 A.2d 1227 (Sup. Ct. 1988).
4. The court found "that Melissa's (Baby M's) best interests will be served by unsupervised, uninterrupted, liberal visitation with her mother." 542 A.2d 52, 53 (1988). The court reinforced the Supreme Court's determination of the parties' roles when it stated that there is "no longer a termination of parental rights or an adoption case and it no longer matters how Melissa was legally conceived. She and her mother have the right to develop their own special relationship." Id.
5. *In re Baby M*, 109 N.J. 396, 537 A.2d 1227 (Sup. Ct. 1988).
6. Malcolm, "Steps to Control Surrogate Births Stir Debate Anew," *N.Y. Times*, June 26, 1988, §1, at 21, col. 1.
7. 109 N.J. at 454, 537 A.2d at 1257.

8. Id. at 440, 537 A.2d at 1249.

9. Id. at 411, 537 A.2d at 1234, emphasis added. The author, surrogate mother Elizabeth Kane, now believes that "[s]urrogate parenthood is nothing more than reproductive prostitution. It's still rich men using a poor woman's body. . . . " Quoted in Malcolm, "Steps to Control Surrogate Births Stir Debate Anew," *N.Y. Times*, June 26, 1988, §1, at 1, col. 6.

10. 109 N.J. at 469, 537 A.2d at 1264.

11. Id. at 411, 537 A.2d at 1235.

12. N.J.S.A. 9:3–54. See 109 N.J. at 433, 537 A.2d at 1240, n. 4.

13. Id. at 437–38, 537 A.2d at 1247.

14. 109 N.J. at 439, 537 A.2d at 1249.

15. See Gladwell and Sharpe, "Baby M Winner," 196 *The New Republic*, (February 16, 1987), 15–18, for a revealing portrayal of the founder of the surrogacy business, attorney Noel P. Keane.

16. 109 N.J. at 439, 537 A.2d at 1249.

17. Id. at 469, 537 A.2d at 1264.

18. Prior to the Supreme Court's Baby M decision, legislative proposals were more evenly balanced between regulation and prohibition: 14 states presented 26 bills regulating surrogacy contracts, and 17 states introduced 25 bills prohibiting or declaring surrogacy contracts void and unenforceable. None of the bills to regulate surrogacy passed. National Conference of State Legislatures, *Status Report of Bill Introductions in 1988 Legislative Sessions Relating to Surrogacy Contracts* (July 19, 1988) (hereinafter "National Conference"). See Appendix II of this book.

19. Michigan allows medical expenses related to pregnancy; see 1988 Mich. Pub. Acts 199. Florida allows adoption fees and perhaps reasonable surrogate living expenses; see 1988 Fla. Laws 143.

20. See National Conference, supra note 18.

21. 1988 Fla. Laws 143, Ind. Code Ann. tit. 31 § 8–2–1 (Burns Supp. 1988), Ky. Rev. Stat. Ann. § 199.590 (Baldwin Supp. 1988), 1988 Mich. Pub. Acts 199, Neb. Rev. Stat. §25–21,200 (Supp. 1988).

22. Ky. Rev. Stat. Ann. § 199.990 (Baldwin Supp. 1988), 1988 Mich. Pub. Acts 199.

23. Florida appears to penalize violations of its new preplanned adoption law equally between brokers and contract participants. See National Conference, supra note 18.

24. However, doctors and psychologists as well as attorneys may receive reasonable compensation for their professional services. 1988 Fla. Laws 143.

25. Ky. Rev. Stat. Ann. § 199.590 (Baldwin Supp. 1988).

26. 1988 Mich. Pub. Acts 199.

27. Id. Effective September 1, 1988, a surrogate contract is void and unenforceable as contrary to public policy.

28. *Balt. Sun*, Sept. 20, 1988, § A, at 2, col 4.

29. Id.

30. Id.

31. *Balt. Sun*, Sept. 20, 1988, § A, at 2, col 4.

32. See Jordan, "Investigation of Surrogacy Business Sought," *L.A. Daily Journal*, April 7, 1988, at 2, col. 1.

33. Malcolm, *N.Y. Times*, June 26, 1988, §1, at 21, col. 1. Indicative of the "moral" backlash, two books highly critical of surrogacy have recently been published. P. Chester, *Sacred Bond: The Legacy of Baby M* (1988), and E. Kane, *Birth Mother: The Story of America's First Legal Surrogate Mother* (1988).

34. See Katz, "Surrogate Motherhood and the Baby-Selling Laws," 20 *Colum. J.*

L. & Soc. Probs., 1, 8–9, n.34 (1986) (state statutes prohibiting payment for adoption listed). See also National Conference, supra note 18.

35. See Katz, "Surrogate Motherhood and the Baby-Selling Laws," 20 *Colum. J. L. & Soc. Probs.*, 1, 8–9 n.34. See also Cohen and Friend, "Legal and Ethical Implications of Surrogate Mother Contracts," 14 *Clinics in Perinatology*, 281, 284 (1987).

36. The president of Surrogate Parenting Associates, the subject of a protracted legal battle in Kentucky, was a physician who was "paid a fee by the biological father for selection and artificial insemination of the surrogate mother. . . . " See Surrogate Parenting Associates, Inc. v. Commonwealth ex rel. Armstrong, 704 S.W.2d 209, 211 (Ky. 1986); see also Karnezis, "Criminal Liability of One Arranging for Adoption of Child through Other Than Licensed Child Placement Agency ('Baby Broker Acts')," 3 *ALR* 4th 468; Montana Dept. of Social & Rehab. Services v. Angel, 577 P.2d 1223 (Mont. 1978) (physician enjoined from placing children for adoption without a license, but court did not discuss criminal liability for baby-selling).

37. For a general discussion of contractual fee provisions and the potential pressures imposed, see Office of Technology Assessment, U.S. Congress, BA-358, *Infertility: Medical and Social Choices* 275–77 (1988) (hereinafter "OTA").

38. According to Harriet Blankfeld of the Infertility Associates International, "Banning surrogacies is going in the wrong direction. It won't stop the practice; it'll just create an even more secret and dangerous one as we did with abortions." quoted in Malcolm, *N.Y. Times*, June 26, 1988, § 1, at 21, col. 1.

39. See e.g., National Conference of Commissioners of Uniform State Laws, "Uniform Status of Children of Assisted Conception Act," which proposes both Alternative A, which outlines extensive regulatory provisions, and Alternative B, which declares surrogacy agreements void. (Approved and recommended for enactment at the Annual Conference of the National Conference of Commissioners of Uniform State Laws, July 29–August 5, 1988).

40. Predominant trends for physician participation emerged. At court hearings to approve surrogacy agreements, physicians may be asked to file affidavits regarding several aspects of the particular surrogacy arrangement: (1) TESTING—that intended mother is sterile; that at time of physical examination surrogate is likely to be fertile, absence of sexually and genetically transmitted diseases and perhaps demonstration that she is not likely to be pregnant already; and that the natural father has been tested for sexually and genetically transmitted diseases. For example, Rh compatibility testing for both biological parents was a requirement mentioned in several bills (H. 1140, 105th Gen. Assem., 2d Reg. Sess. Ind. (1988); H. 1561, 84th. Leg., 2d Reg. Sess. Mo. (1988), H. 4753, 84th Leg., Reg. Sess. Mich. (1988), A. 827, 1987–88 Wis. Leg. (1988)). Paternity testing by blood or tissue typing was often required (H. 649, 1988 Md. Sess. (1988), H. 6109, Feb. Sess. A. D. Conn. (1988), H. 4753, 84th Leg. Reg. Sess. Mich. (1988), H. 1140, 105th Gen. Assem., 2d Reg. Sess. Ind. (1988), H. 1561, 84th Leg. 2d Reg. Sess. Mo. (1988)). Paternity testing was occasionally made necessary if requested (S. 493, Ga. Sess. (1988), A. 827, 1987–88 Wis. Leg. (1988)). (2) COUNSELING—To establish informed consent, all parties receive counseling concerning effects of surrogacy from qualified health care professional who files conclusions with the court about the capacity of parties to enter into and fulfill contract. The Georgia bill required counseling only after initial appearance at court hearing (S. 493, Ga. Sess. (1988)), while a New Jersey proposal stipulated psychological or psychiatric evaluations preceding counseling (S. 2468, 203d Leg. 1st Ann. Sess. N.J. (1988)). A Maryland proposal allowed for requests by the natural father or his spouse for pre-insemination evaluation and post-insemination counseling (H. 649, 1988 Md. Sess. (1988); H. 4753, 84th Leg., Reg. Sess.

Mich. (1988)). Other proposals specifically considered evaluation of physical and mental fitness of the intended parents (H. 6109, Feb. Sess. A.D. Conn. (1988); H. 1561, 84th Leg. 2d Reg. Sess. Mo. (1988)).

B. INSEMINATION PROCEDURE—Insemination by a licensed physician is mandatory, with possible additional requirements for signing affidavit that informed surrogate of all instructions (H. 4753, 84th Leg., Reg. Sess. Mich. (1988)), that spouse of natural father acknowledged his sperm as being used (H. 649, 1988 Md. Sess. (1988)), that recognized prohibition on genetic materials of intended providers who are related by blood (H. 1529, 50th Leg. Reg Sess., Wash. (1988)).

C. MEDICAL DECISION-MAKING BY SURROGATE—Proposed legislative language typically established the surrogate as controlling all medical decisions relating to pregnancy. A Wisconsin bill provided for an exception if otherwise stipulated in the contract (A. 827, 1987–88, Wis. Leg. (1988)). Connecticut and Maryland proposals required the surrogate to adhere to all medical instructions given to her by the inseminating physician as well as her doctor (H. 6109, Feb. Sess. A. D. Conn. (1988), and H. 649, 1988 Md. Sess. (1988)). Very few proposals explicitly stated that the surrogate was the sole source of consent regarding the clinical management of the pregnancy, including pregnancy termination (H. 1140, 105th Gen. Assem., 2d Reg. Sess. Ind. (1988), H. 1561, 84th Leg., 2d Reg. Sess. Mo. (1988)).

D. MISCELLANEOUS—Administrative duties required of the physician included the sending of surrogate's genetic screening information to the intended parents (H. 1140, 105th Gen. Assem., 2d Reg. Sess. Ind. (1988), H. 649, 1988 Md. Sess. (1988)), certifying and filing with the Registrar of Vital Statistics the surrogate husband's consent to insemination and donor and surrogate signatures agreeing that the donor shall be the legal father (H. 1529, 50th Leg., Reg. Sess. Wash. (1988)), sending medical records and copy of contract to health department, S. 2468, 203rd Leg. 1st Ann. Sess. N.J. (1988). Indiana delineated numerous responsibilities, subject to potential physician liability (H. 1140, 105th Gen. Assem., 2d Reg. Sess. Ind. (1988)).

41. In fact, the court specifically acknowledged that many of these briefs were helpful in resolving the issues. 109 N.J. at 419, 537 A.2d at 1238.

42. ACOG Statement of Policy, "Ethical Issues in Surrogate Motherhood," May, 1983; American Medical Association, Report of the Judicial Council, Report B, (I-84) and related documentation; American Fertility Society, "Surrogate mothers," Chapter 25 of "Ethical Considerations of the New Reproductive Technologies," 46 *Fertility and Sterility*, Supp. 1, 62S–68S (1986). See Appendix IV in this book.

43. See Letter from James H. Sammons, M.D., AMA Executive Vice President, to Robert Robinson, Chairman, Drafting Committee on "Status of Children of the New Biology" (Sept. 22, 1987).

44. ACOG Statement of Policy, supra note 42.

45. Id.

46. Id.

47. See Gladwell and Sharpe, "Baby M Winner," 196 *The New Republic* (February 16, 1987), 15–18, for examples of broker practices creating potential liabilities for physicians.

48. ACOG Statement of Policy, supra note 42.

49. See American Fertility Society "Surrogate Mothers," supra note 42.

50. Id. at 67S.

51. Id. at 68S.

52. See supra note 42. See also possibilities proposed by various state legislatures supra note 40.

53. See generally, Rothenberg, "Baby M, The Surrogacy Contract, and the Health Care Professional: Unanswered Questions" 16 *Law, Medicine and Health Care* 113 (1988).

54. 109 N.J. at 436, 537 A.2d at 1247.

55. 217 N.J. Super. at 343, 525 A.2d at 1142.

56. Id.

57. Id.

58. 109 N.J. at 436–37, 537 A.2d at 1247.

59. Id.

60. Id. at 436, 537 A.2d at 1247.

61. Id. at 437, 537 A.2d at 1247–48.

62. Id. at 437, 537 A.2d at 1247.

63. 109 N.J. at 471, 537 A.2d at 1266, Appendix A, "Surrogate Parenting Agreement," para. 6, emphasis added.

64. In 1987, of the 13 commercial surrogate matching services surveyed, at least 10 performed some sort of psychological screening before any inseminations. OTA, supra note 37 at 272. See also, supra note 40 for examples of recent legislative proposals suggesting such a role.

65. 109 at 439, 537 A.2d at 1248.

66. OTA, supra note 37, Table 14–1, at 274.

67. On average, these women were between 26 and 28 years of age, almost all heterosexual, and approximately 60 percent of them married. According to the surrogate agencies reporting, almost 90 percent of the women were non-Hispanic whites, approximately two-thirds Protestant and nearly one-third Catholic. While this survey did not specify how many children surrogates already had, previous studies report surrogates as having one or two children. Socioeconomically, agencies overall reported that fewer than 35 percent of the women had ever attended college and only 4 percent had pursued graduate study. Six of the 13 agencies responding stated that women on welfare and women who are not financially independent are ineligible to contract. OTA, supra note 37 at 273–74.

68. Selection requirements may include good health, a stable relationship, prior conception, economic independence, 21–35 years of age, and some level of psychological screening or counseling. OTA, supra note 37 at 270.

69. See, e.g., Parker, "Surrogate Motherhood, Psychiatric Screening and Informed Consent, Baby Selling, & Public Policy," 12 *Bull. Am. Acad. Psychiatry Law* 21 (1984). See also, OTA, Table 14–1, "Demographic Survey of Surrogate Mothers" at 274.

70. 109 N.J. at 437, 537 A.2d at 1248.

71. *Tarasoff v. Regents of the University of California,* 17 Cal. 3d 425, 551 P.2d 334, 131 Cal Rptr. 14 (1977).

72. See OTA, supra note 37 at 272.

73. 109 N.J. at 435, 537 A.2d at 1247, n. 9.

74. Id. at 478, 537 A.2d at 1273, Appendix B, "Agreement," para. 10.

75. At least one broker/agency has been involved in four lawsuits for breach of contract. See Gladwell and Sharpe, "Baby M Winner," 196 *The New Republic,* 15–18 (suits for failure to provide adequate medical information, for failure to have a signed contract before insemination, for approval despite a history of heart disease, and for use of fertility drugs to induce ovulation in a woman still nursing her own baby).

76. 109 N.J. at 478, 537 A.2d at 1273, Appendix B, "Agreement," para. 11.

77. 217 N.J. Super. at 356, 525 A.2d at 1149.

78. Id.

79. Id.

80. 109 N.J. at 473, 537 A.2d at 1268, Appendix A, para. 17.

81. Id. at 437, 537 A.2d at 1248.

82. Id. at 437, 537 A.2d at 1248.

83. For a recent article summarizing legislative proposals introduced prior to the final Baby M decision, see Note, "Surrogate Motherhood Legislation: A Sensible Starting Point," 20 *Ind. L. Rev.* 879, 892–94 (1987). See also National Conference, supra note 40, for a summary of 1988 legislative proposals which failed to win approval by session's end.

84. H. 6109, Feb. Sess. Conn. (1988).

85. See generally King, "Reproductive Technologies," 1 *BioLaw* 113, 115–117, 122–124 (1986). See also OTA, supra note 37 Table 13–1 "State Statutes—Artificial Insemination" at 243.

86. OTA, supra note 37, Table 13–1, "State Statutes—Artificial Insemination" at 243. See also Ga. Code § 43–34–42 (1982).

87. 109 N.J. at 470, 537 A.2d at 1265, Appendix A, para. 3, emphasis added.

88. Generally, artificial insemination by donor statutes do not address a physician's duty to screen donors to prevent transmission of sexually transmitted diseases. Only Idaho and Ohio require physicians to quarantine frozen semen and to screen donors for the AIDS virus. OTA, supra note 37 at 248.

89. A physician-patient relationship may be established between the embryo and the physician. The Louisiana IVF statute, La. Civ. Code Ann. art. 9:124 (West Supp. 1988), grants in-vitro embryos the right to bring suit through a legal guardian and assigns specific responsibilities to doctors to guard the embryo from harm. These legal rights are traditionally only available to live born children. OTA, supra note 37 at 272.

90. OTA, supra note 37 at 244.

91. Alternative reproductive techniques, such as in-vitro fertilization, embryo transfer, and gamete intrafallopian transfer (GIFT), present an even more difficult problem for applying the standard of care. These procedures are complex, relatively new, and practices vary widely. OTA, supra note 37 at 175.

92. Standard provisions prevent the surrogate from smoking, drinking alcohol, or taking illegal drugs. Some contracts regulate diet and level of exercise. OTA, supra note 37 at 277–79.

93. Id. at 277–78.

94. 109 at 473, 537 A.2d at 1268, Appendix A, para. 13.

95. Id., 537 A.2d at 1268.

96. Typically, surrogates agree contractually to abide by "her physician's" orders. Often contracts allow the client (natural father) control in deciding on whether the surrogate undergoes particular procedures (e.g., chorionic villi sampling, amniocentesis, abortion). Such provisions clash with issues of personal autonomy, yet provide clout to grant injunctive relief or to claim breach of contract. OTA, supra note 37 at 278.

97. 217 N.J. Super at 346, 525 A.2d at 1143.

98. 109 N.J. at 471, 537 A.2d at 1267, Appendix A, para. 10.

99. Id., 537 A.2d at 1267.

100. Id. at 473, 537 A.2d at 1268.

101. 217 N.J. Super at 375, 525 A.2d at 1159.

102. 410 U.S. 113 (1973).

103. 217 N.J. Super at 375, 525 A.2d at 1159.

104. 109 N.J. at 473, 537 A.2d at 1268, Appendix A, para. 15.

105. One might find this analogous to the situation which led to the distinction

between the duties of "treating" and "examining" physicians in some jurisdictions. See, e.g., Ahnert v. Wildman, 376 N.E.2d 1182 (Ind. App. 1978).

106. 109 N.J. at 473, 537 A.2d at 1268, Appendix A, para. 15.

107. See ACOG Statement of Policy, supra note 42 and accompanying text.

108. Maternal-fetal conflicts may also arise for the physician trying to respect both the surrogate's wishes and the broad contractual provisions for obstetrical intervention for the fetus. See generally Mayo, "Medical Decision Making during a Surrogate Pregnancy," 25 *Hous. L. Rev.* 599, 623–28 (1988).

109. 109 N.J. at 471, 537 A.2d at 1266, Appendix A, para. 4(c) (1).

110. Id. at 414, 537 A.2d at 1236.

111. Id. at 472, 537 A.2d at 1267.

112. Id. at 414, 537 A.2d at 1236.

113. *N.Y. Times,* January 23, 1983, §1, at 19, col. 1. In fact, it was this case that may have motivated the AMA and ACOG to first address the issue.

114. See, e.g., "Model Human Reproductive Technologies & Surrogacy Act," 72 *Iowa L. Rev.* 943, 960–62 (1987); 1987 Mich. H-4573. This Michigan proposal, which did not pass, provided for consent revocation up to twenty days after childbirth.

115. See, e.g., National Commissioners on Uniform State Laws, "Uniform Status of Children of Assisted Conception Act" (1988), Alternative A, which recommends that a surrogate may terminate the agreement by filing written notice within 180 days after the last insemination.

116. See Areen, "Handicapped Child Becomes 'Damaged Goods'," 121 *N.J.L.J.* (Feb. 18, 1988), 25, 26 ; Krimmel, "The Case against Surrogate Parenting," *Hastings Center Report* 35 (Oct. 1983).

117. No pre-insemination screening for HIV infection was performed. It was not until the fifth month of pregnancy that the surrogate was tested. Neither the natural father nor his wife was aware that her sister-in-law, the surrogate, had been an intravenous drug user for five years. Frederick, Delapenha, Gray, et al., "HIV Testing on Surrogate Mothers," 317 *New Eng. J. Med.* (Nov. 19, 1987), 1351. See also Areen, supra note 116.

SURROGACY

A Preferred Treatment for Infertility?

Nadine Taub

No matter what one's position, *Baby M* is a difficult case. Once a child of contract parenthood has come into being, sorting out the competing claims that changed intentions produce is inevitably a troubling process. Even when taken in the abstract, surrogacy arrangements raise disturbing questions: Can we expand the available options for forming families without risking sex, race, and class exploitation? Can we address the pain experienced by those unable to conceive and bear children without commodifying human life? Whatever our views of surrogacy, we cannot hope to resolve the dilemmas it poses without acknowledging and seeking to address the pain of infertility.

Given what we know about infertility, is commercial surrogacy—however troublesome—an appropriate response? Even with only partial information before us, the answer would seem to be a fairly clear no. Surrogacy is at best an after-the-fact accommodation to the problem of infertility, available only to those with substantial financial resources. A remedy only for infertile couples whose problems can be attributed solely to the woman, it does nothing to treat or prevent the causes of infertility. And, particularly if access is restricted by regulation to conventional heterosexual families, it is one that reinforces society's message that raising one's own genetic children (or as close an approximation as possible) within a nuclear unit is a crucial experience. In this way, it stands to exacerbate, rather than alleviate, the pain of infertility.

The astonishing energies and attention that the surrogacy question has thus far attracted would have a much greater pay-off if aimed more directly at the causes of infertility and its attendant pain. To achieve this pay-off, the effort must inevitably be multifaceted. Resources must be mobilized to understand and eliminate the physical causes of infertility, impaired fecundity, and infant mortality. The social pressures and behaviors that both create the expectation that one will have one's own biological family and that make it difficult to do so must be identified and diminished. And the legal system must be subjected to scrutiny and correction to ensure that it does not contribute either to the fact or to the pain of infertility.

The starting point for devising more appropriate approaches to alleviating the pain of infertility must be an accurate assessment of the problem as a physical and social phenomenon. This article, therefore, begins with a look at the extent of infertility and the demand for infertility services. It then turns to a consideration of the factors that contribute to the problem of infertility and identifies policy measures and legal concerns pertinent in addressing these factors. The article concludes with a brief discussion of broader societal changes that will help remedy the pain of infertility.

THE PROBLEM OF INFERTILITY

Information on the extent of infertility nationally comes from surveys conducted by the National Center for Health Statistics. The most recent statistics are based on a weighted national sampling of married couples dating from 1982.[1] Those data show that 2.4 million or 8.5 percent of married couples were infertile, where infertility was defined as twelve months or more of unprotected intercourse without a pregnancy. Of these, approximately 1.0 million were childless, and the other 1.4 million had one or more children prior to becoming infertile. The 1982 survey also found that 4.5 million women (including the unmarried as well as the married) suffered from impaired fecundity, that is, difficulty in conceiving or in carrying a pregnancy to term.

Infertility occurs with greater frequency among certain groups. In 1982, black couples were one and a half times more likely to be infertile than white couples.[2] Infertility is also more common among the less educated.[3] Although there is some controversy over the specifics, it appears that infertility increases with age. The national survey in 1982 found, for example, that (excluding the surgically sterile) 14 percent of married couples with wives aged thirty to thirty-four were infertile, while for couples with wives aged thirty-five to thirty-nine the figure was 25 percent.[4]

Despite the attention infertility is now receiving, available data suggest that overall infertility rates have not increased significantly in recent years. As demographer William D. Mosher wrote in 1987, "Overall, American couples are no more likely to be infertile today than in 1965—in fact they are less likely to be infertile."[5] Studies comparing a national survey conducted in 1965 with the 1982 national survey actually show a drop in the percentage of infertile married couples, from 11 to 8.5 percent. However, the drop is attributable to the rise of surgical sterilization among those who already had at least one child. Since "infertility" was defined as the unsuccessful attempt to get pregnant, sterilized couples were not counted as infertile. When sterilized couples are excluded from the base, there is an apparent relative increase in infertility rates, particularly among childless couples, but the increase is not a statistically significant one. The one age group that has experienced a significant increase in rate is that in which the wife is between twenty and twenty-four.

What, then, explains the current preoccupation with infertility and the emotional pain it causes? Several explanations have been offered. One obvious factor is that the actual number of the primary infertile doubled from 1965 to 1982, as the baby-boom generation reached the child-bearing years and many more people attempted to have their first baby. The increase in infertility among this younger group is attributed primarily to sexually transmitted disease, but may also be due to exposure to occupational hazards and environmental toxins. Additionally, as couples have postponed child-bearing, they have become more vulnerable to the age-related biologic risks of infertility. At the same time, their period for attempting reproduction has been condensed into a shorter interval, while conception—for those who have been taking oral contraceptives—is likely to take longer.[6]

But this increase in the number of infertile couples does not entirely explain the dramatic rise in the demand for infertility services. The estimated number of visits to private physicians' offices for infertility-related consultations rose from about 600,000 in 1968 to over 900,000 in 1972 to about 2 million in 1983, dropping back to 1.6 million in 1984.[7] The relative share of infertility-related visits among all visits has also increased, from 95.6 per 100,000 in 1976 to 101.9 per 100,000 in 1980. Factors contributing to this growth include couples' increased concern with infertility, their increased awareness of possible treatments, and the greater proportion of couples in higher socio-economic brackets experiencing infertility problems.[8]

The dramatic drop in the demand for obstetrical services and the greater incidence of infertility in upper-income populations have also stimulated physicians' interest in infertility problems. In addition, the demand for services has been fed by the extensive media attention that improvements in diagnostic techniques and the development of technology-intensive treatments, ranging from fertility-enhancing drugs to in vitro fertilization and microsurgery, have attracted. Moreover, adoption has become a less feasible alternative for white couples seeking to imitate a genetic nuclear family, as the supply of white infants has decreased. Concern about infertility has also grown as the conservative pro-family movement of the Reagan years superseded the more liberal sexual climate of the 1960s and early 1970s.[9]

Pain is not an inevitable response to the fact of infertility. As the increase in the demand for infertility services suggests, a physical reality takes on significance in a particular social context. Failing to get pregnant must have been a very different experience in the late 1960s and early 1970s, when the *New York Times* spotlighted Zero Population Growth and the Nonparents League,[10] as compared to the present time, when the same paper runs articles with titles like "In TV and Films, as in Life, Babies Are in Fashion Again."[11] Thus, in seeking remedies for the pain of infertility, we must be sensitive to social as well as physical factors.

Addressing the Causes of Infertility

Our knowledge of the causes of infertility is far from complete. Reproductive biology is only partially understood, and multiple factors may contribute to infertility in any one case. Clinical studies of infertile patients are limited to those who appear for evaluation and whose condition is not explained by such obvious causes as surgical sterility. Having used survey techniques rather than physical examinations or tests, the large national studies did not explore the etiology of infertility. Yet the available data do suggest the importance of certain causal factors that could and should be addressed.

Pelvic Inflammatory Disease

There is widespread agreement that pelvic inflammatory disease, often attributable to sexually transmitted infections, is a major cause of infertility and impaired fecundity in women.[12] Though less is known about the effect of sexually transmitted diseases on men, there is reason to suspect an adverse impact on male fertility as well.[13] Public health initiatives directed at the identification and elimination of sexually transmitted diseases such as gonorrhea and chlamydia are therefore key to any effort to prevent infertility. The Office of Technology Assessment of the U.S. Congress has identified five areas for such initiatives: education of patients and public health professionals; definition of the diseases, including their long-term sequelae; optimal treatment and improved clinic services; patient counseling and partner tracing; and research into the social, psychological, and biological aspects of sexually transmitted diseases.[14]

Undertaking such efforts is largely a matter of mobilizing the necessary resources. Care, however, must be taken in the way services are made available. For example, health education and treatment programs that tie services for minors to parental notice requirements, that limit the provision of services to certain religious groups, or that link health services to criminal sanctions are both unwise and arguably unconstitutional. State and federal requirements that have conditioned public funding for contraceptive services provided to minors on parental notification or consent have been criticized as counterproductive and invalidated as contrary to federal law.[15] Through the Adolescent Family Life Act, which requires the involvement of particular sorts of religious groups, the federal government has supported misinformation on the prophylaxis of sexually transmitted disease, quite probably in violation of the First Amendment's prohibition on establishment of religion.[16] Similarly, requirements that health care professionals report youngsters seeking reproductive health care to state officials appear to violate the right to privacy, at least as guaranteed by certain state constitutions.[17]

Iatrogenic Infertility

Improper treatment also contributes to infertility. Medical professionals as well as activists in the women's health movement have drawn attention to the problem of iatrogenic infertility.[18] It is now well known that certain drugs and devices to assist or control reproduction have caused infertility. These, of course, include DES (diethylstilbestrol)[19] and the IUD.[20] Perhaps less well known is the link between adhesions and pelvic inflammatory disease due to pelvic operations such as appendectomies and dilation and curettage.[21] Eliminating unwanted infertility resulting from such causes will require both consumers and providers to be actively aware of the possible consequences of treatments.

A number of legal provisions are relevant to establishing the proper climate of care. Stringent informed-consent requirements will help ensure that risks are carefully identified and evaluated by medical professionals and patients. Such requirements must ensure that patients are provided with both adequate information and the opportunity to consider it fully. Legally mandated informed-consent standards requiring discussion of all forms of treatment may be a useful mechanism in improving the provision of information to patients.[22] Requirements that providers inform patients of their own track records on the use of key procedures are another.[23] Informed-consent standards that specify that, where feasible, consent must be obtained outside the hospital or outside particularly stressful settings within the hospital would help ensure that patients can weigh the available alternatives and discuss their decisions with family and friends.

The defensive practice of medicine has also contributed to the overuse of surgical interventions. Thus, limiting iatrogenic infertility will require finding means to incorporate a greater concern for excessive and destructive treatment into the malpractice system. Statutes and common law doctrines that specify that informed refusal of treatment provides a defense to malpractice actions may be a useful means of doing so.[24] Of course, care must be taken to ensure that the "informed" portion of the informed-refusal requirement is enforced vigorously.

To reduce infertility caused by treatment also requires holding manufacturers of drugs and devices accountable for the harm caused by their products. Doing so will entail full and fair enforcement of applicable crimi-

nal laws to those involved in developing and marketing injurious products,[25] as well as holding the line against current efforts to limit
manufacturers' civil products liability.[26] Efforts to ensure that manufacturers are not able to use bankruptcy laws to avoid civil liability may prove
equally important.[27]

Surgical Sterilization

Surgical sterilization is another important factor in explaining infertility.[28]
An impressive percentage of those sterilized have later expressed a desire
for more children, while a smaller, though still significant, percentage have
reported they would seek to reverse the procedure if it could be done safely.
Thus, the National Center for Health Statistics reports that in 1982, 26
percent of those who had "chosen" to be sterilized indicated they would
like to have more children. Ten percent responding to the survey indicated
that they would have the procedure reversed if it were possible.[29]

Rooted in the eugenics movement that developed with liberal and pro-
gressive support at the turn of the century, sterilization abuse has had a
long and unfortunate history in this country. By the 1930s, thirty states
had adopted laws authorizing sterilization of certain criminals and those
considered mentally incompetent.[30] In the early 1970s, an estimated 100,000
to 150,000 women were sterilized annually under federally funded programs.[31] Revelations of sterilization abuse in the 1970s involved both health
care providers and government officials. Certain Southern doctors required
poor black patients to submit to sterilization as a condition of receiving
medical assistance with pregnancy and childbirth.[32] Public hospitals in
California obtained consent for sterilization procedures from Mexican-
American women while they were in labor.[33] A 1972 study by Planned
Parenthood indicated that 94 percent of the obstetrician-gynecologists surveyed favored compulsory sterilization or withholding of welfare support
for additional children born to recipients of public assistance.[34] Particularly
shocking abuses by government officials involved threats of terminating
welfare benefits to force two young Alabama girls to accept sterilization.[35]
Involuntary sterilization in recent years has been the product of misinformation as well as of explicit coercion. One study reported, for example,
that 59 percent of the sterilized Hispanic women interviewed did not know
the procedure was irreversible.[36]

Preventing unwanted sterility will require effective informed-consent
procedures, accompanied by effective monitoring mechanisms to ensure
that reproductive choice is preserved. Like the informed-consent provisions
applicable in other medical matters, informed-consent standards for sterilization must guarantee access to adequate information and ensure sufficient opportunity to consider it. New York City's health and hospital
regulations, later enacted into law by the New York City Council, are a

helpful model. These regulations require, among other things, a thirty-day waiting period and a minimum age of twenty-one, and stipulate that the patient not be hospitalized at the time consent is given. Stringent monitoring of these providers has been important in the regulations' implementation.[37]

Environmental and Workplace Hazards

Toxins in living and work environments have also been linked to infertility.[38] Although research to date has been inadequate to quantify the risks posed by such hazards, the Office of Technology Assessment has already identified eight metals, twenty-four groups of chemicals, and five types of undefined industrial exposures that may affect reproductive health. Four health hazards—ionizing radiation, lead, ethylene oxide, and dibromochloropropane—have been regulated at least in part because of their effects on the reproductive system.[39] Greater exposure to environmental hazards is one of the factors offered to explain the higher rate of infertility experienced by black couples.[40]

Expanding our understanding of these factors is a crucial first step in controlling them. Additional research is obviously essential to taking that step. But even to undertake that research, it will be necessary to disabuse ourselves of the conviction that women are entirely responsible for reproduction and that the fetus is always hypersusceptible. Without an appreciation of the male role in reproduction and its vulnerability, hazards will continue to be minimized or ignored unless they endanger pregnant women, and sex-based "fetal protection" policies that exclude women of child-bearing age from the workplace are likely to remain the sole response to the problem. Often based on preliminary, inconclusive, and sometimes speculative information,[41] such policies have a harsh impact on women.[42]

With a changed perception of the problem, it will become possible to enact and enforce legal provisions barring discriminatory worker-exclusion policies and requiring those responsible to make work and living environments safe for persons of both sexes. As a long-term goal, such changes could include amendment of federal laws regulating workplace health and safety and the use of toxic substances, and prohibiting employment discrimination to clarify and expand existing protections so as to ensure complete protection of all workers. More immediate efforts might appropriately be aimed at enacting legislation on the state and local level to develop workable models that could then be implemented more broadly.[43]

Lack of Prenatal and Neonatal Care

Infertility as it is generally understood extends beyond the technical definition used by demographers. People who are unable to conceive children, who are unable to carry children, and whose infants are unable to sustain life are all equally of concern. It is no secret that maternal and infant mortality in the United States far exceeds that in other industrialized countries. It has recently been reported, for example, that

> the U.S. infant mortality rate is almost twice the rate of Finland, Japan and Sweden; the maternal mortality rate is 60–70 percent higher than in Canada and most Scandinavian countries and the percentage of newborns weighing under 2500 g. . . . is twice as high in the United States as in Norway.[44]

The link between those rates and health care is well documented.[45] Yet, as has also been reported recently, the crazy quilt of programs and policies by which maternity care is provided in the United States leaves a substantial number of expectant mothers without services. Thus, more than half a million women who give birth each year (representing 15 percent of the annual births) lack private or public insurance coverage.[46]

Addressing the problem of infertility fully, then, must include massive efforts to make adequate prenatal and neonatal care available. This is, of course, primarily a question of allocating the necessary resources and seeing that they are distributed in an effective, nondiscriminatory manner.[47] Such efforts may take a variety of forms. They may, for example, be part of an overall effort to ensure access to comprehensive health care services as part of a state or national health plan,[48] or they may be targeted directly at mothers and infants.[49] Making the necessary services available, however, may require eliminating legal constraints on midwives and other care providers who meet consumer preferences in a cost-effective way.[50]

Postponed Child-Bearing

Medical researchers have devoted considerable attention to the connection between a woman's age and her fertility. Although there is some disagreement over the specifics, the fact that a woman's fertility declines with age is now well established.[51] Researchers and policymakers may not, however, adequately appreciate the connection between women's opportunities and the difficulties they experience in handling work and family responsibilities in the face of current social arrangements. Addressing infertility due to delay in child-bearing may thus require more basic societal reorganization. Many women, correctly perceiving the difficulties posed by the lack of child care facilities and the continuing division of labor along gender lines, postpone having children until an age at which they are more likely to experience difficulty conceiving and bearing children.

If we are to reduce infertility due to postponed child-bearing, it may thus be necessary for us to think in terms of basic societal changes as well as conventional public health initiatives.[52] Evening out child-rearing responsibilities may reduce the pressure somewhat, but more fundamental changes to allow the integration of family and work life will probably be required to affect behavior patterns significantly. Shorter and more flexible work hours, more generous leave policies, and high-quality child care options near the home and at the place of work must become a reality. Antidiscrimination laws[53] and mandated nurturing leaves[54] may provide sticks, while tax benefits and governmental subsidies[55] may provide carrots to bring such changes about.

ADDRESSING THE PAIN OF INFERTILITY

There are, then, clear and sensible steps that we can take to address the physical causes of infertility. But more should be done to address the social pain of infertility. To the extent that that pain is due to a sense that one has failed at a task that should come naturally and easily to any living being, we must combat that cultural expectation. To the extent that it is due to a sense of missing out on the experience of caring for children through thick and thin, we must make plain that adoption, foster care, stepparenthood, and numerous less formal arrangements offer equivalent possibilities. And to the extent that it is due to the inability to make contact with children in a social world organized around nuclear families, we must open up the opportunities to be aunts, uncles, godparents, special friends, and honorary kin by fostering an inclusive, rather than an exclusive, notion of family.

CONCLUSION

In challenging our assumptions about family and parenthood, the case of *Baby M* has already proved both important and fascinating. It has succeeded in drawing our attention and sympathy to the pain of infertility. Its most important legacy, however, may be the motivation it has given us to address that problem in constructive and far-reaching ways.

REFERENCES

1. W. D. Mosher, "Fecundity and Infertility in the United States," *American Journal of Public Health*, 78 (Feb. 1988): 181–82.

2. W. F. Pratt et al., "Infertility—United States, 1982," *Morbidity and Mortality Weekly Reports*, 34 (1985): 197–99. Figures from 1976 suggest that black infertility rates were twice that of whites. S. D. Aral and W. Cates, Jr., "The Increasing Concern with Infertility: Why Now?," *Journal of the American Medical Association*, 78 (Nov. 1983): 2327–31.

3. Mosher, supra note 1.
4. Id.
5. Id.
6. Aral and Cates, supra note 2.
7. U.S. Congress, Office of Technology Assessment, *Infertility: Medical and Social Choices* (1988), 51 (hereafter cited as "OTA, *Infertility*").
8. Aral and Cates, supra note 2.
9. Id.
10. Id.
11. *New York Times*, Oct. 12, 1987, sec. B5. The connection between the appearance of articles about the loss women without children feel and the movement of women into the traditionally male public sphere in the late 1960s and 1970s has probably not been traced. The relationship is worth examining, however, just as the relationship between women's wartime role and the 1950s' cultural emphasis on femininity is worth examining.
12. Aral and Cates, supra note 2; J. Menken et al., "Age and Infertility," *Science*, 233 (1986): 1389–94. Pratt, supra note 2 (sexually transmitted diseases account for an estimated 30 percent of infertility in some high-risk U.S. populations).
13. E. Megary et al., "Infections and Male Fertility," *Obstetrical and Gynecological Scrutiny*, 42 (1987): 283–90.
14. OTA, *Infertility*, supra note 7, at 87.
15. See, e.g., Jane Does 1–4 v. Utah Department of Health, 776 F.2d 253 (10th Cir. 1985) (Utah's parental consent requirement for contraceptive services provided to minors in publicly funded clinics conflicted with Title X of the Public Health Services Act, 42 U.S.C.A. §3100 et seq.); Planned Parenthood Association of Utah, 810 F.2d 984 (10th Cir. 1987) (Utah law requiring providers to obtain written parental consent in order to obtain Medicaid reimbursement for contraceptive services for unemancipated minors violates the federal Medicaid statute); Planned Parenthood v. Heckler, 712 F.2d 650 (D.C. Cir. 1983) (federal regulations requiring Title X-funded family planning services to notify a parent of an unemancipated minor within ten days of providing prescription contraceptives and mandating compliance with all state parental-consent requirements impermissibly conflicts with Title X). For arguments regarding the unconstitutionality of such provisions, see E. Paul and D. Klassel, "Minor's Right to Confidential Contraceptive Services: The Limits of State Power," *Women's Rights Law Reporter*, 10 (Spring 1987): 45–64.
16. In *Kendrick v. Bowen*, (657 F. Supp. 1547 [D.D.C. 1987]), the Adolescent Family Life Act (42 U.S.C. §300z et seq.) was found to constitute an establishment of religion, and the requirement that applicants involve religious organizations was enjoined. Vacating the injunction on direct appeal, the Supreme Court reversed and remanded for a determination as to whether the AFLA is currently being administered impermissibly and, if so, the appropriate remedy. (Bowen v. Kendrick, 57 U.S.L.W. 4818, June 29, 1988.) The teachings of the Family of America's Foundation illustrate the misinformation disseminated by programs funded under the statute. In addition to teaching the ineffective Billings ovulation method of family planning, "because it helps realize that the family is an integral part of the church," FAF taught adolescents that condoms are "a pollution of their own bodies" and were "messy and unnatural," caused "irritations," and were "never" recommended. Brief of the American Public Health Association et al. as Amici Curiae, Bowen v. Kendrick, U.S. Supreme Court, October term, 1987, Nos. 87–253, 87–431, 87–462, 87–775 at 22.
17. See, e.g., Planned Parenthood Affiliates of California v. Van de Kamp, 226 Cal. Rpt. 361 (Cal. App. 1986), app. den. (state attorney general's interpretation of

Child Abuse Reporting Law as requiring reporting to the state of all adolescents under fourteen seeking reproductive health care violates privacy guarantee in California state constitution).

18. See, e.g., W. Keye, "Strategy for Avoiding Iatrogenic Infertility," *Contemporary OB/GYN,* 19 (March 1982): 185–95.

19. S. Musaker, J. Garcia, and H. Jones, "Experience with Diethylstilbestrol-Exposed Infertile Women in a Program of in Vitro Fertilization," *Fertility & Sterility,* 42 (1984): 20–24.

20. OTA, *Infertility,* supra note 7, at 67–68.

21. See id.: 73–74.

22. Consideration should perhaps be given to developing legislation similar to New York's Public Health Law §2404, McKinney's 1988 Supplement, mandating the commissioner of health to develop an informed-consent standard that specifies all forms of treatment for use in obtaining consent in breast cancer cases.

23. See, e.g., Bill A.3821, now before the New York State Legislature, which would mandate reporting of hospitals' Cesarean rates.

24. See J. Gallagher, "Fetus as Patient," in S. Cohen and N. Taub, eds., *Reproductive Laws for the 1990s* (forthcoming) [hereafter cited as *"Reproductive Laws"*].

25. See, e.g., "Professor Is Charged with Lying for Maker of Birth Control Device," *New York Times,* March 4, 1988, sec. A1.

26. See, e.g., H. R. 1115, "The Uniform Product and Safety Act," now pending in Congress. H. R. 1115 would eliminate all existing and future state grounds for recovery by victims of defective products and replace them with four narrowly tailored state grounds. The bill would also add several new federal defenses and immunities, permit states to develop additional protections, and limit the availability of punitive damages.

27. Serious questions have been raised, for example, about the use of Chapter 11 bankruptcy proceedings by the A. H. Robins Company to limit its liability for the injuries suffered by users of the Dalkon Shield. See "Women Urged to Reject Robins Plan," *Washington Post,* May 3, 1988, sec. C3; "A Legal and Medical Tangle," *Washington Post,* May 4, 1988, sec. B3.

28. In 1982, 9.4 million single women and couples reported that they had "elected" to be sterilized. S. Henshaw and S. Singh, "Sterilization Regret among U.S. Couples," *Family Planning Perspectives,* 18 (Sept./Oct. 1986): 238.

29. Id.

30. P. Friedman, *The Rights of Mentally Retarded Persons* (1976), pp. 115–16.

31. Relf v. Weinberger, 372 F. Supp. 1196, 1199 (D.D.C. 1974).

32. Walker v. Pierce, 560 F.2d 609 (4th Cir. 1977).

33. Madrigal v. Quilligan, U.S. Dist. Ct., C.D., Calif., No. CV-75–2057-JNC (June 30, 1978).

34. *Family Planning Digest,* 1 (Jan. 1972): no. 1 p. 3.

35. *Relf v. Weinberger,* supra note 31.

36. A. Clarke, "Subtle Forms of Sterilization Abuse: A Reproductive Rights Analysis," in R. Arditti, R. D. Klein, and S. Minden, eds., *Test-Tube Women* (1984), 195.

37. See Rodriguez-Trias, "A Model for Advocacy from Proposal to Policy," in *Reproductive Laws,* supra note 24.

38. U.S. Congress, Office of Technology Assessment, *Reproductive Health Hazards in the Workplace* (1985).

39. OTA, *Infertility,* supra note 7, at 69.

40. Id.: 51.

41. See, e.g., Brief Amicus Curiae on Behalf of the American Public Health As-

sociation et al., International Union, UAW v. Johnson Controls, U.S. Ct. App., 7th Cir., No. 88–1308.

42. See J. Bertin, "Reproductive Hazards in the Workplace," in *Reproductive Laws*, supra note 24.

43. Id.

44. *Blessed Events and the Bottom Line: Financing Maternity Care in the United States*, A Study by The Alan Guttmacher Institute, 1987, p.2.

45. See, e.g., U.S. Congress, Office of Technology Assessment, *Healthy Children: Investing in the Future* (1988).

46. See, e.g., R. Gold, A. Kenney, and S. Singh, "Paying for Maternity Care in the United States," *Family Planning Perspectives*, 19 (Sept./Oct. 1987): 190–211.

47. Id.

48. See, e.g., "Massachusetts Passes State Health Insurance," *Nation's Health* (May-June, 1988): 1, describing that state's newly enacted plan offering universal health insurance to every citizen in the state.

49. See, e.g., Office of Technology Assessment, *Healthy Children*, supra note 45, discussing, *inter alia*, expansion of Medicaid benefits and federal grants for improving newborn screening.

50. See, e.g., Note, "Childbearing & Nurse-Midwives: A Woman's Right to Choose," *N.Y.U. Law Review*, 58 (1983): 661; and "U.S. Limits Stays of Foreign Nurses," *New York Times*, April 10, 1988, p. 1.

51. See, e.g., OTA, *Infertility*, supra note 7, at 52.

52. N. Wikler and M. Fabe, *Up Against the Biological Clock* (1979).

53. See Abraham v. Graphic Arts Int'l Union, 660 F.2d 811 (failure to provide adequate leave policy having a disparate impact on women violates Title VII of the Civil Rights Act of 1964); De la Cruz v. Tormey, 582 F.2d 45 (9th Cir. 1978) (college's failure to provide day care facilities for students having a disparate impact on women violates Title IX of the Education Act Amendments of 1972).

54. The Family and Medical Leave Act—which is now pending in Congress and which would provide job guarantees for employees of both sexes who take disability (including pregnancy) leaves and/or dependent care leaves—might be a start. See H. R. 925 and S. 249.

55. See, e.g., Select Committee on Children, Youth, and Families, U.S. House of Representatives, *Families and Child Care: Improving the Options* (98th Cong., 2d Sess., Sept. 1984).

CASE REVIEW ESSAYS

The New Jersey Supreme Court
Baby M Decision

THE CASE OF BABY M
Love's Labor Lost

George P. Smith, II

AN EXPRESSION OF LOVE OR
COMMON SENSE?

It has been estimated that in the United States some twenty thousand babies are born through artificial insemination by donor (AID) each year.[1] With the startling new advances in reproductive technology, or what has been termed "collaborative conception,"[2] it is now possible for a child to have up to five "parents": an egg donor, a sperm donor, a surrogate mother who gestates the fetus, and the couple who actually raises the child.[3] What we now face, then—not only in considering the New Jersey Supreme Court's decision *In re Baby M*[4] but in the whole area of the "new" reproductive biology—is, in the words of a popular columnist, a "mess."[5]

Interestingly, the enormity of this complex, multiparent scenario—which seems to be on its way to becoming a reality with *Baby M* and its anticipated progeny—was totally lost on Mary Beth Whitehead. "I just can't see how four people loving [Baby M], five people loving her, can hurt her,"[6] she said recently. Ms. Whitehead's rather simplistic response to this "love scenario" was perhaps underscored by an equally legerdemanic New Jersey Supreme Court. The court called upon the parties to let their "undoubted love" and "good faith" settle the vexatious issue of visitation "in the best interest of the child."[7] To be effective, law must operate within a rational structure and not a vortex of sentimentality.[8]

More than love is needed to settle this dilemma; common sense—devoid of exaggerated emotionalism and imbued with an appreciation of hard facts and realities—is required. For example, how will the court draw up or supervise the complicated arrangements to share the child, arrange visits with her, and see that her needs are placed above those of the party litigants? How can the court gauge the attitudes of Ms. Whitehead's two sons, aged twelve and thirteen, toward their new half-sister? To what extent will Ms. Whitehead's divorce and her new marriage to Mr. Gould confuse Baby

M and her sense of identity? Will exposure to Ms. Whitehead's parents add an unsettling dimension to the child's "best interests"?

Finally, how will Baby M be affected by the legions of inquiring journalists who will be following this lead story over the years, as she moves through childhood and into the stresses of adolescence? The ABC television network's recent production of "Baby M"[9] will surely be playing the rerun circuit as Baby M Stern grows older, with updates on how she is relating to her two sets of parents. Given Ms. Whitehead's background and temperament, front-page news stories about her "struggles" to visit her child (and possibly to revise the custody decree) can be anticipated over the years ahead—and this, all in the "best interests" of the child! Instead of promoting tranquility, the judiciary has agreed to preside over an "obvious human muddle" that will preserve the current "emotional shambles" for years to come.[10]

Parental Fitness

The trial court did not find Ms. Whitehead to be an "unfit mother"[11]; indeed, it recognized her as a "good mother to her [two previous] children."[12] Yet her numerous failings of character (i.e., domineering attitude, impulsiveness, dishonesty, selfishness, and insensitivity),[13] together with her financial instability, the modest employment opportunities of her husband, and his alcoholism, combined to create a "vulnerable household."[14] The court concluded that in it "the prospects for a wholesome independent psychological growth and development would be at serious risk."[15]

Although the court acknowledged that Ms. Whitehead was capable of showing love and affection for Baby M,[16] this—in itself—was insufficient to vitiate the weaknesses of the Whitehead household. As the New Jersey Supreme Court concluded correctly, the application of the best-interest test "boils down" to a judgment call regarding the "likely future happiness of a human being."[17]

What I find disconcerting—given the tone of this analysis by the court—is the insistence that visitation rights should be considered for Ms. Whitehead. Factors judged undesirable and a threat to Baby M's "likely future happiness" when considering custody rights should also be of importance when considering visitation rights. The long-range influence and impact of Ms. Whitehead's contact with Baby M will be devastating for the child's psychosocial development.

The Supreme Court of New Jersey appears to be mystically devoted to the "sacredness" of biological motherhood—without a dispassionate and objective examination of the totality of the circumstances that give rise to it and the "benefits" of allowing it to continue and develop through visitation.

Toward a New Right of Familial Procurement

The courts have slighted or even refused to recognize the mental elements of procreation. Rather, they consider the biology of reproduction dominant over the psychology and, indeed, have traditionally given little consideration to the motivations of initiating parents.[18] Thus, as might be expected, final decisions in surrogacy cases have failed to include accurate assessments of either the child's best interests or of adequate care for the child.[19] Adequate care should be but a complement to best interests, not a separate standard. With this approach, the "mentally conceiving" (or "initiating") parents would be recognized, of necessity, as holding the priority of right to raise the child,[20] without extra-custodial visitation rights from the birthing mother. Admittedly, before this approach could be validated, a new right of "familial procurement" would have to be structured. Judicial protection of the choice to procreate[21] would be recognized as but a logical analogue to the "recognition of a fundamental interest in procuring assistance to overcome a personal inability to procreate."[22] Absent the wide acceptance of this new or coordinate right, the best-interests test must, however, remain controlling.

Determining Best Interests

How should the test for the best interests of the child be developed and—for that matter—applied? Obviously, the test is fact-sensitive and defies a uniform standard of application. Yet a core set of factors may reasonably be employed to test the extent to which the best interests of the disputed child would be advanced in a given environment.[23] These are: the economic, physical, mental, social, psychological, or ethical harm that would befall or threaten the infant in either family; the social values that would be reinforced or impaired with placement of the child in either family; the suitability of the character of the opposing parties; the economic or social burden that custodial or visitation rights would impose on the parties *and* on the infant; and the practicability of the ultimate action (i.e., the ease of enforcement if the parties are in different jurisdictions).[24]

Middle-class standards should never be considered a handicap or a negative value for a court to consider in determining who can give a child the most adequate care, which, in turn, will ensure that its best interests are advanced. Parents with good educations, attractive jobs, and financial security should—in the normal course of affairs—be able to afford a child better care and better opportunities for growth than would a less advantaged family. It really is that simple.

If the goal of law is to maximize the welfare or utility of all human beings, a prima facie case could be posited for according children some measure of legal protection against their parents or those who would assert custodial rights.[25] Efficiency, emotional stability, and security are minimal investments for a child's development.[26]

A JUDICIAL QUANDARY

New Jersey Chief Justice Wilentz expressed fear about the long-term negative psychological impact of surrogacy on the child, the natural mother, the natural father, and the adoptive mother. His solution was to hold surrogacy contracts for money invalid and unenforceable. Yet by condoning visitation rights for Ms. Whitehead, the chief justice has given the traumas permission to build. The Sterns' parental authority will surely be undermined, and the stability and security the child so desperately needs will be jeopardized.[27]

It was for these very reasons that Baby M's guardian ad litem—relying on the testimony of a number of her experts—recommended that Ms. Whitehead's visitation rights be suspended, with a re-evaluation after five years. Subsequently, without further expert testimony, she revised her position and argued that visitation should be suspended until the child attains majority. The court opined that the testimony of the guardian's experts was undeveloped on the issue of visitation, "really derivative of their views about custody and termination." Thus it decided that the kind, the conditions if any, and the circumstances of visitation should be determined on remand.[28]

Seeking a Unity of Understanding

The New Jersey Supreme Court failed to consider surrogacy, the termination of parental rights, and custody and visitation rights as complementary or even inextricably linked issues. Rather than combining the testimony and other evidentiary proofs into one unified approach to the problem, the court segmented the proofs and did not build upon them. Such a synthesis would have avoided the confusion surrounding a "new" application and development of the best-interest test for visitation rights.

The child's adequate care and best interest are the paramount issues. There should be a unity of understanding on this point. Children have an interest not only in their legitimation (whether or not the surrogacy is validated) but also in the extent of their parents' custody and visitation rights. Courts must seek, when presented with cases such as Baby M, to achieve the proper balance of competing interests among the parents and the child. While it may well be "desirable for the child to have contact with both parents,"[29] the issue must be settled by application of the standard of reasonableness—not by a "standard" of emotionalism. If the court had employed this principle, it would have upheld Dr. Stern's adoption of Baby M, not overturned it.

My argument is simple and straightforward: the court should have realized that the evidentiary considerations and judicial analysis it used in awarding custody to Mr. Stern also supported the termination of Ms. Whitehead's parental rights altogether and the foreclosure of visitation until the child attained majority.

The court recognized the controlling mandate of the New Jersey statutes that premise such drastic action on a showing of "forsaken parental obligation" and either a "continuous neglect or failure to perform the natural and regular obligations of care and support of a child."[30] The caselaw shows that the health and development of a child must be at risk of serious impairment by a continuation of the parental relationship before termination will be ordered.[31]

It is a common canon of statutory interpretation that statutes should be construed liberally so as to promote the ends of justice.[32] Here, justice clearly demands assurance that the child's health and development will not be jeopardized or compromised. It is not an improper crossover or linkage to urge the courts to recognize this fundamental ideal. They should endeavor to develop and apply *uniformly* the test for the best interests of the child to cases involving termination of parental rights, custody, visitation, and the validity of surrogacy contracts.

The major—if not the sole—task for contemporary judges is to avoid the infusion of extra-constitutional *moral* and *political* norms into their deliberations. Rather, they should seek to translate the legislative morality of a questioned statute into a *practical* rule[33]—i.e., reasonable implementation of the best-interests test. This should be the standard by which pertinent statutes in this field as well as general policy issues should be determined by the courts.

There is an obvious need to reform existing law in order—depending upon one's persuasion—to accommodate or to forbid artificial conception. More fundamental, however, is the need to equip the legal system to deal adequately now and in the future with the vexatious *human* problems entailed by the new reproductive technologies.[34]

STRUCTURING A NEW FRAMEWORK

Since surrogate parenting is the biological counterpart of artificial insemination by donor (AID)—with the surrogate being thus equivalent to the semen donor—one might hope that the current laws controlling AID would provide a basis for regulating parenthood arrangements in surrogacy. Such is not the case, however.[35]

Existing statutory distinctions allow AID donors to be paid for sperm but deny payment to surrogate mothers. They thus may well be challenged as an unconstitutional denial of equal protection.[36] Further distinction might be found in separating cases

> involving surrogating practices when there will be no genotypical relationship between the child and the individuals seeking its procreation and those cases in which a womb is "borrowed" to carry a child conceived by persons who will be the biological parents and who propose to integrate fully the child into their family.[37]

Twenty-three jurisdictions currently prohibit financial compensation to surrogates, except for certain specific expenses, under state adoption laws.[38] A Michigan court has ruled payment to a surrogate based upon a contract to perform services invalid, deeming it a contract to sell a baby.[39] The Kentucky Supreme Court reached the opposite conclusion, based on constitutional grounds. It reasoned that surrogacy was not baby-selling, because the biological father had already established a legal relationship with the child.[40]

Legislative Reforms

State legislatures are currently considering a number of proposals to legalize and/or regulate surrogate motherhood.[41] In its 1988 mid-year meeting, the Family Law Section of the American Bar Association approved a Model Surrogacy Act that not only makes surrogacy contracts enforceable but also destroys the common-law presumption that the woman who bears a child is its legal mother. The model act approves a range of payments to the surrogate mother, from $7,500 to $12,500.[42]

Outlawing surrogacy and creating stringent enforcement mechanisms would have the obvious effect of forcing a powerful black market to develop—particularly since the process of becoming a surrogate mother is not an exceptionally difficult one to master. A ban on surrogate motherhood in all forms would also be difficult and distasteful to enforce. Many enforcing agents might find it awkward to exact a penalty from a woman for becoming a mother, or to impose a prison sentence on those who promoted the pregnancy's advancement and implementation. Such measures would be offensive to basic public policy, which recognizes the family as the bulwark of society.[43]

A second approach would be for states to structure a licensing procedure for surrogacy. Such a program would seek to protect the health and well-being of the child, together with the safety of the surrogate. It would define the contracting parents' rights and determine the extent of their potential liabilities as well as define the responsibilities of any intermediaries (doctors, lawyers, or family friends). A licensing board empowered to set, enforce, and implement standards could make any necessary administrative decisions.[44]

Any comprehensive regulatory approach should have as its goal the greater protection of the children born with the new reproductive technologies.[45] Some have suggested that nothing less than a *new framework* is necessary, in order to correct the growing incoherence of legal mismatching by the courts that gives every indication of worsening as more and more "crafted," fact-sensitive opinions are made.[46]

The dilemma we face is that a legislative framework for surrogacy may cause the number of such arrangements to increase alarmingly, with the risk that—absent statutory organization of the area—our chief goal of protecting the children will suffer. Because of the political volatility of the issue, proposals to validate surrogacy contracts or to provide for their execution by legislation may meet strong opposition.[47]

In the absence of a controlling statute, the courts should take an expansive view of the elements of adequate care as a complement to maintenance and promotion of the child's best interests and furthermore, when possible, steer clear of making custodial decisions on the basis of contract theory.[48]

Toward a Delicate Balance

Although I find nothing abhorrent about the development of legislation validating surrogate contracts, I find greater comfort in having the courts seek a reasonable balance of competing interests in determining where the disputed child's best interests truly lie. The framework for principled decision-making that I have posited is more adaptable to the needs of equity than is contract law. Granted, a contract is the memorialization of the participating parties' intent and their operative standard of reasonableness. Yet flexibility must be assured, which can only be accomplished by applying the test for the best interests of the child, guided by rationality instead of emotionalism.

In the final analysis, the question remains: How can we achieve a balance between the benefits that the new reproductive technologies offer infertile couples and the risks of abuse inherent in the "solution"? This problem can only be addressed "when society decides what its values and objectives are in this troubling, yet promising area."[49]

References

1. Lori Andrews, *New Conceptions* (New York: Ballantine, 1984).

2. John Robertson, "Procreative Liberty and the Control of Conception, Pregnancy and Childbirth," *Virginia Law Review*, 69 (1983): 405, 424–26.

3. Lori Andrews, "The Stork Market: The Law of the New Reproductive Technologies," *American Bar Association Journal*, 70 (1984): 50, 56; see Smith, "Intimations of Life: Extracorporeality and the Law," *Gonzaga Law Review*, 21 (1986): 395.

4. In re Baby M, 14 Fam. L. Rep. (BNA) 2007 (1988).

5. Goodman, "In the Swirl of Surrogacy," *Washington Post*, Feb. 6, 1988, sec. A23.

6. Id.

7. *Baby M*, supra note 4, at 2027; William and Elizabeth Stern agreed to seek an out-of-court settlement on visitation rights for Ms. Whitehead. She, in turn, agreed to start using the Sterns' name for the child, Melissa, rather than continuing to use the name she had chosen, Sara. "Couple Seeks Agreement on Baby M Visits," *Washington Post*, Feb. 14, 1988, sec. A9.

8. R. Posner, *Economic Analysis of Law*, 2d ed. (Boston: Little, Brown, 1977), 190.

9. "Couple," supra note 7.

10. Goodman, supra note 5.

11. In re Baby M, 217 N.J. Super. 313, 525 A.2d 1128 (N.J. Super. Ct. Ch. Div. 1987).

12. *Baby M*, supra note 4, at 2019.

13. Id.: 2023.

14. Id.

15. Id.: 2024.

16. Id.: 2023.

17. Id.: 2024; see, gen., J. Goldstein, A. Freud, and A. Solnit, *Beyond the Best Interests of the Child* (New York: Free Press, 1973).

18. Note, "Redefining Mother: A Legal Matrix for New Reproductive Technologies," *Yale Law Journal*, 96 (1986): 187, 194, 195.

19. Id.: 206.

20. Id.: 208, n. 1.

21. Griswold v. Connecticut, 381 U.S. 479 (1965).

22. Note, "Redefining Mother," supra note 18, at 198, 199; See Walter Wadlington, "Artificial Conception: The Challenge for Family Law," *Virginia Law Review*, 69 (1983): 465, 508–9.

23. *Restatement (second) of Torts* §§827(a), 828(a) (1977).

24. Id.: §§827(a), 828(a).

25. Posner, supra note 8, at 111.

26. Id.: 117.

27. *Baby M*, supra note 4, at 2018.

28. Id.: 2026.

29. Id.

30. Id.: 2013.

31. Id., citing New Jersey Div. of Youth & Family Servs. v. A. W., 103 N.J. 591 (1986).

32. Llewellyn, "Remarks on the Theory of Appellate Decision and the Rules or Canons about How Statutes Are to Be Construed," *Vanderbilt Law Review*, 3 (1950): 395, 402.

33. R. Bork, "Tradition and Morality in Constitutional Law," Francis Boyer Lec-

ture on Public Policy (Washington, D.C.: American Enterprise Institute, December 1984), 3, 11.

34. Wadlington, supra note 22, at 467. See Smith, "Procreational Autonomy v. State Intervention: Opportunity or Crisis for a Brave New World?," *Notre Dame Journal of Law, Ethics & Public Policy,* 2 (1986): 635.

35. John Robertson, "Surrogate Mothers: Not So Novel after All," *Hastings Center Report* (Oct. 1983): 28; Smith, "The Razor's Edge of Human Bonding: Artificial Fathers and Surrogate Mothers," *Western New England Law Review,* 5 (1983): 639, 649. See also Chief Justice Wilentz's distinction in *Baby M,* supra note 4, at 2021.

36. Coleman, "Surrogate Motherhood: Analysis of the Problems and Suggestions for Solutions," *Tennessee Law Review,* 50 (1982): 71, 81–82. For a more complete historical analysis of the AID cases, see Smith, "Through a Test Tube Darkly: Artificial Insemination and the Law," *Michigan Law Review,* 67 (1968): 127; Wadlington, "Artificial Insemination: The Dangers of a Poorly Kept Secret," *Northwestern University Law Review,* 64 (1970): 777.

37. Wadlington, supra note 22, at 502.

38. See, e.g., Ala. Code §26–10–8 (1977); Ariz. Rev. Stat. Ann. §8–126(c) (1974); Cal. Penal Code §273(a) (West 1970); Colo. Rev. Stat. §19–4–115 (1986); Del. Code Ann. tit. 13 §928 (1981); Fla. Stat. Ann. §63.212(1)(b) (West Supp. 1983) (exempts stepparents); Ga. Code Ann. §74–418 (Supp. 1984); Idaho Code §18–1511 (1979); Ill. Rev. Stat. ch. 40 §§1526, 1701, 1702 (1981); Ind. Code Ann. §35–46–1–9 (West Supp. 1984–85); Iowa Code Ann. §600.9 (West 1981); Ky. Rev. Stat. §199.590(2) (Supp. 1986); Md. Ann. Code §5–327 (1984); Mass. Ann. Laws ch. 210 §11A (Michie/Law. Coop. 1981); Mich. Comp. Laws Ann. §710.54 (West Supp. 1983–84); Nev. Rev. Stat. §127.290 (1983); N.J. Stat. Ann. §9:3–54 (West Supp. 1984–85) (exempts stepparents); N.Y. Soc. Serv. Law §374(6) (McKinney 1983); N.C. Gen. Stat. §48–37 (1984); Ohio Rev. Code Ann. §3107.10(A) (Baldwin 1983); S.D. Codified Laws Ann. §25–6–4.2 (1984); Tenn. Code Ann. §36–1–135 (1984); Utah Code Ann. §76–7–203 (1978); Wis. Stat. Ann. §946.716 (West 1982). See also, Katz, "Surrogate Motherhood and the Baby Selling Laws," *Columbia Journal of Law & Social Problems,* 20 (1986): 1.

39. Doe v. Kelly, 106 Mich. App. 169, 307 N.W.2d 438 (1981), cert. denied, 459 U.S. 1183 (1983). See, gen., Johnson, "The Baby M Decision: Specific Performance of a Contract for Specially Manufactured Goods," *Southern Illinois University Law Journal,* 11 (1987): 1339, 1342.

40. Surrogate Parenting Assoc., Inc. v. Kentucky, 704 S.W.2d 209 (Ky. 1986).

41. Alexander Capron, "Alternative Birth Technologies: Legal Challenges," *University of California at Davis Law Review,* 20 (1987): 679, 695; Comment, "Surrogate Motherhood Legislation: A Sensible Starting Point," *Indiana Law Review,* 20 (1987): 879, 891–98; Wadlington, supra note 22, at 482–86.

42. Moss, "Guidelines for Surrogacy," *American Bar Association Journal,* 74 (1988): 137. See also "Model Human Reproductive Technologies and Surrogacy Act: An Act Governing the Status of Children Born Through Reproductive Technologies and Surrogacy Arrangements," *Iowa Law Review,* 72 (1987): 1015.

43. Smith, "Razor's Edge," supra note 35, at 662, 663. See Smith and Iraola, "Sexuality, Privacy and the New Biology," *Marquette Law Review,* 67 (1984): 63. See, gen., Erickson, "Contracts to Bear a Child," in G. Smith, ed., *Ethical, Legal and Social Challenges to a Brave New World* (New York: Associated Faculty Press, 1982), 98.

44. Smith, "Razor's Edge," supra note 35, at 663; see Bitner, "Womb for Rent: A Call for Pennsylvania Legislation Legalizing and Regulating Parenting Agreements," *Dickinson Law Review,* 90 (1985): 227.

45. Wadlington, supra note 22, at 511.

46. Note, "Redefining Mother," supra note 18, at 192. See, gen., Robertson, "Embryos, Families and Procreative Liberty: The Legal Structure of the New Reproduction," *Southern California Law Review*, 59 (1986): 939.

47. Capron, supra note 41, at 697.

48. Id.: 700.

49. *Baby M*, supra note 4, at 2027. See Smith, "The Perils and Peregrinations of Surrogate Mothers," *International Journal of Medicine & Law*, 1 (1982): 325.

SOLOMON WOULD WEEP
A Comment on *In the Matter of Baby M* and the Limits of Judicial Authority

Randall P. Bezanson[1]

In commenting on the New Jersey Supreme Court's decision in the Baby M case, I will focus on the result of the court's decision and what it implies about the limits of judicial power, not on the court's opinion. The reason is that, excepting the court's basic premises, I can find little in the opinion to criticize. My difficulty, instead, is with the premises from which the court approached the case, and what they imply about the capacity of courts to construct legal doctrine on the basis of largely, if not wholly, unexplored social and cultural values. The result reached in the Baby M case—that Mr. Stern is Baby M's legal father and Ms. Whitehead her legal mother—is, in my judgment, surely the worst result possible. That it was indisputably the logical, reasoned, and straightforward result of existing legal concepts of parenthood, adoption, baby-selling, and the like, as the New Jersey court so well opined, is hardly reassuring.

The surrogacy dispute in *Baby M* provided the court with an issue as to which there is *no* law. Existing statutory provisions and common law doctrines are relevant to the surrogacy question only as they are grounded on assumptions about parentage, family, and the reproductive process. But these assumptions are simply irrelevant to the dilemmas posed by surrogacy arrangements, and by many other reproductive technology issues as well. There was no right or wrong answer in the Baby M case, but there is a lesson to be learned. Courts are not equipped to create fundamental social policy. Our society's basic moral and ethical values must be shaped and expressed through the pluralistic legislative process, not in court. The *Baby M* court should have decided *only* the question of Baby M's custody, based on its determination of the child's best interests.

OLD QUESTIONS IN NEW
CONTEXTS

The New Jersey Supreme Court disposed of Baby M's fate with apparent legal ease. It did this by treating the existing statutes, judicial interpretations, and surrounding public policies applicable to baby-selling, adoption, termination of parental rights, and best interests as both applicable and dispositive of the case. In accepting these premises—as the district court did not—the court left in its wake a series of unanswered questions that go to the very basis upon which it made its decision, including the meaning of "mother," the meaning of "parent," and the meaning of "family" in a new social and technological setting.[2] I wish to explore these concepts in this essay—not with the purpose of providing definitions or answers but, rather, with a view toward explaining *why* they are ambiguous in the surrogacy setting, and why the court ought not to have decided them, even by silent implication.

We need not look too deeply into history to understand that technology consistently places old questions in new contexts. Technology usually unsettles settled expectations; it often jars and frightens; it has a way of disorienting us by wresting away our confident assumptions from a simpler past. Occasionally, it forces us to rethink our very moral fabric, or at least to explore our values anew to determine how they apply in wholly unprecedented contexts.

So it is, in my judgment, with surrogacy.[3] Surrogacy is a change—a technological change, in large part—that so departs from the contexts in which our deepest values have been shaped that the issues it presents cannot be addressed without re-examining those values and ascertaining anew their definition and application to current technology. Courts cannot give surrogacy social and legal meaning simply by operating in their usual Aristotelian fashion, applying norms and values drawn from the past and present to current social problems, without remaking the very character of those values. When the limits of existing values—constitutional, cultural, social, and moral—provide no clear guidance, when the very moorings of existing social values have no clear application, courts should not act unless expressly empowered to do so.

The role of these limitations in the surrogacy problem can be expressed through a single example. The example departs from the facts of the Baby M case in order more clearly to make a point that applies to *Baby M* as well, and to focus attention on the rigid and broad holding of the New Jersey Supreme Court with respect to the invalidity of surrogacy arrangements.

Let us assume that a married couple, Mr. and Ms. A, want to have a child and wish the child to be biologically related to them. Mr. and Ms. A can both provide gametes, but Ms. A is medically unable to carry and deliver a child. Mr. and Ms. A therefore contract with Ms. B, who is also married, to have the As' fertilized ovum implanted in Ms. B and borne by her. Mr. and Ms. B both agree to this arrangement, and agree as well to relinquish the resulting child, C, to the As after its birth. After C's birth, Mr. and Ms. B change their mind and want to keep C as their child. The question posed by this situation is, of course, "Who are the parents?"[4]

This question involves a broad array of issues. One set of issues involves, generally, a group of scientific, medical, and ethical problems. For example, should the As' interest in a biologically related child be respected and even encouraged? Is a surrogacy arrangement medically necessary and emotionally advisable? Do all parties to the arrangement appreciate its implications? Even if they do, should we recognize consent in such a situation? And, would the As or the Bs be fit and proper parents for C? This list only begins to suggest the exceedingly complex legal, medical, emotional, genetic, and psychological implications of such arrangements.

There is, however, a set of more fundamental antecedent questions that depend for their answer on basic cultural and moral values rather than on judgments about the implications of such arrangements for the parties to it and for the child. For example, in our case we have no legal or pre-existing social referent for deciding who is the mother. Our experience has always endorsed the unimpeachable premise that the woman who gives birth is the mother—genetically, physiologically, and emotionally. In other words, biology has always provided us with a point of reference on this most basic question, and has allowed us to avoid re-examining the nature and meaning of motherhood from a moral and cultural standpoint.

In our case, however, biology does not answer the question, for both Ms. A, the genetic parent, and Ms. B, who carried the child in her body, are biologically,[5] physiologically, and emotionally related to the child. Without the comforting moorings of our past experience, we have to think beyond biology to determine who is—or to put it more accurately, who *should be*—the mother. The sources often looked to in exploring issues of this kind—history and evolving cultural values[6]—seem unlikely to provide guidance on the wholly new issue of the competing claims of two "biologically" related mothers. For answers, we must look forward, not backward.

The same type of issue is presented with respect to the father, but here we at least have some experience to draw upon. The biological ambiguities of paternity have always existed—although technology is having the opposite effect on paternity by making it possible to be more confident of biological relatedness than we have been in the past. Jurisdictions that have explored the question of paternity have often concluded—through legislation, it should be noted—that biology should not always be determinative. For example, the husband of a woman who gives birth in wedlock is legally presumed to be the father of the child—in our case, Mr. B. would be the presumed father of the child, C—unless the paternity of another is proven by clear and convincing evidence.[7] In other words, our society has decided that Mr. B should be C's father, whether he is biologically related to C or not, with only a narrow exception.[8]

When we begin to appreciate the ultimately obscure, if not ambiguous, nature of parental relationships in cases such as that which I have posited, we begin to appreciate that parenthood is, in the end, largely a construct of the law. The law, in turn, is but a construct of our collective moral, social, and cultural values and attitudes. It should come as no surprise that in other nations and in other cultures the concept of parenthood has been, and is today, very different from our own. It was not, after all, very long ago in Anglo-American law that many of the rights and responsibilities of parenthood, including custody, flowed through the father. Today, many courts give preference in custody determinations to the mother.[9] Whether this rule was right or wrong, or whether today's attitudes are better, is beside the point. The point is that there are no absolutely right answers for all places and times. But there are right places from which such answers emerge, and there are wrong places. Courts are the wrong places for such answers to be developed in the first instance.

I have posited a case that makes my point most easily. It is a case that makes obvious the fundamental ambiguity in the surrogacy setting of our notions of motherhood, fatherhood, and ultimately of "family," itself a culture-bound concept. One might well accept my premises in this case but dispute their application in the Baby M case, for there the historically based biological premise of maternity applies. Yet my case simply illustrates more clearly the point also raised by the Baby M case. Even there, we must come to grips with the meaning of family and parentage in new arrangements that involve from the outset the potential struggle of multiple parties. The Baby M case involved four, not two, participants from the outset, and all surrogacy arrangements involve and require at least two, and perhaps as many as five, knowing and active participants in the creation of a new life. The adjustment of these peoples' potentially conflicting interests, as well as the ascertainment of the resulting child's best interests, simply cannot be resolved through legal concepts that reflect other moral consenses, and whose application is therefore problematic if not altogether irrelevant.

To apply existing law in wooden fashion neither achieves justice nor avoids the underlying moral and cultural problems. Justice is not achieved because justice is a product of moral and cultural consensus, which in this setting does not exist. The moral and cultural problems cannot be escaped by simply applying statutory law, for that law reflects values, even if silently, and thus necessarily imposes them on the future. If a court applies existing law to an unprecedented case, in other words, it evades the imperative that the appropriate institutions address core questions anew. The absence of action leaves intact a set of values that were not the product of any deliberative scrutiny and that would not have been selected were such scrutiny applied.

This is precisely what the New Jersey Supreme Court did. The values the court selected, notwithstanding its protestations to the contrary, were that reproduction by marriage partners and without assistance should be heavily preferred, that biology should conclusively determine parentage, and that the value of biological parentage almost conclusively outweighs the costs to a child of having parentage split from the outset. These are understandable values, but they are far from obviously correct ones.

Setting Limits on Judicial Authority

The New Jersey Supreme Court should not have addressed the Baby M case in such a way as to resolve, even by implication, the parentage and family issues raised by surrogacy. The court simply had no law on which to draw in resolving surrogacy's challenge to our society's moral and cultural view of maternity, paternity, and family. The statutes and common law doctrines dealing with parentage, custody, and the like were not crafted and did not evolve with surrogacy in mind.

Other sources of law—such as the respect accorded by the Constitution and the common law to procreative decisions, family choices, and personal values—provide, as the New Jersey Supreme Court rightly observed, essentially no guidance.[10] For every privacy or liberty claim that one of the parties could make, an equivalent claim could be made by another party. The child's interests are equally incommensurate if they are defined in terms of the privacy interests of the contending parents. Finally, history and evolving cultural values, the sources from which the United States Supreme Court has frequently sought guidance in ruling on procreative and related privacy issues, are largely useless in dealing with surrogacy.[11]

Courts do not, and should not, lightly abdicate authority. They have successfully extended that authority to address the issue of procreative liberty, as the most obvious and contemporaneous example. But the privacy cases, which range from contraception to health care decisions,[12] differ from the surrogacy problem on two grounds. First, in most such cases the Constitution weighs in on one side of the conflict, expressing existing cultural norms with ascertainable historical roots. In other such cases, a countervailing social interest has been established and expressed in relevant and applicable form. In contrast, surrogacy involves directly competing constitutional interests of the same order, with no textual guidance as to their respective weight. The intended parents' claims of privacy and procreative liberty do not have clear textually based priority over the surrogate's claim of procreative liberty and private choice. Moreover, because surrogacy raises fundamental questions about cultural values that have not been explored and that are not resolved in existing statutory policy or common law, there exists no ascertainable social consensus to be added into the equation.

A Preferred Approach to the Baby M Case

It will not do to assert simply that the New Jersey court should not have decided Baby M's fate. The refusal to decide would have constituted a decision, and in any event the court would rightly claim that it had jurisdiction in the case and thus had a clear obligation to decide it. The court, therefore, had to decide the case. But *how*—by what method—should it have been decided?

The court, I feel, could have resolved the dispute while declining to address the surrogacy problems in any way. At the same time it could have exercised the equitable power—often used in custody cases—to do justice in the best interests of *this* child. The decision would not have set any precedent for the validity of surrogacy arrangements nor implied that the child's best interests were governed by legal concepts of parenthood. The court could have stated, in short, that on the *surrogacy* issues there was simply no law to apply and that, given the nature of the issues presented, a court should have no power to create law.

Stripped of the surrogacy issues, the case consists of only a bundle of competing claims to the child, involving the legal forms of parentage, custody, support, visitation, and the like. But the existing body of law on such matters is properly inapplicable. These claims should be resolved as the *result of*, rather than as the reason for, a decision about the child's best interests. The custody decision should, in short, flow from the court's inescapable duty to protect the best interests of the child.

This suggestion carries the implicit assumption that one or more of the competing claimants should be awarded custody. This is not inconsistent with my view of the problems that surrogacy arrangements pose for the courts. Courts seeking to resolve the competing parentage claims of the parties to the arrangement have no ascertainable moral or cultural guide. In contrast, existing law and clear and applicable cultural values do reject the possibility of a court (in the absence of an independent adoption procedure) roaming beyond this limited group to find parents who have no connection to the surrogacy arrangement or whose involvement is incidental only. Adoption, not a judicial custody proceeding, is the place for such matters.

A determination of custody in the child's best interests, as suggested, would be difficult but would not, in its essence, be unfamiliar to a state court that regularly exercises equitable authority in custody cases. In the absence of legislative guidance, future cases would also be resolved on their facts alone.

Such a decision would have at least two salutary effects. It would be more likely to lead to a *result* that is, and appears to be, just to the child. For my part, I would hope that such a decision would not divide Baby M's parentage between two families. Even if that result were reached, however, I would find more satisfying an opinion that explained how it served the *child*'s interests, rather than why the parent's status or conduct dictated the child's fate. Such a decision would also place squarely upon society the duty to shape moral values in regard to surrogacy, and it would not allow indifference or the lack of necessity to serve as an excuse for legislative inattention.

REFERENCES

1. The author is a member of the drafting committee of the Uniform Status of Children of Aided Conception Act, of the National Conference of Commissioners on Uniform State Laws. The views expressed here are those of the author and do not reflect the views of the drafting committee or the Conference.

As part of a seminar offered at the Iowa Law School, a group of law students drafted a "Model Reproductive Technologies and Surrogacy Act" that addresses many of the issues raised by surrogacy arrangements. The Model Act has been published as the "Model Reproductive Technologies and Surrogacy Act," *Iowa Law Review*, 72 (1987): 943.

2. The very ambiguity of the terms "family," "mother," and "father" in the surrogacy context would ordinarily counsel against their use, for the terms themselves carry connotations of our current preconceptions about the applicable legal and social arrangements. I will use them in this essay despite the confusion they engender, however, for I am not prepared to burden this short discussion with a new set of terms.

In the October 1984 issue of *Law, Medicine & Health Care*, Alexander Capron made the terminological point nicely:

> [M]any of the new reproductive possibilities remain so novel that terms are lacking to describe the human relationships they can create. For example:
> ·What does one call the woman who bears a child conceived from another woman's egg? Is she the "carrying mother" (as the British say)? Or the "gestational mother" (which might be a better reminder of the active—and very important—*developmental process* in which she is an essential participant)? . . .
> ·How does one describe the relationship between the husband of a surrogate mother (who has been inseminated by another man's sperm) and the resulting child? Or the relationship between that child and other children born to the surrogate mother?
> In fact, it is not even clear what we should call the area under inquiry. (Alexander Capron, "The New Reproductive Possibilities: Seeking a Moral Basis for Concerted Action in a Pluralistic Society," *Law, Medicine & Health Care*, 12 [1984]: 192.)

3. For the purposes of this essay, I use the term "surrogacy" to include agreements with a person or persons by which a woman agrees to bear a child conceived through assisted reproduction and to relinquish the child to that other person(s) upon the child's birth.

Another definition, which is both more restrictive and more expansive, can be found in the "Model Human Reproductive Technologies and Surrogacy Act," supra note 1, at 952:

> "Surrogacy" or "Surrogacy Arrangement" means any arrangement by which a woman agrees to be impregnated by noncoital means, using either the intended father's sperm or the intended mother's egg, or both, with the intent that the intended parents are to become the parents of the resulting child after the child's birth.

4. See supra, note 2.

5. I am using the term "biologically" in a loose sense, but I intend by it to indicate that both Ms. A, a genetic parent, and Ms. B, who carried the child in her womb and provided it sustenance, protection, and much more, are physically related to the child in clear and unbreakable ways.

6. See Olmstead v. United States, 277 U.S. 438, 478 (Brandeis, J., dissenting); Thornburgh v. American College of Obstetricians & Gynecologists, 106 S. Ct. 2169, 2187 (Stevens, J., concurring); Griswold v. Connecticut, 381 U.S. 479 (1965); Roe v. Wade, 410 U.S. 113 (1973).

7. Uniform Parentage Act sec. 4, 9A Unif. Laws Ann. 587 (1979). The presumption of paternity under the Uniform Act is strong and difficult to overcome. See id., comment to sec. 4; sec. 6–7.

8. Indeed, in cases of assisted reproduction, the paternity of a husband who is known not to be the genetic father is conclusive if he consented to paternity at the time of an insemination. Uniform Parentage Act, sec. 5, 9A Uniform Laws Ann. 587 (1979).

9. See Henry Foster, A "Bill of Rights" for Children (Springfield, Ill.: Thomas, 1974); Hazel Fredericksen and R. A. Mulligan, The Child and His Welfare (San Francisco: Freeman, 1972).

10. See Griswold v. Connecticut, 381 U.S. 479 (1965); Pierce v. Society of Sisters, 268 U.S. 510 (1925); Roe v. Wade, 410 U.S. 113 (1973); Village of Belle Terre v. Boraas, 416 U.S. 1 (1974).

11. See cases cited supra, note 10.

12. See, e.g., Matter of Conroy, 98 N.J. 321, 486 A.2d 1209 (1986); Griswold v. Connecticut, 381 U.S. 479 (1965); Roe v. Wade, 410 U.S. 113 (1973).

APPENDIXES

APPENDIX I

EXCERPTS FROM THE DECISION OF THE
NEW JERSEY SUPREME COURT
IN THE CASE OF BABY M
Delivered by Chief Justice Wilentz

. . . . .

We invalidate the surrogacy contract because it conflicts with the law and public policy of this State. While we recognize the depth of the yearning of infertile couples to have their own children, we find the payment of money to a "surrogate" mother illegal, perhaps criminal, and potentially degrading to women. Although in this case we grant custody to the natural father, the evidence having clearly proved such custody to be in the best interests of the infant, we void both the termination of the surrogate mother's parental rights and the adoption of the child by the wife/stepparent. We thus restore the "surrogate" as the mother of the child. . . .

We find no offense to our present laws where a woman voluntarily and without payment agrees to act as a "surrogate" mother, provided that she is not subject to a binding agreement to surrender her child. Moreover, our holding today does not preclude the Legislature from altering the current statutory scheme, within constitutional limits, so as to permit surrogacy contracts. Under current law, however, the surrogacy agreement before us is illegal and invalid.

. . . . .

II.
Invalidity and Unenforceability
of Surrogacy Contract

We have concluded that this surrogacy contract is invalid. Our conclusion has two bases: direct conflict with existing statutes and conflict with the public policies of this State, as expressed in its statutory and decisional law.

One of the surrogacy contract's basic purposes, to achieve the adoption of a child through private placement, though permitted in New Jersey "is very much disfavored." . . . Its use of money for this purpose—and we have no doubt whatsoever that the money is being paid to obtain an adoption and not, as the Sterns argue, for the personal services of Mary Beth Whitehead—is illegal and perhaps criminal. . . . In addition to the inducement of money, there is the coercion of contract: the natural mother's irrevocable agreement, prior to birth, even prior to conception, to surrender the child to the adoptive couple. Such an agreement is totally unenforceable in private placement adoption. . . . Even where the adoption is through an approved agency, the formal agreement to surrender occurs only *after* birth . . . , and then, by regulation, only after the birth mother has been counseled. . . . Integral to these invalid provisions of the surrogacy contract is the related agreement, equally invalid, on the part of the natural mother to cooperate with, and not to contest, proceedings to terminate her parental rights, as well as her contractual concession, in aid of the adoption, that the child's best interests would be served by awarding custody to the natural father and his wife—all of this before she has even conceived, and, in some cases, before she has the slightest idea of what the natural father and adoptive mother are like.

. . . . .

A. CONFLICT WITH STATUTORY PROVISIONS

The surrogacy contract conflicts with: (1) laws prohibiting the use of money in connection with adoptions; (2) laws requiring proof of parental unfitness or abandonment before termination of parental rights is ordered or an adoption is granted; and (3) laws that make surrender of custody and consent to adoption revocable in private placement adoptions.

(1) Our law prohibits paying or accepting money in connection with any placement of a child for adoption. . . . Violation is a high misdemeanor. . . . Excepted are fees of an approved agency . . . and certain expenses in connection with childbirth. . . .

Considerable care was taken in this case to structure the surrogacy arrangement so as not to violate this prohibition. The arrangement was structured as follows: the adopting parent, Mrs. Stern, was not a party to the surrogacy contract; the money paid to Mrs. Whitehead was stated to be for her services—not for the adoption; the sole purpose of the contract was stated as being that "of giving a child to William Stern, its natural and biological father"; the money was purported to be "compensation for services and expenses and in no way . . . a fee for termination of parental rights or a payment in exchange for consent to surrender a child for adoption"; the fee to the Infertility Center ($7,500) was stated to be for legal representation, advice, administrative work, and other "services." Nevertheless, it seems clear that the money was paid and accepted in connection with an adoption.

The Infertility Center's major role was first as a "finder" of the surrogate mother whose child was to be adopted, and second as the arranger of all proceedings that led to the adoption. Its role as adoption finder is demonstrated by the provision requiring Mr. Stern to pay another $7,500 if he uses Mary Beth Whitehead again as a surrogate, and by ICNY's agreement to "coordinate arrangements for the adoption of the child by the wife." The surrogacy agreement requires Mrs. Whitehead to surrender Baby M for the purposes of adoption. The agreement notes that Mr. *and Mrs.* Stern wanted to have a child, and provides that the child be "placed" with Mrs. Stern in the event Mr. Stern dies before the child is born. The payment of the $10,000 occurs only on surrender of custody of the child and "completion of the duties and obligations" of Mrs. Whitehead, including termination of her parental rights to facilitate adoption by Mrs. Stern. As for the contention that the Sterns are paying only for services and not for an adoption, we need note only that they would pay nothing in the event the child died before the fourth month of pregnancy, and only $1,000 if the child were stillborn, even though the "services" had been fully rendered. Additionally, one of Mrs. Whitehead's estimated costs, to be assumed by Mr. Stern, was an "Adoption Fee," presumably for Mrs. Whitehead's incidental costs in connection with the adoption.

Mr. Stern knew he was paying for the adoption of a child; Mrs. Whitehead knew she was accepting money so that a child might be adopted; the Infertility Center knew that it was being paid for assisting in the adoption of a child. The actions of all three worked to frustrate the goals of the statute. It strains credulity to claim that these arrangements, touted by those in the surrogacy business as an attractive alternative to the usual route leading to an adoption, really amount to something other that a private placement adoption for money.

. . . . .

Baby-selling potentially results in the *exploitation* of all parties involved.
. . . Conversely, adoption statutes seek to further humanitarian goals, foremost
among them the best interests of the child. . . . The negative consequences of baby
buying are potentially present in the surrogacy context, especially the potential for
placing and adopting a child without regard to the interest of the child or the natural
mother.

. . . . .

[(2)] In this case a termination of parental rights was obtained not by proving the
statutory prerequisites but by claiming the benefit of contractual provisions. From
all that has been stated above, it is clear that a contractual agreement to abandon
one's parental rights, or not to contest a termination action, will not be enforced
in our courts. The Legislature would not have so carefully, so consistently, and so
substantially restricted termination of parental rights if it had intended to allow
termination to be achieved by one short sentence in a contract.

Since the termination was invalid, . . . it follows, as noted above, that adoption
of Melissa by Mrs. Stern could not properly be granted.

(3) The provision in the surrogacy contract stating that Mary Beth Whitehead
agrees to "surrender custody . . . and terminate all parental rights" contains no
clause giving her a right to rescind. It is intended to be an irrevocable consent to
surrender the child for adoption—in other words, an irrevocable commitment by
Mrs. Whitehead to turn Baby M over to the Sterns and thereafter to allow termination of her parental rights. The trial court required a "best interests" showing as
a condition to granting specific performance of the surrogacy contract. . . . Having
decided the "best interests" issue in favor of the Sterns, that court's order included,
among other things, specific performance of this agreement to surrender custody
and terminate all parental rights.

Mrs. Whitehead, shortly after the child's birth, had attempted to revoke her
consent and surrender by refusing, after the Sterns had allowed her to have the
child "just for one week," to return Baby M to them. The trial court's award of
specific performance therefore reflects its view that the consent to surrender the
child was irrevocable. We accept the trial court's construction of the contract; indeed
it appears quite clear that this was the parties' intent. Such a provision, however,
making irrevocable the natural mother's consent to surrender custody of her child
in a private placement adoption, clearly conflicts with New Jersey law.

B. PUBLIC POLICY CONSIDERATIONS

The surrogacy contract's invalidity, resulting from its direct conflict with the above
statutory provisions, is further underlined when its goals and means are measured
against New Jersey's public policy. The contract's basic premise, that the natural
parents can decide in advance of birth which one is to have custody of the child,
bears no relationship to the settled law that the child's best interests shall determine
custody. . . .

The surrogacy contract guarantees permanent separation of the child from one
of its natural parents. Our policy, however, has long been that to the extent possible,
children should remain with and be brought up by both of their natural parents. . . . While not so stated in the present adoption law, this purpose remains
part of the public policy of this State. . . . This is not simply some theoretical ideal
that in practice has no meaning. The impact of failure to follow that policy is nowhere better shown than in the results of this surrogacy contract. A child, instead
of starting off its life with as much peace and security as possible, finds itself
immediately in a tug-of-war between contending mother and father. . . .

The surrogacy contract violates the policy of this State that the rights of natural parents are equal concerning their child, the father's right no greater than the mother's. . . . The whole purpose and effect of the surrogacy contract was to give the father the exclusive right to the child by destroying the rights of the mother.

. . . . . .

Under the contract, the natural mother is irrevocably committed before she knows the strength of her bond with her child. She never makes a totally voluntary, informed decision, for quite clearly any decision prior to the baby's birth is, in the most important sense, uninformed, and any decision after that, compelled by a pre-existing contractual commitment, the threat of a lawsuit, and the inducement of a $10,000 payment, is less than totally voluntary. Her interests are of little concern to those who controlled this transaction.

Although the interest of the natural father and adoptive mother is certainly the predominant interest, realistically the *only* interest served, even they are left with less than what public policy requires. They know little about the natural mother, her genetic makeup, and her psychological and medical history. Moreover, not even a superficial attempt is made to determine their awareness of their responsibilities as parents.

Worst of all, however, is the contract's total disregard of the best interests of the child. There is not the slightest suggestion that any inquiry will be made at any time to determine the fitness of the Sterns as custodial parents, of Mrs. Stern as an adoptive parent, their superiority to Mrs. Whitehead, or the effect on the child of not living with her natural mother.

This is the sale of a child, or, at the very least, the sale of a mother's right to her child, the only mitigating factor being that one of the purchasers is the father. Almost every evil that prompted the prohibition of the payment of money in connection with adoptions exists here.

The differences between an adoption and a surrogacy contract should be noted, since it is asserted that the use of money in connection with surrogacy does not pose the risks found where money buys an adoption. . . .

First, and perhaps most important, all parties concede that it is unlikely that surrogacy will survive without money. Despite the alleged selfless motivation of surrogate mothers, if there is no payment, there will be no surrogates, or very few. That conclusion contrasts with adoption; for obvious reasons, there remains a steady supply, albeit insufficient, despite the prohibitions against payment. The adoption itself, relieving the natural mother of the financial burden of supporting an infant, is the equivalent of payment.

Second, the use of money in adoptions does not *produce* the problem—conception occurs, and usually the birth itself, before illicit funds are offered. With surrogacy, the "problem," if one views it as such, consisting of the purchase of a woman's procreative capacity, at the risk of her life, is caused by and originates with the offer of money.

Third, with the law prohibiting the use of money in connection with adoptions, the built-in financial pressure of the unwanted pregnancy and the consequent support obligation do not lead the mother to the highest paying, ill-suited, adoptive parents. She is just as well off surrendering the child to an approved agency. In surrogacy, the highest bidders will presumably become the adoptive parents regardless of suitability, so long as payment of money is permitted.

Fourth, the mother's consent to surrender her child in adoptions is revocable, even after surrender of the child, unless it be to an approved agency, where by regulation there are protections against an ill-advised surrender. In surrogacy, consent occurs so early that no amount of advice would satisfy the potential mother's need, yet the consent is irrevocable.

The main difference, that the plight of the unwanted pregnancy is unintended while the situation of the surrogate mother is voluntary and intended, is really not significant. Initially, it produces stronger reactions of sympathy for the mother whose pregnancy was unwanted than for the surrogate mother, who "went into this with her eyes wide open." On reflection, however, it appears that the essential evil is the same, taking advantage of a woman's circumstances (the unwanted pregnancy or the need for money) in order to take away her child, the difference being one of degree.

In the scheme contemplated by the surrogacy contract in this case, a middle man, propelled by profit, promotes the sale. Whatever idealism may have motivated any of the participants, the profit motive predominates, permeates, and ultimately governs the transaction. The demand for children is great and the supply small. The availability of contraception, abortion, and the greater willingness of single mothers to bring up their children has led to a shortage of babies offered for adoption. . . . The situation is ripe for the entry of the middleman who will bring some equilibrium into the market by increasing the supply through the use of money.

Intimated, but disputed, is the assertion that surrogacy will be used for the benefit of the rich at the expense of the poor. . . . In response it is noted that the Sterns are not rich and the Whiteheads not poor. Nevertheless, it is clear to us that it is unlikely that surrogate mothers will be as proportionately numerous among those women in the top twenty percent income bracket as among those in the bottom twenty percent. . . . Put differently, we doubt that infertile couples in the low-income bracket will find upper income surrogates.

. . . . . .

The point is made that Mrs. Whitehead *agreed* to the surrogacy arrangement, supposedly fully understanding the consequences. Putting aside the issue of how compelling her need for money may have been, and how significant her understanding of the consequences, we suggest that her consent is irrelevant. There are, in a civilized society, some things that money cannot buy. In America, we decided long ago that merely because conduct purchased by money was "voluntary" did not mean that it was good or beyond regulation and prohibition. . . . Employers can no longer buy labor at the lowest price they can bargain for, even though that labor is "voluntary," . . . or buy women's labor for less money than paid to men for the same job, . . . or purchase the agreement of children to perform oppressive labor, . . . or purchase the agreement of workers to subject themselves to unsafe or unhealthful working conditions. . . . There are, in short, values that society deems more important than granting to wealth whatever it can buy, be it labor, love, or life. Whether this principle recommends prohibition of surrogacy, which presumably sometimes results in great satisfaction to all of the parties, is not for us to say. We note here only that, under existing law, the fact that Mrs. Whitehead "agreed" to the arrangement is not dispositive.

The long-term effects of surrogacy contracts are not known, but feared—the impact on the child who learns her life was bought, that she is the offspring of someone who gave birth to her only to obtain money; the impact on the natural mother as the full weight of her isolation is felt along with the full reality of the sale of her body and her child; the impact on the natural father and adoptive mother once they realize the consequences of their conduct. . . .

The surrogacy contract creates, it is based upon, principles that are directly contrary to the objectives of our laws. . . . It guarantees the separation of a child from its mother; it looks to adoption regardless of suitability; it totally ignores the child; it takes the child from the mother regardless of her wishes and her maternal fitness; and it does all of this, it accomplishes all of its goals, through the use of money.

Beyond that is the potential degradation of some women that may result from this arrangement. In many cases, of course, surrogacy may bring satisfaction, not only to the infertile couple, but to the surrogate mother herself. The fact, however, that many women may not perceive surrogacy negatively but rather see it as an opportunity does not diminish its potential for devastation to other women.

In sum, the harmful consequences of this surrogacy arrangement appear to us all too palpable. In New Jersey the surrogate mother's agreement to sell her child is void. . . . Its irrevocability infects the entire contract, as does the money that purports to buy it.

. . . . .

IV.
Constitutional Issues

Both parties argue that the Constitutions—state and federal—mandate approval of their basic claims. The source of their constitutional arguments is essentially the same: the right of privacy, the right to procreate, the right to the companionship of one's child, those rights flowing either directly from the fourteenth amendment or by its incorporation of the Bill of Rights, or from the ninth amendment, or through the penumbra surrounding all of the Bill of Rights. They are the rights of personal intimacy, of marriage, of sex, of family, of procreation. Whatever their source, it is clear that they are fundamental rights protected by both the federal and state Constitutions. . . . The right asserted by the Sterns is the right of procreation; that asserted by Mary Beth Whitehead is the right to the companionship of her child. We find that the right of procreation does not extend as far as claimed by the Sterns. . . .

. . . The right to procreate very simply is the right to have natural children, whether through sexual intercourse or artificial insemination. It is no more than that. Mr. Stern has not been deprived of that right. Through artificial insemination of Mrs. Whitehead, Baby M is his child. The custody, care, companionship, and nurturing that follow birth are not parts of the right to procreation; they are rights that may also be constitutionally protected, but that involve many considerations other than the right of procreation. To assert that Mr. Stern's right of procreation gives him the right to the custody of Baby M would be to assert that Mrs. Whitehead's right of procreation does *not* give her the right to the custody of Baby M; it would be to assert that the constitutional right of procreation includes within it a constitutionally protected contractual right to destroy someone else's right of procreation.

We conclude that the right of procreation is best understood and protected if confined to its essentials, and that when dealing with rights concerning the resulting child, different interests come into play. There is nothing in our culture or society that even begins to suggest a fundamental right on the part of the father to the custody of the child as part of his right to procreate when opposed by the claim of the mother to the same child. We therefore disagree with the trial court: there is no constitutional basis whatsoever requiring that Mr. Stern's claim to the custody of Baby M be sustained. Our conclusion may thus be understood as illustrating that a person's rights of privacy and self-determination are qualified by the effect on innocent third persons of the exercise of those rights. . . .

V.
Custody

Having decided that the surrogacy contract is illegal and unenforceable, we now must decide the custody question without regard to the provisions of the surrogacy contract that would give Mr. Stern sole and permanent custody. (That does not mean that the existence of the contract and the circumstances under which it was entered may not be considered to the extent deemed relevant to the child's best interests.) With the surrogacy contract disposed of, the legal framework becomes a dispute between two couples over the custody of a child produced by the artificial insemination of one couple's wife by the other's husband. Under the Parentage Act the claims of the natural father and the natural mother are entitled to equal weight, *i.e.*, one is not preferred over the other solely because it is the father or the mother. . . . The applicable rule given these circumstances is clear: the child's best interests determine custody.

. . . . . .

The circumstances of this custody dispute are unusual and they have provoked some unusual contentions. The Whiteheads claim that even if the child's best interests would be served by our awarding custody to the Sterns, we should not do so, since that will encourage surrogacy contracts—contracts claimed by the Whiteheads, and we agree, to be violative of important legislatively-stated public policies. Their position is that in order that surrogacy contracts be deterred, custody should remain in the surrogate mother unless she is unfit, regardless of the best interests of the child. We disagree. Our declaration that this surrogacy contract is unenforceable and illegal is sufficient to deter similar agreements. We need not sacrifice the child's interests in order to make that point sharper. . . .

. . . . . .

It seems to us that given her predicament, Mrs. Whitehead was rather harshly judged—both by the trial court and by some of the experts. She was guilty of a breach of contract, and indeed, she did break a very important promise, but we think it is expecting something well beyond normal human capabilities to suggest that this mother should have parted with her newly born infant without a struggle. Other than survival, what stronger force is there? We do not know of, and cannot conceive of, any other case where a perfectly fit mother was expected to surrender her newly born infant, perhaps forever, and was then told she was a bad mother because she did not. We know of no authority suggesting that the moral quality of her act in those circumstances should be judged by referring to a contract made before she became pregnant. We do not countenance, and would never countenance, violating a court order as Mrs. Whitehead did, even a court order that is wrong; but her resistance to an order that she surrender her infant, possibly forever, merits a measure of understanding. We do not find it so clear that her efforts to keep her infant, when measured against the Sterns' efforts to take her away, make one, rather than the other, the wrongdoer. The Sterns suffered, but so did she. And if we go beyond suffering to an evaluation of the human stakes involved in the struggle, how much weight should be given to her nine months of pregnancy, the labor of childbirth, the risk to her life, compared to the payment of money, the anticipation of a child and the donation of sperm?

. . . . . .

We have a further concern regarding the trial court's emphasis on the Sterns' interest in Melissa's education as compared to the Whiteheads'. That this difference is a legitimate factor to be considered we have no doubt. But it should not be overlooked that a best-interests test is designed to create not a new member of the intelligentsia but rather a well-integrated person who might reasonably be expect to be happy with life. "Best interests" does not contain within it any idealized lifestyle; the question boils down to a judgment, consisting of many factors, about the likely future happiness of a human being. . . . Stability, love, family happiness, tolerance, and, ultimately, support of independence—all rank much higher in predicting future happiness than the likelihood of a college education. . . . We do not mean to suggest that the trial court would disagree. We simply want to dispel any possible misunderstanding on the issue.

. . . . .

Conclusion

This case affords some insight into a new reproductive arrangement: the artificial insemination of a surrogate mother. The unfortunate events that have unfolded illustrate that its unregulated use can bring suffering to all involved. Potential victims include the surrogate mother and her family, the natural father and his wife, and most importantly, the child. Although surrogacy has apparently provided positive results for some infertile couples, it can also, as this case demonstrated, cause suffering to participants, here essentially innocent and well-intended.

We have found that our present laws do not permit the surrogacy contract used in this case. Nowhere, however, do we find any legal prohibition against surrogacy when the surrogate mother volunteers, without any payment, to act as a surrogate and is given the right to change her mind and to assert her parental rights. Moreover, the Legislature remains free to deal with this most sensitive issue as it sees fit, subject only to constitutional constraints.

If the Legislature decides to address surrogacy, consideration of this case will highlight many of its potential harms. We do not underestimate the difficulties of legislating on this subject. In addition to the inevitable confrontation with the ethical and moral issues involved, there is the question of the wisdom and effectiveness of regulating a matter so private, yet of such public interest. Legislative consideration of surrogacy may also provide the opportunity to begin to focus on the overall implications of the new reproductive biotechnology—*in vitro* fertilization, preservation of sperm and eggs, embryo implantation and the like. The problem is how to enjoy the benefits of the technology—especially for infertile couples—while minimizing the risk of abuse. The problem can be addressed only when society decides what its values and objectives are in this troubling, yet promising, area.

. . . . .

Appendix II

STATUS OF STATE LEGISLATION PROPOSED OR ENACTED THROUGH OCTOBER 5, 1988

Compiled by Marilyn Adams for the National Conference of State Legislatures, 1050 17th Street, Denver, Colorado 80265, 303/623-7800

During the 1987 legislative sessions, approximately 72 surrogacy bills were introduced in 26 states and the District of Columbia. The bills fall generally into three separate categories: (1) bills that would regulate surrogate contracts, establish standards or make specific provisions for these contracts; (2) bills that would prohibit surrogacy contracts or declare such contracts unenforceable or to be contrary to public policy and null and void; and (3) bills which would establish a task force, interim study committee, joint legislative committee, or commission to study the issue of surrogate parenthood. Several states introduced legislation in more than one category.

In the 1987 sessions, 13 states and the District of Columbia introduced 26 bills that would regulate surrogacy contracts, and 17 states introduced 25 bills that would prohibit surrogacy contracts or declare such contracts null, void and contrary to public policy. Fifteen states also introduced 21 bills to set up study commissions or task forces to study the issues surrounding surrogate motherhood.

During the 1987 sessions, no legislation was enacted to regulate surrogacy contracts. Although Arkansas' bill passed both houses of the Assembly, the Governor vetoed the legislation because it did not provide for a court hearing on the contract. Nevada also passed legislation to amend its adoption statutes. This legislation does not specifically address the issue of regulation of surrogacy contracts or make provisions for those contracts, but it does include a reference to "lawful surrogate contracts," and some analysts have interpreted this statute as permitting surrogacy arrangements. Louisiana passed a law which declares surrogacy contracts null, void, unenforceable, and contrary to public policy. This law, however, does not provide for penalties for violation. In addition, Delaware, Indiana, Louisiana, North Carolina, Rhode Island, and Texas established special commissions to study surrogate motherhood.

Again in 1988, surrogate parenting bills were introduced in a number of state legislatures throughout the country. As of October 5, 16 states had introduced 22 bills to regulate surrogacy; 18 states had introduced, or carried forward from 1987, 31 bills to prohibit these contracts; and nine states were considering establishment of study committees. Of these legislative initiatives, none has passed which would regulate surrogacy contracts.

During the 1988 legislative sessions, several states passed legislation that provides that surrogacy contracts are contrary to public policy and void. Following the "Baby M" decision by the New Jersey Supreme Court, the legislation passed during the 1988 sessions focused on the issue of compensation to the surrogate mothers and to third party surrogate brokers, to make such compensation unlawful.

Florida's preplanned adoption law provides penalties for violation of its provisions, making the violations a felony of the third degree with penalties of imprisonment of up to five years and/or a fine not to exceed $5,000. The Florida bill does not completely prohibit informal surrogacy arrangements, but it does provide that contracts for surrogate parenthood arrangements involving compensation to any party (over and above actual costs and fees for adoption) for the purchase, sale, or transfer of custody or parental rights in connection with any child, or in connection with any fetus yet unborn, are void and unenforceable; however, if a preplanned adoption arrangement is entered into, it must be based upon an agreement containing certain minimum terms. While the contract is not enforceable, the agreement will provide evidence of the parties' intent. Under Florida's new law, surrogate arrangements are defined as "pre-planned adoption arrangements" and the rights of the parties are to be decided pursuant to the Florida Adoption code.

In March, 1988, Indiana passed a law declaring any surrogacy agreement involving compensation to be unlawful, including verbal and unwritten agreements. Any existing surrogacy contract involving compensation over and above actual medical expenses of the surrogate mother is now unenforceable in any court in Indiana. If payment of fees is involved, then violation of the new surrogacy law is a Class D felony punishable by up to two years imprisonment and/or a $10,000 fine. Penalties for violations are set under the child selling statutes. In Indiana, preplanned adoptions are also unlawful and adoption agreements may only be made after the birth of the child. The surrogacy law does not prohibit surrogacy itself but makes contracts involving compensation void and unenforceable in the Indiana courts.

Kentucky also enacted a law making contracts providing for compensation for surrogate mothers and surrogate brokers prohibited and unenforceable. However, according to a spokesperson in the legislative office, if there is no compensation to any party, and no written contract, but simply a verbal agreement, then the surrogacy arrangement would seem to be permitted. Kentucky's surrogacy statute amends KRS 199.590, but penalties for violation are provided in KRS 199.990 under the child selling statutes. Penalties for violations are set at not less than a $500, or more than a $2,000, fine and six months imprisonment, or both.

Michigan's surrogacy bill was signed into law on June 27, 1988. This law makes it a crime to enter into, or assist in the formation of, a surrogate parentage contract for compensation. The law provides penalties for violations of up to five years imprisonment and a maximum $50,000 fine for persons acting as surrogate brokers. It also provides for misdemeanor penalties of a fine of not more than $10,000 or imprisonment for not more than one year, or both, for anyone who engages in a surrogacy contract involving any compensation over and above the actual medical expenses of a surrogate mother or surrogate carrier.

Nebraska's surrogacy law enacted in February, 1988, makes surrogate parenthood contracts void and unenforceable if compensation is involved. Surrogate parenthood contracts are defined as those contracts whereby a woman is compensated for bearing a child of a man who is not her husband. However, the bill does not provide for penalties for violation, and the law does not prohibit surrogacy contracts that do not involve compensation. It does, however, act as a barrier to court enforcement of the provisions of contracts involving compensation should a dispute arise among the parties to the contract. The law does not prohibit the practice of surrogacy itself, and does not provide for a penalty for entering into a surrogacy contract if there is no compensation to any of the parties involved.

In the following summary, bills that have been signed into law, and study resolutions adopted, are indicated by an asterisk (*). The status indicated is based on the latest information available from the bill tracking service (State Net) as of October 5, 1988.

(1) Bills that would prohibit surrogacy contracts

A. Bills enacted:

FL S-9* Same as H-1633. (See also S-29 in previous section.) Relates to preplanned adoption arrangements. Provides that contracts for the purchase, sale, or transfer of custody or parental rights in connection with a child intended to be born of a proposed pregnancy is unlawful. Provides penalties. Provides that parties may enter into a preplanned adoption arrangement and that the arrangement shall be based upon a nonbinding preplanned adoption agreement which shall contain certain terms. 7/1/88: Signed by Governor.

IN S-98* Johnson. (317/232-9400) Establishes a moratorium on the civil enforcement of various provisions of a surrogate agreement. Provides that evidence of a surrogate agreement may not be considered by a court to decide an issue concerning child custody, child visitation, child support, or other related issues absent fraud, duress, or misrepresentation, urges the legislative council to establish a study committee to study aided conception. 1/29/88 To House. To House Committee on Judiciary. 3/5/88: To Governor. Signed by Governor. Title 31, Article 8.

KY BR-219 S-4* Travis. (502/564-8100) Prohibits contracts which would compensate a woman for her artificial insemination and subsequent termination of parental rights to a child born as a result of that artificial insemination; makes void any contracts entered into in violation of such provisions. 3/18/87: Prefiled for 1988. 1/5/88: Introduced. To Senate Committee on Judiciary-Civil. 3/11/88: Signed by Governor. Acts. Chapter 52.

MI S-228* Binsfeld (517/373-2413) Establishes surrogate parentage contracts as contrary to public policy and void; prohibits surrogate parentage contracts for compensation; provides for children conceived, gestated, and born pursuant to a surrogate parentage contract; sets penalties; provides that surrogate and husband are legal parents. 6/9/88: Passed House. 6/9/88: To Governor for signature. 6/27/88: Signed by Governor. Public Act 199 of 1988.

NE LB-674* Chambers. (402/471-2612) Relates to surrogate parenthood contracts; to declare such contracts void and to provide rights and obligations; and to define a term. 1/22/88: Amended on Legislative floor. 2/10/88: Signed by Governor. LB-674.

B. Bills defeated or awaiting further action:

FL H-1633 Committee on Judiciary. Relates to preplanned adoption arrangements. Provides that contracts for the purchase, sale, or transfer of custody or parental rights in connection with a child intended to be born of a proposed pregnancy is unlawful. Provides penalties. Provides that parties may enter into a preplanned adoption arrangement and that the arrangement shall be based upon a nonbinding preplanned adoption agreement which shall contain certain terms. 5/6/88 Introduced.

GA S-421 Kidd. (404/656-5040) Relates to unlawful advertisements and inducements with respect to adoptions, so as to authorize the payment of lost wages or living expenses of an expectant mother during a certain period of pregnancy. 1/29/88: To House. To House Committee on Judiciary.

KS S-620 Winter. (913/296-7364) Renders void and unenforceable agreements for services of a surrogate mother for consideration; renders void agreements for services of surrogate mother without consideration. 3/3/88: Re-referred to Senate Committee on Judiciary.

MD H-1479 Kreamer. (301/858-3289) Establishes that a surrogate mother agreement requiring exchange of consideration is void and against public policy; prohibits a person from procuring, acting as agent for, facilitating or assisting in the carrying out of such an agreement for consideration; authorizes the sister-in-law of a birth father to act as a surrogate mother and accept reasonable compensation for expenses; prohibits court enforcement of oral or written surrogate mother agreements. 3/21/88: From House Committee on Judiciary: Reported unfavorably.

MD S-795 Stone. (301/858-3587) Prohibits a person from being a party to an agreement in which a woman agrees to conceive a child through artificial insemination and agrees voluntarily to relinquish her parental rights; provides a misdemeanor penalty of a fine of up to $10,000, imprisonment of up to one year or both. 3/25/88: To House Committee on Judiciary.

MN H-1701 Rest. (612/296-4176) Makes surrogate mother agreements void and unenforceable as contrary to public policy. Prohibits advertising for persons to act as surrogate mothers and procuring or inducing formation of surrogate mother agreements. 10/12/87: Prefiled. 3/14/88: From House Committee on Judiciary: Do pass as amended.

MN S-1660 Brandl. (612/296-4837) Prohibits surrogate mother contracts and related activities. 2/11/88: Introduced. To Senate Committee on Judiciary.

MS S-2157 Miller. (601/359-3770) Provides that contracts for surrogate motherhood shall be absolutely null, void and unenforceable as contrary to public policy, and to define contracts for surrogate motherhood. 1/19/88: Introduced. To Senate Committee on Judiciary. 3/21/88: To House Committee on Judiciary A. 4/13/88: Rereferred to House Committee on Judiciary A.

NH S-281 Hounsell. (603/271-3420) Prohibits surrogate parenting. 1/26/88: From Senate Committee on Judiciary: Refer to Interim Study. To Interim Study.

NJ A-13 Kavanaugh. (602/292-4840) Prohibits surrogate parenting agreements for consideration as a crime of the third degree. 1/13/88: Introduced. To Assembly Committee on Judiciary.

NY A-10851 Weinstein. (518/455-5462) Declares surrogate parenting contracts void and unenforceable. Prohibits compensation in connection with such contracts except for certain medical and legal fees. Provides for certain rights of birth mothers in legal proceedings. 5/14/88: Introduced. To Assembly Committee on Judiciary.

NY A-8852 Proud. (518/455-4527) Prohibits the practice of surrogate motherhood, whether accomplished by artificial insemination or in vitro fertilization wherein the surrogate mother agrees to surrender the child, regardless of consideration or the lack of it. 1/28/88: Introduced. To Assembly Committee on Judiciary.

NY A-9882 Faso. (518/455-5314) Declares surrogate parenting to be against public policy and makes any agreement or contract providing therefore void and unenforceable. 3/16/88: Introduced. To Assembly Committee on Judiciary.

NY A-11607 Committee on Rules. Defines "surrogate parenting contract" and prohibits its formation. Penalizes violations for arranging or assisting in the formation of such contracts. Makes such contracts void as contrary to public policy. 5/26/88: Introduced. To Assembly Committee on Judiciary.

NY S-6891 Marchi. (518/455-3215) Prohibits the practice of surrogate motherhood, whether accomplished by artificial insemination or in vitro fertilization wherein the surrogate mother agrees to surrender the child. 2/2/88: Introduced. To Senate Committee on Judiciary.

NY S-9134 Marchi. (518/455-3215) Declares surrogate parenting contracts void and unenforceable. Prohibits compensation in connection with such contracts except for certain medical and legal fees. Provides for certain rights of birth mothers in legal proceedings. 7/12/88: Introduced. To Senate Committee on Judiciary.

UT H-201 Atkinson. (801/533-5801) Relates to surrogate parenthood; provides that specified contracts for surrogate parenthood arrangements are null and void; provides a criminal penalty for violation. 1/22/88: Introduced. 2/16/88: Amended on House floor. Failed to pass House.

VA H-237 Melvin. (804/786-6888) Makes contracts for surrogate motherhood unenforceable. 1/21/88: From House Committee on Health, Welfare and Institutions: Reported favorably. To House Committee on Courts of Justice. 3/18/88: Carried over to 1989. In House Committee on Courts of Justice.

WA H-2030 Padden. (206/786-7984) Prohibits surrogate parenting. Nullifies and voids surrogate parenting contracts, written or unwritten and as defined, whether with or without valuable consideration. 2/8/88: Introduced. To House Committee on Health Care.

(2) Bills that would regulate contracts

AZ S-1378 Brewer. (602/255-4136) Includes in articles on adoption various definitions relating to surrogate-parent agreements, and laws on central adoption registry, petition for custody by spouse of natural parent and money paid in connection with adoption. 2/9/88: To Senate Committee on Health and Welfare, then to Committee on Judiciary. 4/14/88: From Joint Committee on Judiciary: Reported favorably.

CT H-6109 Committee on Judiciary. Concerns surrogate parenthood. 3/15/88: Introduced. To Joint Committee on Judiciary.

FL S-29 Frank. (904/487-5075) Creates Surrogate Parenthood Act. Prohibits contracting, procuring, inducing or agreeing to surrogate parenthood arrangement, except as specified. Requires written contract and specifies contract provisions, including provisions for establishing parental rights and responsibility for child support. Restricts certain intestate inheritance. Declares certain contracts void. Prohibits certain implantations of human egg. Provides criminal penalties. 4/5/88: Introduced. To Senate Committee on Judiciary-Civil, then to Senate Committee on Judiciary-Criminal. Died in committee. (See S-9 in section on prohibiting surrogacy contracts.)

GA S-493 Barnes. (404/656-5040) Relates to the parent and child relationship generally, so as to regulate surrogate parenting and the rights, responsibilities, and agreements relating thereto. 1/25/88: Introduced. To Senate Committee on Children and Youth. 2/12/88: Failed to pass Senate.

IA H-2052 Teaford. (515/281-3221) Regulates the practice of surrogate parenting. 1/18/88: Introduced. To House Committee on Human Resources.

IA H-2279 Hammond. (515/281-3221) Regulates the practice of surrogate parenting. 2/19/88: Introduced. To House Committee on Human Resources.

IA SCR-120 Committee on Human Resources. Relates to new reproduction technologies. 3/3/88: Introduced.

IN H-1140 Bayliff. (317/232-9600) Regulates aided conception and reproductive service agreements. Provides for criminal penalties for noncompliance with statutory requirements. Changes references to natural parent, biological parent, and adoptive parent to parent. 1/6/88: Introduced. To House Committee on Judiciary.

MA S-717 Bertanazzi. (617/722-1420) Relates to surrogate motherhood. 1/6/88: Introduced. To Joint Committee on the Judiciary. 5/16/88: Failed to pass Senate.

MD H-649 Athey. (301/858-3469) Sanctions surrogate mother agreements under specified circumstances. Exempts surrogate mother agreements from designated legal presumptions of paternity. Prohibits agreements that do not comply with the Act. Requires agreements to include specified provisions. Establishes parental obligations of a surrogate, a birth father and the spouse of a birth father. Requires the surrogate's written consent relinquishing parental rights. Requires the agreement to be filed with the birth certificate. 1/29/88: Introduced. To House Committee on Judiciary. 3/21/88: From House Committee on Judiciary: Reported unfavorably.

MD S-436 Hoffman. (301/858-3648) Relates to surrogate motherhood; permits an interested party in an adoption matter to pay reasonable expenses associated with the pregnancy of a natural mother if authorized by the court for good cause shown; and requires that the expenses be certified. 3/4/88: To House. To House Committee on Judiciary.

MI H-5725 Honigman. (517/373-1799) Eliminates adoption consent in certain circumstances if paternity has been acknowledged. 6/2/88: Introduced. To House Committee on Judiciary.

MO H-1561 Shear. (314/751-4163) Enacts the "Surrogate Parenting Act." 1/26/88: To House Committee on Judiciary.

NH H-1108 M. Jones. (603/271-2548) Requires probate court approval of surrogate parenting arrangements. 1/6/88: Introduced. To House Committee on Judiciary. 2/17/88: To Interim Study.

NH H-1139 Price. (603/271-2548) Relates to surrogate parenting agreements. 1/6/88: Introduced. To House Committee on Judiciary.

NJ A-593 Haytaian. (609/292-4840) Amends various fees charged by surrogates. 2/1/88: From Assembly Committee on County Governing and Regional Authorities.

NJ A-956 Kern. (609/292-4840) Provides requirements for surrogate parenthood contracts. 1/12/88: Introduced. To Assembly Committee on Judiciary.

NJ S-2468 Costa. (609/292-4840) Provides requirements for surrogate gestation contracts. 5/2/88: Introduced. To Senate Committee on Judiciary.

NY A-5529 Schmidt. (518/455-5668) Prohibits any consideration for a surrogate parenting agreement but permits payments by the intended parents of all reasonable, actual and necessary expenses of the surrogate mother rendered in connection with the birth of the child or incurred as a result of her pregnancy. 1/20/88: Amended on Assembly floor. Recommitted to Assembly Committee on Judiciary.

VT H-549 Fortna. (802/828-2247) Relates to surrogate parenting. 1/5/88: Introduced. To House Committee on Judiciary.

WA H-1529 Braddock. (206/786-7980) Relates to becoming parents. 1/20/88: Introduced. To House Committee on Health Care.

AL H-172 McKee. (205/261-7707) Provides that a contract for surrogate motherhood shall be absolutely null, void, and unenforceable as contrary to public policy. 3/22/88: From Senate Committee on Health: Reported favorably.

AL S-664 Sanders. (205/261-7800) Provides that a contract for surrogate motherhood shall be absolutely null, void, and unenforceable as contrary to public policy. 4/11/88: Introduced. To Senate Committee on Judiciary.

CA A-2403 Longshore. (916/445-7333) Specifies that a biological parent may not voluntarily relinquish the custody and control of his or her child except pursuant to specified procedures for adoption or for the establishment of a guardianship or conservatorship. 1/30/88: From Assembly Committee on Judiciary: Filed with Chief Clerk pursuant to Joint Rule 56. Died.

CA A-2404 Longshore. (916/445-7333) Relates to certain contracts which are contrary to public policy and are void. Includes among those categories of contracts those whereby a woman receives consideration for an agreement to undergo specified prenatal diagnostic testing or procedures for other than stated purposes and those whereby a woman receives consideration for an agreement to abort, or consent to the abortion of, her child. 1/30/88: From Assembly Committee on Judiciary: Filed with Chief Clerk pursuant to Joint Rule 56. Died.

CA A-3200 Mojonnier. (916/445-2112) Provides for criminal sanctions for specified actions relating to contracts to bear a child. Provides that certain contracts are contrary to public policy and are void. Includes among those categories of contracts, contracts to bear a child, as defined. Fiscal impact. 2/18/88: To Assembly Committee on Judiciary. 5/12/88: In Assembly. Read third time and amended. Returned to third reading. 6/2/88: To Senate Committee on Judiciary. 6/30/88: From Senate Committee on Judiciary with author's amendments. Read second time and amended. Re-referred to committee. 6/30/88: In Senate Judiciary Committee. 6/30/88: From Senate Committee on Judiciary with author's amendments. Read second time and amended. Re-referred to committee.

CA S-2635 Watson. (916/445-5965) Expresses the intent of the Legislature with regard to providing certainty of the parent and child relationship; provides that it is a misdemeanor for any person or agency to offer to pay money or anything of value for a woman to conceive a child for a husband and wife, thereby imposing a new crime. Fiscal impact. 4/4/88: From Senate Committee on Judiciary with author's amendments. Read second time and amended. Re-referred to Committee. 4/14/88: In Senate. Joint Rule 61(b) (5) suspended.

FL H-747 Canady. (904/488-9890) Defines the term "mother" for purposes of the Florida Adoption Act; prohibits contracts for the transfer of parental rights in connection with any child, in return for consideration. 4/5/88: Introduced. To House Committee on Judiciary.

WI A-827 Magnuson. (608/266-5342) Establishes laws on surrogate parenting. 1/14/88: Introduced. To Assembly Committee on Children and Human Services.

(3) Bills that would establish a study commission or task force

A. Bills enacted:

CA ACR-171* Mojonnier. (916/445-2112) Creates the Joint Committee on Surrogate Parenting, and directs and authorizes the Joint Committee to ascertain, study and critically analyze facts relating to commercial and noncommercial parenting. The Joint Committee would be required to report its findings to the Legislature, including findings on specified issues, no later than December 31, 1989. 9/15/88: Resolution Chapter 150, Statutes of 1988.

NH H-1098* McGovern. (603/271-2548) Establishes a committee to study surrogate parenting. 1/6/88: Introduced. To House Committee on Judiciary. 2/18/88: To Senate Committee on Public Institutions, Health and Human Services. 4/27/88 Became law without Governor's signature.

RI S-2413* Carlin. (401/277-6655) (Joint Resolution) Extends the reporting date of the special legislative commission on surrogate mother contracts. 2/24/88: To House Committee on Judiciary. 5/25/88: Became law without Governor's signature.

UT H-17* Protzman. (801/533-5801) Relates to state affairs in general. Establishes a committee to study and recommend legislation regarding surrogate parenthood. 1/28/88: From House Committee on Health: Reported favorably. 3/14/88: To Governor. Signed by Governor. Chapter 94.

B. Bills awaiting further action:

MA H-2712 Bartley. (717/722-2356) Provides for an investigation and study by a special commission relative to the need to regulate contracting for surrogate parenthood. 2/2/88: Introduced. To Joint Committee on Judiciary. 5/12/88: From Joint Committee on Judiciary with S-1706.

MA H-1146 Clapprood. (617/722-2356) Provides for an investigation and study by a special commission relative to the need to regulate contracting for surrogate parenthood. 1/22/88: Introduced. To Joint Committee on Judiciary. 5/12/88: From Joint Committee on Judiciary with S-1706.

NC S-1583 Rand. Extends the life of the adoptions and surrogate parenthood study commission and makes an additional appropriation therefor. 6/8/88: Introduced. To Senate Committee on Appropriations.

NH H-751 Green. (603/271-2548) Relates to surrogate parenting contracts. 2/17/88: To Interim Study.

NJ AJR-5 Felice. (609/292-4840) Creates a commission to study the subject of surrogate parenthood. 1/13/88: Introduced. To Assembly Committee on Judiciary.

NJ S-1242 Feldman. (609/292-4840) Creates the New Jersey Commission on Surrogate Parenthood and appropriates $90,000. 1/12/88: Introduced.

VA HJR-11 Keating. (804/786-7294) Creates a joint subcommittee to study the legal issues involved in the use of procreative technology. 1/18/88: Introduced. To House Committee on Rules.

VA HJR-65 Cohen. (804/786-7253) Establishes a joint subcommittee to study surrogate parenting. 1/25/88: Introduced. To House Committee on Rules.

VA HJR-106 Maxwell. (804/786-7192) Establishes a joint subcommittee to study surrogate motherhood. 1/26/88: Introduced. To House Committee on Rules.

VA HJR-118 Callahan. (804/786-6991) Establishes a joint subcommittee to study surrogate parenting. 1/26/88: Introduced. To House Committee on Rules. 3/3/88: House concurred with Senate amendments.

VA SJR-3 Michie. (804/786-6887) Requests a study of surrogate mothering. 1/13/88: Introduced. To Senate Committee on Rules. 3/12/88: Senate concurred in House amendments.

WI AJR-71 Tesmer. (608/266-8588) Provides for Legislative Council study of surrogate motherhood. 3/23/88: Amended on Senate floor. Passed Senate. 4/21/88: To Assembly for concurrence. Assembly concurred in Senate amendments.

Sources

State Net, A Service of Information for Public Affairs, Inc.
1900-14th Street
Sacramento, CA 95814
Updated through October 5, 1988

1987 The National Directory of State Agencies
Bethesda, Maryland 20816

State contacts for information on 1988 surrogacy laws passed

Florida, SB9, Deborah Kearney, Staff Attorney, Committee on Judiciary, Florida House of Representatives, 904/488-1663.

Indiana, S-98, Robin Winten, Senate Research, 317/232-9539.

Kentucky, S-4, Robert Sherman and Glenn Osborn, Legislative Research, 502/564-8100.

Michigan, S-228, Daryl Homes, Senator Connie Binsfield's Office, 517/373-2413.

Nebraska, Susan Gillen, Legislative Research, 402/471-2221.

Appendix III
Model Surrogacy Acts

A. Section of Family Law of the American Bar Association

Introduction—not to be Considered Part of the Act

While surrogacy poses potential problems in the areas of class, eugenics and race, surrogacy will be used, and therefore, it is necessary to control these potential problems and provide for the best interests of children born out of the use of such services.

MODEL SURROGACY ACT

[Sections in brackets have not been included in this Appendix.—Ed.]

Section 1. Purposes. Medical knowledge and technology combined with the lack of infants readily available for adoption have created an increasing demand for surrogacy. The purposes of this act are to:

(a) Facilitate the creation of a parent/child bond;

(b) Facilitate private reproductive choices by effectuating the parties' intentions while minimizing the risks to the parties;

(c) Facilitate informed and voluntary decision making;

(d) Define and delineate the rights and responsibilities of the intended parent or parents, the providers of genetic materials, the surrogate, and her husband, if any.

Comments on Section 1. This act overrules the common law presumption that she who bears a child is presumed to be its mother and provides that a surrogacy agreement shall govern.

Section 2. Definitions.

(a) *Agreement or Surrogacy Agreement:* An agreement that meets the requirements of Section 5 of this act.

(b) *Genetic Materials:* The sperm, ovum, and embryo.

(c) *Intended Parent:* The individual or individuals who enter into a surrogacy agreement with a surrogate with the intent to become the legal parent or parents of the child born to the surrogate.

(d) *Providers of Genetic Materials:* The persons who, pursuant to the terms of the agreement, provide the sperm and ovum from their bodies that are planned to be used ultimately to create the child.

(e) *Qualified Facility:* A facility that meets the requirement in Section 16 of this act.

(f) *Parties:* The parties to the agreement are: the intended parent or parents, the surrogate, and the surrogate's husband, if any.

(g) *Surrogate:* The gestational carrier of any embryo, a fetus, or a child.

(h) *Related:* A surrogate is related to the intended parents if the child born of the surrogacy agreement and the surrogate would stand in relation to each other as grandchild and grandparent; as niece or nephew and aunt or uncle; or as siblings.

Comments on Section 2.

(a) *Agreement or Surrogacy Agreement:* See Section 5 of this act.

(b) *Genetic materials:* By including embryo in the definition of genetic materials, the committee intended to permit embryo transfer.

(c) *Intended parent:* The committee defined intended parent in the singular or the plural to avoid prohibiting an unmarried person from employing the services of a surrogate.

(d) *Providers of Genetic Materials:* This definition is intended to exclude a physician, geneticist, or licensed facility from being considered as the provider of genetic materials unless he or she contributes either sperm or an ovum from his or her body. This definition may include: a surrogate who, in addition to being the gestational carrier, provides the ovum from her body; an intended parent who provides the ovum from her body; or an intended parent who provides the sperm from his body.

(e) *Qualified facility:* See Section 16 for comments.

(f) *Parties:* Although the committee decided that a surrogate's husband who does not currently reside with her may be difficult to locate, because of the common law presumption of paternity and because of the possibility that the husband may return during the period of fertility, the committee decided to require that the surrogate's husband be a party to the agreement.

(g) *Surrogate:* Nothing in this definition is intended to change the legality of terminating a pregnancy under state law.

Section 3. Legality of Surrogacy Agreement.

(a) An agreement for surrogacy in compliance with Section 5 below shall be valid as a matter of public policy.

(b) The payment of a fee to the surrogate for her services as a surrogate is authorized. The minimum and maximum fee to be paid to the surrogate shall be determined by an administrative body of three persons, called the [Name of State] Surrogacy Fee Agency. The [Name of State] Surrogacy Fee Agency shall not set the minimum fee at less than [$7,500]. The maximum fee shall not be more than 150% of the minimum fee. To assure that fair compensation will be paid to surrogates for their services, the agency shall determine the minimum and maximum fee every two years taking into consideration any relevant changes during the past two years, including, but not limited to, any changes in the services rendered by surrogates and any changes in the consumer price index or other indicia of the cost of living. Each two years the governor shall appoint one member of the agency and each house of the legislature shall appoint one member.

(c) The surrogacy agreement may, however, waive the payment of a fee, or provide for a lesser fee, if the surrogate is related to the intended parents or if the surrogate and intended parents have known each other for a period of more than three years before the agreement is signed.

(d) No minor may be a party to an agreement for surrogacy.

(e) The transfer of genetic materials to the surrogate shall be permitted and shall not constitute an experiment as prohibited under _____ .

(f) Prior to entering into any surrogacy agreement all parties must have full and informed consent. Informed consent consists of all parties being apprised of their rights and liabilities under the agreement by legal counsel; all parties being apprised of the medical risks involved by a licensed physician; all parties being apprised of psychological risks by a licensed registered mental health practitioner; and that the surrogate has a previous history of childbirth.

Comments on Section 3.

Legality. Section 5 of this act sets forth the contents of a surrogacy agreement. Paragraph e of Section 5 requires that the agreement state the compensation, if any, to the providers of genetic materials and to the surrogate. Under present law, a child born to a surrogate can only become the legal child of the intended parents through adoption proceedings. All adoption acts prohibit the sale of a child for adoption. Most jurisdictions allow only the payment of the medical expenses for the birth mother and child. The major policy argument for prohibiting payment to a birth parent is to assure that the adopting parents do not coerce the birth parents who, typically, did not plan to have a child and who, sometimes, lack sufficient resources to provide for a child themselves. This policy argument does not apply to payment to a surrogate. A surrogate plans to have a child and, assuming the contract was entered into at arm's length, she would not be the victim of coercion. This act, therefore, does not prohibit payment to the surrogate for her services. *See, Surrogate Parenting Associates v. Kentucky,* 407 S. W. 2d 209, 213 (Ky, 1986).

Set Amount of Compensation. The committee determined that the amount of compensation should be within state guidelines.

No Experiment. A woman may be unable to carry a child but able to produce ova. If she and her physician wish to employ in vitro fertilization and transfer the resulting embryo into a surrogate, Paragraph (d) of this Section is intended to clarify that such techniques do not constitute experimentation with human embryos. *See, Smith v. Hartigan,* 556 F. Supp. 157 (N.D. Ill. 1983).

Section 4. Required Examinations—and Health Care Provider Responsibilities.

(a) *Physician's Responsibilities and Required Examination.*

(1) *Examination of Providers of Genetic Materials.* Before the insemination and not more than one year before the insemination, a physician or physicians licensed in this jurisdiction shall examine or have tests performed on the surrogate and the providers of genetic materials to determine to a reasonable degree of medical certainty his, her, or their opinion regarding the examined or tested person's:

(A) general physical health,

(B) fertility,

(C) sexually transmitted diseases,

(D) mental health and whether there is any significant mental disease in the examined or tested person's history that more likely than not will be inherited by a child born of the prospective surrogate;

(E) all other tests or examinations recommended by the American Fertility Society.

In arriving at an opinion regarding whether the examined person has a mental disease that will be inherited by a child born of the prospective surrogate, a physician may rely on test results performed by a person with a doctorate in clinical psychology who is certified or licensed in this state.

(2) *Summary Attached to Surrogacy Agreement.* The physician or physicians shall summarize the results of any test or examination made pursuant to this paragraph in writing. All summaries shall be attached to the Surrogacy Agreement. Any physician who has provided a written summary for the purposes of inclusion in a surrogacy agreement shall be required to promptly disclose to the intermediary agency any relevant changes discovered by such physician. In such an instance, the doctor/patient privilege shall not apply. The physician's disclosure to the intermediary agency shall be in writing.

(3) *Prohibited Combinations of Genetic Materials.* No physician or any other person shall cause a surrogate to be artificially inseminated with any of the following prohibited combinations of genetic materials:

(A) The combination of sperm and ovum from an ancestor and a descendant, a brother and a sister, whether the relationship is by half or whole blood;

(B) The combination of sperm and ovum of an uncle and a niece of an aunt and nephew, whether the relationship is by half or whole blood; and

(C) The combination of sperm and ovum of cousins of the first degree.

(b) *Required Examination by Licensed or Registered Mental Health Practitioner.*

(1) *Examination of Surrogate.* Before the insemination and not more than 18 months before the insemination, the surrogate shall be examined by a licensed or registered mental health practitioner. If a psychiatrist's services are employed, then he or she shall be a physician board certified in psychiatry and licensed to practice medicine. If a psychologist is employed, then such person shall have a doctorate in clinical psychology and have state certification or licensing. The licensed or registered mental health practitioner shall examine the surrogate to determine whether, to a reasonable degree of psychiatric or psychological certainty, the surrogate:

(A) has any psychosis or mental disability that would prevent her from understanding and fulfilling her responsibilities under a surrogacy agreement;

(B) is mentally and emotionally capable of entering into a surrogacy agreement.

(2) *Summary Attached to Surrogacy Agreement.* The psychiatrist or psychologist shall summarize the results of any test or examination made pursuant to this paragraph in writing. All summaries shall be attached to the Surrogacy Agreement. Any psychiatrist or psychologist who has provided a written summary for the purposes of inclusion in a surrogacy agreement shall be required to promptly disclose to the intermediary agency any relevant changes discovered by such mental health professional. In such an instance, the mental health carer provider/patient privilege shall not apply. The disclosure to the intermediary agency shall be in writing.

(c) *Required Examinations by Social Worker and Counseling.*

(1) *Examination of Surrogate.* Before the insemination and not more than one year before the insemination, the surrogate shall be examined by a social worker who shall obtain a complete social history of the prospective surrogate and determine whether the prospective surrogate appears to be suited to being a surrogate.

(2) *Examination of Intended Parents.* Before the insemination and not more than one year before the insemination, the intended parents shall be examined by a social worker who shall obtain a complete social history of the intended parents and determine whether the intended parents appear to be suited to going through the process of having a child through surrogacy and raising a child born of a surrogacy agreement.

(3) *Recommendations Attached to Surrogacy Agreement.* The social worker or workers shall state in writing their recommendation regarding the person or persons they have examined. For the surrogate, the social worker or workers shall state whether the prospective surrogate appears to be suited to being a surrogate. For the intended parents, the social worker or workers shall state whether they appear to be suited to the process of having a child through surrogacy and raising a child born of a surrogacy agreement. All recommendations shall be attached to the Surrogacy Agreement. Any social worker who has provided a written summary for the purposes of inclusion in a surrogacy agreement shall be required to promptly disclose to the intermediary agency any relevant changes discovered by such social worker. In such an instance, any privilege shall not apply. The disclosure to the intermediary agency shall be in writing.

(4) *Counseling.* If the surrogate's attorney or intended parents' attorney requests, or if the intermediary agency requests, the licensed social worker shall counsel the various parties as deemed necessary by the social worker.

(d) *Attachments Made Part of the Agreement and Part of Petition.* All attachments to the Surrogacy Agreement shall be part of the Agreement for all purposes.

Comments on Section 4.

American Fertility Society Standards. The American Fertility Society currently has no standards for testing a surrogate; however, the society has standards for testing and examinations of artificial insemination donors and for *in vitro* fertilization involving fertilization of ova removed from the woman in whom they are to later be placed. If legislation is passed regarding surrogacy and reference is made to the American Fertility Society, it is assumed that the American Fertility Society will develop standards for surrogacy.

Required Examination by Two Mental Health Professionals. Not only is a psychologist's examination required, but a social worker's examination is also required.

Mandatory Counseling. This provision insures that any one who is believed to require counseling will obtain it. If the intended parents' attorney believes that the surrogate needs counseling, then the surrogate must attend counseling. If the surrogate's attorney believes that the intended parents need counseling, then the intended parents must attend counseling. If the intermediary agency believes that each of the parties needs counseling, then everyone must attend counseling. There is, however, no penalty provided for in the statute for failure to attend counseling.

Section 5. Content of Surrogacy Agreement and Disclosure of Court Records. The surrogacy agreement shall be in writing and signed by the parties and shall:

(a) State that the surrogate and her husband, if any, agree that they have no parental or custodial rights or obligations of any child conceived pursuant to the terms of the surrogacy agreement and full and immediate physical custody of the child shall go to the intended parents upon birth.

(b) State that, before the surrogacy agreement was signed, the proposed providers of genetic materials and the surrogate were examined by a licensed physician for the Rh factor compatibility and sexually transmitted diseases as required by Section 4 of this act.

(c) State that the intended parents shall pay the medical expenses arising out of the performance of the surrogacy agreement for the surrogate's services during insemination, pregnancy and a post partum period, but the obligation for such post partum expenses shall be limited to expenses incurred in the six months following delivery of the child, or fetus, or involuntary termination of pregnancy.

(d) Provide for:

(1) Term life insurance for the period from insemination through the sixth month after the birth of the child with minimum death benefits of $100,000 the life of the surrogate and with beneficiaries as the surrogate selects. If the condition of health of the surrogate makes the premiums for such a policy extraordinarily expensive, the amount of death benefits may be reduced so that the premium would be approximately what would be paid for $100,000 of death benefits for a healthy person of the same age as the surrogate and otherwise similar to the surrogate.

276   APPENDIXES

(2) Term life insurance for the period from insemination through certification of parentage of a minimum amount of $100,000 on the life or lives of the intended parent or parents with the child or a trust for the sole benefit of the child as beneficiary;

(3) Adequate health insurance for the surrogate, with at least eighty percent coverage of the expenses listed in subsection (c) above. The health insurance may have exclusions for preexisting health conditions of the surrogate. Adequate health insurance shall include coverage through a health maintenance organization.

(e) State the compensation, if any, to the providers of genetic materials and the surrogate.

(f) State that upon execution of the surrogacy agreement and before the surrogate is inseminated, all known and estimated expenses shall be placed in a trust fund to assure payment of such expenses.

(g) State that the intended parent or parents shall take custody of and parental responsibility for any child conceived pursuant to the terms of the surrogacy agreement, regardless of the child's or children's health, regardless of any mental condition or defect, and regardless of whether the child is born alive or stillborn.

(h) Recite that before signing the surrogacy agreement:

(1) The surrogate and the providers of genetic materials have previously authorized the release of a summary of their medical records, but if a summary is not available, the whole record, to the intended parent or parents; however, no such recitation need be made by an intended provider of genetic materials who is also an intended parent;

(2) The records in (1) and (2) above have been released and that the surrogate and the intended parent or parents have received the released records;

(3) The surrogate and her husband, if any, have been informed of and consented to any known and anticipated medical and psychological risks associated with the performance of the surrogacy agreement.

(i) Recite that the intended parent or parents and the surrogate have previously authorized the release of their criminal and civil records—including arrests and convictions for all offenses other than minor traffic offenses—and consenting to the examination of any sealed or impounded records that the intended parent or parents and the surrogate have reviewed the released information before signing the surrogacy agreement or have waived such right.

(j) State that the intended parent or parents shall not be liable for wages, child care, transportation, or any other expenses of the surrogate and her husband, if any, unless expressly provided in the agreement.

(k) State that the surrogate shall be the sole source of consent with respect to the clinical management of the pregnancy, including termination of the pregnancy.

(l) State that the damages for breach and remedies for non-performance shall be as provided in Section 6 below.

(m) State that the surrogate and the providers of genetic materials agree to submit themselves and the child for the performance of blood and tissue typing tests.

(n) State that the surrogate has consulted with a lawyer of her choice and that the fees of the lawyer are to be paid either by the surrogate, or that the intended parents are to pay the surrogate's attorney's fees to a certain maximum amount.

(o) State the intentions of the parties with respect to their rights to know or not know the identity of the other or others and their rights to meet or not meet the other or others. The parties may agree to change their intentions with respect to their choice to know or not to know the identity of the other or others and their ·choice to meet or not to meet the other or others. Such change shall be consented to by all of the parties in a writing signed after the surrogacy agreement and does not require any consideration. There need be no mutuality with the respect to the knowledge of one party's name—the intended parents may agree to disclose their identity without learning the identity of the surrogate and vice-versa. Nothing in this section shall be construed to prohibit an agreement for partial disclosure of identity without full disclosure.

(p) State that the court shall have the authority to modify the approved agreement only as provided in Section 17 of this act.

(q) The surrogate shall be entitled to a summary of the medical records of the providers of genetic materials as relates to sexually transmitted diseases. The surrogate shall also be entitled to access any civil or criminal records relating to the subject of the fitness of the intended parents as custodians of a child.

Section 6. Remedies in the Event of Breach. The parties to a surrogacy agreement shall have the following rights and remedies:

(a) *Voluntary termination or child not genetically related.* If the termination of the pregnancy is the voluntary act of the surrogate and not medically necessary, or if the child is not genetically related to one or both of the providers of genetic materials and the lack or relationship is not due to physician or laboratory error, then the intended parent or parents shall have a cause of action against the surrogate. The action for such damages shall be brought within not more than one year after the termination of pregnancy or birth and may be brought within the certification of parentage proceedings, or such proceedings may be brought as a breach of contract action in such venue as is prescribed for breach of contract actions.

(b) *Involuntary termination.* If the termination of the pregnancy is involuntary, medically necessary, or consented to by all parties, then the surrogate shall be entitled to be paid:

(1) the portion of the total compensation that is in proportion to the total anticipated period of gestation,

(2) medical expenses, if the agreement provides that the intended parent or parents are to pay the medical expenses during the pregnancy, and reasonable attorney's fees and costs to the surrogate for enforcement of her rights.

The action for such damages shall be brought within not more than one year after the termination of the pregnancy and may be brought within the certification of parentage proceedings, or such proceedings may be brought as a breach of contract action in such venue as is prescribed for breach of contract actions.

(c) *Specific Performance.* After the child is born, either of the parties shall have the right to specific performance, that is, the right to have the court order and enforce the delivery of the child to the intended parent or parents. The party who is awarded specific performance shall be awarded reasonable attorney's fees and reasonable costs—such costs shall include not only the costs incurred in connection with the litigation, but also the costs, if any incurred in locating the child. No action for specific performance against a party to the agreement may be brought more than 14 days after the intended parent or parents first learn of the delivery of the child. An action for specific performance may be brought within the certification of parentage proceedings, or such proceedings may be brought as an action at equity in such venue as is prescribed for equity actions. If the action is brought within the certification of parentage proceedings, the hearing on the matter shall be within 7 days of notice to the other party or parties. If the action is brought as an action in equity, then the return date on such summons shall be in seven days and hearing on the petition shall be not more than seven days after the return date on the summons. Unless continued for good cause. The rights to specific performance shall be in addition to the rights at law, except as limited in (a), (b), (c), and the agreement. In proceedings for specific performance under extraordinary circumstances including, but not limited to, circumstances where neither the surrogate nor the intended parents want the child because of a defect, the court may appoint an attorney for the child, with the fees of the attorney to be paid by a party, or the parties, as the court in its discretion determines is equitable.

(d) *Joinder of person with custody of child.* Any person or persons other than the surrogate, her husband, if any, the intended parent or parents (or the survivor of the intended parents if the agreement provided for two intended parents and one of them has died), or the guardian of the child as provided for in the agreement, having actual custody of the child may be joined or named as party defendants and shall be served with process as in other civil cases, except that the return date on such summons shall be in seven days after the return date on the summons unless continued for good cause. No action against such a person or persons for specific performance or for custody may be brought more than fourteen days after the intended parent or parents first learn of the whereabouts of the child. The party who is awarded specific performance or custody or both shall be awarded reasonable attorney's fees and costs—such costs shall include not only the costs incurred in connection with the litigation, but also the expenses, if any, incurred in locating the child. The rights to specific performance and costs shall be in addition to the rights at law.

(e) *Other Actions.* Any cause of action arising from a surrogacy agreement shall be limited to specific performance as provided above only and actions for breach of contract as provided above or otherwise provided by law. Remedies for breach of contract not specified in this section may be brought within the certification of parentage proceedings and shall be limited to money damages in the amounts stated in the agreement, or, if no amount is stated in the agreement for the breach that occurred, then damages shall be limited to the amount that the agreement stated the surrogate was to be paid plus the reasonable attorney's fees and costs in bringing the breach of contract action.

(f) *Surrogate's Option Upon Death of Intended Parents.* If both the intended parents die before they take physical custody of the child, the surrogate may, within three days of the date of the death of the last of the intended parents to survive, exercise an option to retain the child as her own. This option shall be exercised in writing with personal delivery to either the executor or administrator of the estate of the last surviving decedent, or a close relative of such decedent, or if such persons cannot be identified and located within the three day period, then by publishing a notice in a newspaper of general circulation in the county of residence of the intended parents, or if such place of residence is not known, then in the county where the child was delivered. The notice shall be published within fourteen days of the date of the death of the last of the intended parents to survive. Such published notice shall be calculated to give reasonable notice to the personal representative, or relatives of the last surviving decedent, of the surrogate's exercise of the option to retain custody of the child as her own. In addition to the publication of the notice, the surrogate shall mail notice to the attorney, if any, who represented the intended parents in negotiations of the surrogacy agreement by certified mail, return receipt requested. If the surrogate exercises the option, the estates of the intended parents shall remain liable for the fees and expenses pursuant to the surrogacy agreement.

. . . . .

Section 10. Responsibilities of Health Facility or Licensed Person Delivering Child.

(a) Any health facility or person licensed to deliver children from pregnant women in this state shall, upon the request of the surrogate or an intended parent, maintain in its, his, or her records a copy of a surrogacy agreement and shall act in accordance with that agreement. Hospitals and persons licensed to deliver children from pregnant women in this state shall presume that an agreement bearing the names and business addresses of the lawyer representing the surrogate and the lawyer representing the intended parents is valid and requires them to treat it as valid.

(b) Upon release of a child to the intended parent or parents, the health facility or person licensed to deliver children from pregnant women shall report the release to the [State Department of Health]. The report shall be on forms supplied by the [Department]. In completing the report, the health facility or person licensed to deliver children from pregnant women shall not disclose the identity of the surrogate to the intended parent or parents. Such report shall be transmitted to the intended parents. Such report shall be transmitted to the [Department] within 48 hours from the release of the child from the health facility or, if the child is not born in a health facility, within 72 hours from the birth of the child.

Comments on Section 10. A state agency should create licensing regulations and require the surrogacy be provided only by licensed physicians or licensed facilities. A physician should be involved to show that protocol must be observed to obtain the benefits of the law. *See, Jhordan C. v. Mary K.,* 224 Cal. Rptr. 530 (1986). Although the results in this case are somewhat troubling, the committee determined that by requiring a physician to be involved the people using surrogacy will recognize the seriousness of their actions.

Section 11. Tissue or Blood Typing.

(a) The child and providers of genetic materials who are parties to the contract shall be tested for blood and tissue type within 14 days after receiving notice of that the child may reliably be blood and tissue typed. The blood and tissue typing shall be performed at the expense of the intended parents. Blood and tissue type tests shall not be delayed after the child's own blood and tissue types may be determined unless the tests would pose life threatening danger. The tests shall include the human leukocyte antigen test. In order to avoid certification of parentage, within 14 days after the test results are mailed to the parties, the party or parties seeking to assert that the child is not as intended must file their petition, and mail or otherwise serve notice directly or on the agents of the other parties to the contract.

(b) If the intended parent or parents prove that the child is not as intended, that is, not genetically related to the providers of genetic materials, then the intended parent or parents shall not be required to retain or assume custody of the child or to make any payments pursuant to the terms of the agreement. If, however, the child is not as intended because of physician or laboratory error, then the intended parent or parents shall be required to retain or assume custody and shall be required to make all payments pursuant to the terms of the agreement.

(c) If the surrogate proves that the child is not as intended and that the genetic materials are hers, then the surrogate may assume custody of the child if she chooses. If, however, the child is not as intended due to physician or laboratory error, then the surrogate may not assume custody. The intended parents shall be entitled to damages as specified in Paragraph a of Section 6 for breach of contract if the child is not as intended for reasons other than physician or laboratory error.

(d) It is presumed that the child is as intended and that neither the physician nor the laboratory caused any error. The burden of proof shall be on the party asserting that the child is not as intended or that the physician or lab erred.

(e) The intended parent or parents shall pay for the blood and tissue type testing of the providers of genetic materials and the child.

(f) If no petition is filed or if notice is not mailed or otherwise served within 14 days after the mailing of the test results, then all objections to certification of parentage shall be deemed waived.

. . . . . .

B. National Conference of Commissioners on Uniform State Laws

Uniform Status of Children of Assisted Conception Act

SECTION 1. DEFINITIONS. In this [Act]:
(1) "Assisted conception" means a pregnancy resulting from (i) fertilizing an egg of a woman with sperm of a man by means other than sexual intercourse or (ii) implanting an embryo, but the term does not include the pregnancy of a wife resulting from fertilizing her egg with sperm of her husband.
(2) "Donor" means an individual [other than a surrogate] who produces egg or sperm used for assisted conception, whether or not a payment is made for the egg or sperm used, but does not include a woman who gives birth to a resulting child.
[(3) "Intended parents" means a man and woman, married to each other, who enter into an agreement under this [Act] providing that they will be the parents of a child born to a surrogate through assisted conception using egg or sperm of one or both of the intended parents.]
(4) "Surrogate" means an adult woman who enters into an agreement to bear a child conceived through assisted conception for intended parents.

COMMENT
The definition of "assisted conception" establishes the scope of coverage of this Act. It is intended to be a broad definition. Section 1(1) (i) includes both "traditional"

Uniform Status of Children of Assisted Conception Act, drafted by the National Conference of Commissioners on Uniform State Laws and by it approved and recommended for enactment in all the states at its annual Conference Meeting in its ninety-seventh year, in Washington, D.C., July 29–August 5, 1988. Printed through permission of the NCCUSL. Copies of the complete Act may be ordered at $3.00 each from them at 676 North St. Clair Street, Suite 1700, Chicago, Illinois 60611, 312/915-0195. Due to limitations of space, the Act has been presented here without the prefatory note and comments.

artificial insemination with fertilization occurring inside the woman's body and *in vitro* fertilization in which the joinder of sperm and egg takes place outside the body. Section 1(1) (ii) is designed to include within the definition the situation in which fertilization takes place through sexual intercourse and the resulting embryo is transplanted to the womb of another woman.

The final clause of Section 1(1) purposefully excludes husband-wife procreation from the definition of assisted conception. There are two reasons for this exclusion. First, as a policy matter, the rules pertaining to husband-wife procreation ought to be the same regardless of the means utilized for procreation. Thus, if a husband and wife choose to procreate through *in vitro* fertilization or more traditional artificial insemination, the status of the resulting child should be determined by existing laws, such as the Uniform Parentage Act, which govern the status of children produced by sexual intercourse. Second, the rules of this Act designating parentage and status of children are not always appropriate to husband-wife procreation. For example, a husband ought not be permitted, through the use of artificial insemination, to claim the status of a nonparent donor under Section 4(a) of this Act. As a result of the exclusion in Section 1(1), he will not be permitted to claim that status.

It should be noted that while this Act is intended to govern the status of children of assisted conception, it is *not* intended to establish a regulatory scheme establishing the appropriate methods for the performance of such assisted conception. A jurisdiction may, *e.g.*, choose to enact separate regulations requiring genetic screening when assisted conception is undertaken, requiring that assisted conception be conducted only under certain conditions, etc.

While it may be suggested that the word "donor" ought properly to be limited to those who merely offer genetic material without compensation, Section 1(2) defines the term to include those who receive compensation for their genetic material. The term donor is regularly used to describe those who sell sperm to sperm banks. *See, e.g.*, Curie-Cohen, et. al, *Current Practice of Artificial Insemination by Donor*, 300 N. Eng. J. Med. 585 (1979). Also, those who sell their blood to blood banks are usually referred to as blood donors. *See, e.g., Hillsborough County v. Automated Medical Laboratories*, 471 U.S. 707 (1985).

The bracketed language in Section 1(2) should be enacted only if the adopting jurisdiction selects Alternative A, infra, concerning surrogacy. The exception clause at the end of Section 1(2) makes it clear that a woman whose egg is fertilized through assisted conception and who bears the resulting child is not considered a donor. Under Section 2 of the Act she will be the mother of that child, unless a surrogacy arrangement has been approved under Alternative A.

The bracketed language which appears as Section 1(3) should be enacted only if the adopting jurisdiction selects Alternative A concerning surrogacy.

It should be emphasized that regardless of which alternative treatment of surrogacy agreements is chosen by a particular jurisdiction, Section 1(4) should be enacted. This subsection defines a surrogate. Regardless of what force, if any, an enacting jurisdiction chooses to give to surrogacy agreements, it is necessary to define what is meant by a surrogate.

SECTION 2. MATERNITY. [Except as provided in Sections 5 through 9,] a woman who gives birth to a child is the child's mother.

COMMENT

The unbracketed language in this section codifies existing law concerning maternity and is made necessary only because of the existence and growing use of technology enabling a woman to give birth to a child to which she is not genetically related. This provision makes it clear that unless the enacting jurisdiction has adopted Alternative A, which in some circumstances designates someone other than the woman who gives birth as the mother, the woman who bears a child is the mother of that child. The bracketed language in this section should be enacted only if the adopting jurisdiction selects Alternative A concerning surrogacy.

SECTION 3. ASSISTED CONCEPTION BY MARRIED WOMAN. [Except as provided in Sections 5 through 9,] the husband of a woman who bears a child through assisted conception is the father of the child, notwithstanding a declaration of invalidity or annulment of the marriage obtained after the assisted conception, unless within two years after learning of the child's birth he commences an action in which the mother and child are parties and in which it is determined that he did not consent to the assisted conception.

COMMENT

The presumptive paternity of the husband of a married woman who bears a child through assisted conception reflects a concern for the best interests of the children of assisted conception. Any uncertainty concerning the identity of the father of such a child ought to be shouldered by the married woman's husband rather than the child. Thus, the husband (not someone acting on his behalf such as a guardian, administrator or executor) has the obligation to file an action aimed at denying paternity through lack of consent to the assisted conception rather than the child or mother having an obligation to prove the husband's paternity.

It should be noted, however, that if the nonpaternity action is timely filed and the husband's lack of consent is demonstrated, the child will be without a legally-recognized father because the sperm donor is not the father under Section 4(a) of the Act. Also, because the filing of such a nonpaternity action is permitted within two years of the husband's learning of the child's birth, the period of uncertainty concerning the identity of the child's father will be longer than two years in the relatively rare case where the husband is not immediately made aware of the child's birth.

By designating the husband of a woman who bears a child through assisted conception as the father, it is intended that he will be considered the father for purposes of any cause of action which arises before the birth of the child. Thus, for example, he would be the father under any state law authorizing a wrongful death action for the death of any unborn child during pregnancy.

The bracketed language in this section should be enacted only if the adopting jurisdiction selects Alternative A concerning surrogacy. Under that alternative, under certain circumstances the husband of the woman bearing the child will not be the father of the child. Instead, the man whose sperm was used in the creation of the child usually will be the father in such cases.

SECTION 4. PARENTAL STATUS OF DONORS AND DECEASED INDIVIDUALS. [Except as otherwise provided in Sections 5 through 9:]
(a) A donor is not a parent of a child conceived through assisted conception.
(b) An individual who dies before implantation of an embryo, or before a child is conceived other than through sexual intercourse, using the individual's egg or sperm, is not a parent of the resulting child.

COMMENT

Present statutory law is split concerning the parental status of sperm donors. Fifteen states have statutes, patterned after Section 5(b) of the Uniform Parentage Act, specifying that a donor will not be considered the father of a child born of artificial insemination if the semen was provided to a licensed physician for use in artificial insemination of a married woman other than the donor's wife. Fifteen other statutes do not explicitly limit nonparenthood to situations where the semen is provided to a physician. Instead, they shield donors from parenthood in all situations where a married woman is artificially inseminated with her husband's consent.

Subsection 4(a), when read in light of Section 3, opts for the broader protection of donors provided by the latter group of statutes. That is, if a married woman bears a child of assisted conception through the use of a donor's sperm, the donor will not be the father and her husband will be the father unless and until his lack of consent to the assisted conception is proven within two years of his learning of the birth. This provides certainty for prospective donors. It should be noted, however, that under Section 4(a) nonparenthood is also provided for those donors who provide sperm for assisted conception by unmarried women. In that relatively rare situation, the child would have no legally recognized father. It should also be noted that Section 4(a) does not adopt the UPA's requirement that the donor provide the semen to a licensed physician. This is not realistic in light of present practices in the field of artificial insemination.

In providing nonparenthood for "donors," Section 4(a) includes by reference the definition of donor in Section 1(2) which covers those who provide sperm or eggs for assisted conception. Thus, if a woman provided an egg for assisted conception which resulted in another woman bearing the child, the egg donor would not be the child's mother. This would provide no burden on the child in light of Section 2's general rule declaring that the woman who gives birth to a child is that child's mother.

Subsection 4(b) is designed to provide finality for the determination of parenthood of those whose genetic material is utilized in the procreation process after their death. The death of the person whose genetic material is either used in conceiving an embryo or in implanting an already existing embryo into a womb would end the potential parenthood of the deceased. The latter situation, in which cryopreservation is utilized to "freeze" an embryo which has been created *in vitro,* is already in existence and gave rise to much controversy in Australia in the early 1980's.

A married couple died after having created an embryo through *in vitro* fertilization. Among the many questions raised after their simultaneous death in a plane crash was whether posthumous implantation of the embryo would result in children who would be those of the deceased couple. Under Section 4(b), it would be clear that implantation after the death of any genetic parent would not result in that genetic parent being the legally recognized parent. Clearly, under Section 2 of the Act, the woman who bears the child will be the mother. The paternity of such child would presumptively be that of the mother's husband, if she is married, under Section 3 of the Act. For a discussion of recent Australian legislation in the area, see Corns, *Legal Regulation of In Vitro Fertilisation in Victoria,* 58 L. Inst. J. 838 (1984); Note, *Genesis Retold: Legal Issues Raised by the Cryopreservation of Preimplantation Human Embryos,* 36 Syr. L. Rev. 1021, 1029 n. 49 (1985).

Section 4(b) is the only provision of the Act which would deal with procreation by those who are married to each other. It is designed primarily to avoid the problems of intestate succession which could arise if the posthumous use of a person's genetic material could lead to the deceased being termed a parent. Of course, those who want to explicitly provide for such children in their wills may do so.

The bracketed language at the beginning of this section should be adopted only by those jurisdictions enacting Alternative A concerning surrogacy. Under that provision, certain persons who would otherwise be considered donors will be parents.

ALTERNATIVE A

COMMENT

A state that chooses Alternative A should also consider Section 1(3) and the bracketed language in Sections 1(2), 2, 3, and 4.

[SECTION 5. SURROGACY AGREEMENT.

(a) A surrogate, her husband, if she is married, and intended parents may enter into a written agreement whereby the surrogate relinquishes all her rights and duties as a parent of a child to be conceived through assisted conception, and the intended parents may become the parents of the child pursuant to Section 8.

(b) If the agreement is not approved by the court under Section 6 before conception, the agreement is void and the surrogate is the mother of a resulting child and the surrogate's husband, if a party to the agreement, is the father of the child. If the surrogate's husband is not a party to the agreement or the surrogate is unmarried, paternity of the child is governed by [the Uniform Parentage Act].

COMMENT

Because of the significant controversy concerning the appropriateness of arrangements under which a woman agrees to bear a child on behalf of another woman, this Act proposes two alternatives. Under Alternative A, in Section 5 through 9, the adopting state is offered a framework under which such agreements are given effect under limited and prescribed circumstances. This alternative also outlines the parent-child relationships which are established when such agreements are approved by a court.

Alternative B, consisting of alternative Section 5, declares such agreements to be void and describes the parent-child relationships between any child born pursuant to such agreements and the other parties. The strong desire of some childless couples for a biologically-related child together with the technological capacity to utilize the sperm of a husband in impregnating a woman not his wife and the willingness of others to aid such couples in satisfying those desires creates a strong likelihood that such agreements will continue to be written. Therefore, it is crucially important that a state enacting the Act adopt either Alternative A or Alternative B.

Under Section 5(a) of Alternative A, together with the definition of "intended parents" under Section 1(3), a valid surrogacy agreement requires the participation of two intended parents who are married to each other and a surrogate, who is defined by Section 1(4) as an *adult* woman who agrees to bear a child through assisted conception for the intended parents. If the surrogate is married, her husband must also be a party to the surrogacy agreement. Additional requirements for a surrogate and the intended parents are imposed by Section 6 of Alternative A. It should be noted that Section 5(a) simply authorizes such agreements. It does not give them effect in terms of designating parenthood, etc. In order to become effective in such matters, the agreement must be approved by the appropriate court under Section 6.

Section 5(b) makes clear that agreements which are not approved under Section 6 are void. Nonapproved agreements in a jurisdiction which has adopted Alternative A of the Act have the same effect as all surrogacy agreements under Alternative B. That is, the surrogate is the mother of any child of assisted conception born pursuant to such agreements. Her husband, if he is a party to such agreement, shall be the father. If the surrogate's husband is not a party to such agreement or if she is unmarried, paternity of the child will be left to existing law.

SECTION 6. PETITION AND HEARING FOR APPROVAL OF SURROGACY AGREEMENT.

(a) The intended parents and the surrogate may file a petition in the [appropriate court] to approve a surrogacy agreement if one of them is a resident of this State. The surrogate's husband, if she is married, must join in the petition. A copy of the agreement must be attached to the petition. The court shall name a [guardian ad litem] to represent the interests of a child to be conceived by the surrogate through assisted conception and [shall] [may] appoint counsel to represent the surrogate.

(b) The court shall hold a hearing on the petition and shall enter an order approving the surrogacy agreement, authorizing assisted conception for a period of 12 months after the date of the order, declaring the intended parents to be the parents of a child to be conceived through assisted conception pursuant to the agreement and discharging the guardian ad litem and attorney for the surrogate, upon finding that:

(1) the court has jurisdiction and all parties have submitted to its jurisdiction under subsection (e) and have agreed that the law of this State governs all matters arising under this [Act] and the agreement;

(2) the intended mother is unable to bear a child or is unable to do so without unreasonable risk to an unborn child or to the physical or mental health of the intended mother or child, and the finding is supported by medical evidence;

(3) the [relevant child-welfare agency] has made a home study of the intended parents and the surrogate and a copy of the report of the home study has been filed with the court;

(4) the intended parents, the surrogate, and the surrogate's husband, if she is married, meet the standards of fitness applicable to adoptive parents in this State;

(5) all parties have voluntarily entered into the agreement and understand its terms, nature, and meaning, and the effect of the proceeding;

(6) the surrogate has had at least one pregnancy and delivery and bearing another child will not pose an unreasonable risk to the unborn child or to the physical or mental health of the surrogate or the child, and this finding is supported by medical evidence;

(7) all parties have received counseling concerning the effect of the surrogacy by [a qualified health-care professional or social worker] and a report containing conclusions about the capacity of the parties to enter into and fulfill the agreement has been filed with the court;

(8) a report of the results of any medical or psychological examination or genetic screening agreed to by the parties or required by law has been filed with the court and made available to the parties;

(9) adequate provision has been made for all reasonable health-care costs associated with the surrogacy until the child's birth including responsibility for those costs if the agreement is terminated pursuant to Section 7; and

(10) the agreement will not be substantially detrimental to the interest of any of the affected individuals.

(c) Unless otherwise provided in the surrogacy agreement, all court costs, attorney's fees, and other costs and expenses associated with the proceeding must be assessed against the intended parents.

(d) Notwithstanding any other law concerning judicial proceedings or vital statistics, the court shall conduct all hearings and proceedings under this section in camera. The court shall keep all records of the proceedings confidential and subject to inspection under the same standards applicable to adoptions. At the request of any party, the court shall take steps necessary to ensure that the identities of the parties are not disclosed.

(e) The court conducting the proceedings has exclusive and continuing jurisdiction of all matters arising out of the surrogacy until a child born after entry of
an order under this section is 180 days old.

COMMENT

Section 6, along with Section 8 which deals with parentage under an approved
surrogacy, is the core of Alternative A. It provides for state involvement, through
supervision by a court, in the surrogacy process before the assisted conception.
The purpose of this early involvement is to insure that the parties are appropriate
for a surrogacy arrangement, that they understand the consequences of what they
are about to do and that the best interests of any child(ren) born of the surrogacy
arrangement are considered before the arrangement is authorized.

The forum for state involvement is a petition brought by *all* the parties to the
arrangement (including the surrogate's husband if she is married) in which the
parties seek a judicial order authorizing the assisted conception contemplated by
their agreement. The agreement itself must be submitted to the court. The court
must hold a hearing on the petition and, under Section 6(b), must make ten separate
findings before the surrogacy arrangement will be allowed to proceed. It should
be noted that Section 6(b) (10) requires a finding that the arrangment would not
be "substantially detrimental to the interest of any of the affected individuals." This
insures the court will retain a measure of discretion to consider and utilize all
relevant information.

This pre-conception authorization process is roughly analogous to adoption procedures currently in place in most jurisdictions. Just as adoption contemplates the
transfer of parentage of a child from the natural to the adoptive parents, surrogacy
involves the transfer from the surrogate to the intended parents. Section 6 is designed to protect the interests of the child(ren) to be born under the surrogacy
arrangement as well as the surrogate and the intended parents. It should be noted
that under Section 1(3) at least one of the intended parents will be genetically related
to the child(ren) born of the arrangement.

Section 6 seeks to protect the interests of the child(ren) in several ways. Under
Section 6(a), a guardian ad litem must be appointed to represent the interests of
any child conceived through the surrogacy arrangement. An enacting jurisdiction
may choose either mandatory or optional independent representation for the surrogate. Under Section 6(b) (3), the court will be informed of the results of a home
study of both the intended parents and the surrogate. A study of the surrogate is
required because of the possibility of termination of the agreement under Section
7 in which case the surrogate will be the legally recognized mother.

Further protection of the child is provided by the finding required by Section 6(b)
(4) that both intended parents and surrogate (and her husband, if any) satisfy the
standards of fitness required of adoptive parents. Under Section 6(b) (6), the court
must assure itself, on the basis of medical evidence, that the pregnancy will not be
dangerous to the child. While Section 6(b) (8) does not require any medical or genetic
screening, it does mandate that if such testing is required by the agreement (or
other law) the results will be available to the court and all parties. Section 6(b) (9)
requires assurance that health-care costs during pregnancy have been provided.
The provisions in Section 6(b) (1) and Section 6(e) dealing with exclusive jurisdiction
are designed to minimize the possibility of parallel litigation in different states and
the consequent risk of childnapping for strategic purposes.

The interests of the surrogate are also protected by Section 6. The bracketed
version of Section 6(a) would require appointed counsel to represent her interests
and, at the least, counsel will be permitted for her. The findings required by Section
6(b) (5) and Section 6(b) (7) will protect the surrogate against the possibility of

overreaching or fraud. Under Section 6(b) (6), the court must find that the surrogate has had at least one previous pregnancy and delivery. Presumably such a finding helps insure that the surrogate fully understands the nature and experience of pregnancy. The court must also find the contemplated pregnancy and delivery would not pose unreasonable physical or mental health risks to her. The requirement of assurance of provision for health-care costs until birth imposed by Section 6(b) (9) protects the surrogate. Section 6(c) requires that all costs associated with the hearing be borne by the intended parents, unless otherwise provided in the agreement. If the agreement imposed such costs on the surrogate, the court could find, under Section 6(b) (10), that the agreement was not in the surrogate's interest and refuse to authorize it.

While most surrogacy arrangements apparently involve intended parents and surrogates who have met each other, if the surrogate does not want her identity revealed to the intended parents, she may request (under Section 6(d)) that the court take all steps to insure that anonymity. At any event, Section 6(d) requires all proceedings to be held in camera with sealed records to insure confidentiality. It should be noted that in addition to the protections offered the surrogate by Section 6 at the hearing, she is given the right under Section 7 to terminate the agreement, even after it has been approved.

The major protection of the interests of the child provided by the Act is the authorization procedure itself. By providing for the court order authorizing the assisted conception and the surrogacy arrangement, the Act establishes closely supervised surrogacy as one of the methods to guarantee the security and well being of the child. It is as well an option for those intended parents who are *unable* (see Section 6(b) (2)) to procreate through traditional means and thus some protection for their interests. The requirements of Sections 6(b) (5), (6), and (7) help provide assurance to the intended parents that the surrogate is capable and knowingly enters the surrogacy arrangement. The interest of producing a healthy child is promoted through Section 6(b) (6)'s required finding that a pregnancy by the surrogate will not be unreasonably risky to the child.

Section 6, while constructing a detailed set of requirements for the petition and the findings which must be made before an authorizing order can be issued, nowhere states the consequences of violations of the rules. Because of the variety of types of violations which could possibly occur, it was felt that a bright-line rule concerning the effect of such violations was inappropriate. The question of the consequences of a failure to abide by the rules of Section 6 is left to a case-by-case determination. A court should be guided in making such a determination by the narrow purpose of Alternative A to permit surrogacy arrangements and the equities of a particular situation. Note that Section 7 provides a period for termination of the agreement and vacating of the order. The discovery of a failure to abide by the rules of Section 6 would certainly provide the occasion for terminating the agreement. On the other hand, if a failure to abide by the rules of Section 6 is discovered by a party during a time when Section 7 termination would be permissible, failure to terminate might be an appropriate reason to estop the party from later seeking to overturn or ignore the Section 6 order.

SECTION 7. TERMINATION OF SURROGACY AGREEMENT.

(a) After entry of an order under Section 6, but before the surrogate becomes pregnant through assisted conception, the court for cause, or the surrogate, her husband, or the intended parents may terminate the surrogacy agreement by giving written notice of termination to all other parties and filing notice of the termination with the court. Thereupon, the court shall vacate the order entered under Section 6.

(b) A surrogate who has provided an egg for the assisted conception pursuant to an agreement approved under Section 6 may terminate the agreement by filing written notice with the court within 180 days after the last insemination pursuant to the agreement. Upon finding, after notice to the parties to the agreement and hearing, that the surrogate has voluntarily terminated the agreement and understands the nature, meaning, and effect of the termination, the court shall vacate the order entered under Section 6.

(c) The surrogate is not liable to the intended parents for terminating the agreement pursuant to this section.

COMMENT

Subsections (a) and (b) provide for termination of the surrogacy arrangement after the authorization order in two situations. Under subsection (a), any party or the court for cause may cancel the arrangement before the pregnancy has been established. This provides for a period of cancellation during a time when the interests of the parties would not be unduly prejudiced by such termination. By definition, the procreation process has not begun and, therefore, there is no interest to be asserted on behalf of the child. The intended parents certainly have an expectation interest during this time, but the nature of this interest is little different from that which they would have while they were attempting to create a pregnancy through traditional means.

Subsection (b) gives a surrogate who has provided the egg for the assisted conception 180 days after the last insemination to recant and decide to keep the child as her own. Under most current surrogacy arrangements, the surrogate will have provided the egg. The subsection requires that all parties to the agreement be given notice and that a hearing be held on a filing of an intent to terminate by the surrogate. Such notice, of course, must be provided in a constitutionally acceptable manner. If the court determines that the surrogate's termination is voluntary and she is aware of the consequences of such a termination (see Section 8(b)), it must vacate the authorization order.

This 180-day recantation period can, at one level, be described as a compromise between two polar positions concerning recantation. On one extreme, some argue that once the agreement has been presented to a court which has made the requisite findings under Section 6(b), no recantation should be permitted. After all, the surrogate has entered into an agreement to bear a child for the intended parents and the court has found that she acted knowingly and voluntarily and that she was an appropriate person to fulfill the role of surrogate. It would be argued that the expectation interests of the intended parents ought not be frustrated by the surrogate's unilateral action.

On the other hand, some argue that the surrogate ought to be able to renounce her agreement at any time until after the birth of the child. This position would assimilate the surrogate's rights to those of a birth mother who gives consent to the adoption of her child. Most current adoption statutes provide that valid consent can be given only after birth.

The selection of the 180-day recantation period, however, can be viewed as more than a mere mechanical compromise between the two positions. Instead, this recantation period can be explained by pointing out that the surrogacy arrangement is simply different from both the ordinary contract situation and the ordinary adoption situation and, therefore, ought to be treated differently. Surrogacy is not an ordinary contract because it contemplates the creation of a human being whose interests must be taken into account. It can be argued that the child's interests in a parent-child relationship with his or her biological mother are protected by giving her an extra 180 days to decide if she really wants to give up the child to the intended mother.

On the other hand, surrogacy is different from an adoption and the post-birth consent requirement of adoption is not appropriate for the surrogacy situation. The requirement of post-birth consent in adoption is based on the reality that many birth mothers are young, unmarried women who arrange *during pregnancy* to give their child up for adoption. It is felt that decisions made under such circumstances are often the result of emotional stress created by young women in the midst of an often unwanted pregnancy and, therefore, are pressured in inappropriate ways. Therefore, "pregnant women are irrebuttably presumed incapable of protecting their own interests." Ellman, Kurtz & Stanton, *Family Law: Cases, Text, Problems* 1238 (Michie 1986).

The surrogacy arrangement authorized under this Act is very different. Most importantly, the original decision to give up the child is made *before* the pregnancy by an adult woman who has already experienced a previous pregnancy. It is an arrangement which has been examined and approved by a court under Section 6, with all the protections of the surrogate provided under that section. Any undue pressure which may have been brought to bear on the surrogate to become a surrogate will have been examined at the Section 6 hearing.

Having rejected the contract and adoption analogies, the question of an appropriate time period for recantation remains. Section 7(b)'s 180-day recantation period roughly coincides with the time during which the surrogate has a constitutionally-protected right to terminate the pregnancy. Because the surrogate has this right to choose to *abort*, there is a certain logic in giving the same period in which to decide to *bear* the child and honor her pre-conception agreement. This recantation provision recognizes the right of the surrogate to change her mind well into the pregnancy as well as the interests of the intended parents in the finality of the decision-making process before birth. Note that because the 180-day period begins on the date of the last insemination pursuant to the agreement (a point chosen because of its certainty), it is possible that the recantation period will extend longer than 180 days into pregnancy, if the pregnancy was actually created by an earlier insemination.

A jurisdiction which finds the 180-day period too short can choose not to enact Alternative A at all and opt for Alternative B which provides for no enforcement of surrogacy agreements.

Section 7(c) insures that a recanting surrogate will not be held liable in damages for her recantation, either under subsection (a) or (b). It is intended that no such liability for the surrogate for her recantation can be imposed by the agreement. By creating this immunity for the surrogate, this provision is not intended to *impose* any liability for cost associated with the surrogacy on any other parties to the arrangement. Such obligations, however, may be imposed by the agreement itself, see Section 6(b) (9).

SECTION 8. PARENTAGE UNDER APPROVED SURROGACY AGREEMENT.

(a) The following rules of parentage apply to surrogacy agreements approved under Section 6:

(1) Upon birth of a child to the surrogate, the intended parents are the parents of the child and the surrogate and her husband, if she is married, are not parents of the child unless the court vacates the order pursuant to Section 7(b).

(2) If, after notice of termination by the surrogate, the court vacates the order under Section 7(b) the surrogate is the mother of a resulting child, and her husband, if a party to the agreement, is the father. If the surrogate's husband is not a party to the agreement or the surrogate is unmarried, paternity of the child is governed by [the Uniform Parentage Act].

(b) Upon birth of the child, the intended parents shall file a written notice with the court that a child has been born to the surrogate within 300 days after assisted conception. Thereupon, the court shall enter an order directing the [Department of Vital Statistics] to issue a new birth certificate naming the intended parents as parents and to seal the original birth certificate in the records of the [Department of Vital Statistics].

COMMENT

Under Section 8(a), parentage of the child born pursuant to an approved surrogacy is vested in the intended parents where the order under Section 6 is still in effect. Notice of the birth of the child must be filed by the intended parents and the court, upon receipt of the notice, shall direct the issuance of a birth certificate naming the intended parents as parents. It should be noted that a birth certificate issued under this subsection might later be replaced by a birth certificate naming other individuals as parents of the child if an action to dispute the parentage of the intended parents filed under Section 9(d) is successful.

Section 8(b) deals with parentage where the surrogate has exercised her Section 7(b) right of recantation. It makes clear that the surrogate and her husband, if a party to the agreement, are the parents of the child in such a situation. Where the surrogate is unmarried or her husband was not a party to the agreement, paternity is left to the otherwise relevant state law. It should be noted, however, that if the surrogate has married or remarried since the order authorizing the surrogacy, her husband is not the father of the child. See Section 9(c).

Because under the Act (Section 1(3)) at least one intended parent must be genetically related to the child and Section 7(b) recantation is limited to those surrogates who have provided the egg, in all cases arising under Section 8(b) the intended father will be the genetic father. Thus, the interaction of Section 8(b) and the law of paternity may result in the legally recognized father (the intended father) and the legally recognized mother (the surrogate) being in different households. This situation, while regrettable, is not unique in family law and may precipitate litigation over custody. *See In re Baby M*, 537 A.2d 1227 (N.J. 1988) and the trial court order on remand, 14 Fam. L. Rep. 1276 (1988).

SECTION 9. SURROGACY: MISCELLANEOUS PROVISIONS.

(a) A surrogacy agreement that is the basis of an order under Section 6 may provide for the payment of consideration.

(b) A surrogacy agreement may not limit the right of the surrogate to make decisions regarding her health care or that of the embryo or fetus.

(c) After the entry of an order under Section 6, marriage of the surrogate does not affect the validity of the order, and her husband's consent to the surrogacy agreement is not required, nor is he the father of a resulting child.

(d) A child born to a surrogate within 300 days after assisted conception pursuant to an order under Section 6 is presumed to result from the assisted conception. The presumption is conclusive as to all persons who have notice of the birth and who do not commence within 180 days after notice, an action to assert the contrary in which the child and the parties to the agreement are named as parties. The action must be commenced in the court that issued the order under Section 6.

(e) A health-care provider is not liable for recognizing the surrogate as the mother before receipt of a copy of the order entered under Section 6 or for recognizing the intended parents as parents after receipt of an order entered under Section 6.]

COMMENT

Subsection 9(a) is intended to shield surrogacy agreements which include payment of the surrogate from attack under "baby-selling" statutes which prohibit payment of money to the natural mother in adoptions.

Section 9(b) is intended to acknowledge that the surrogate, as a pregnant woman, has a constitutionally-recognized right to provide for her health care and that of the unborn child.

Section 9(c) makes it clear that a man who marries the surrogate after the surrogacy authorization has been issued is neither a party to the original action nor the father of a resulting child, even if the surrogate exercises her recantation right under Section 7(b). It is felt that since he was not a party to the surrogacy agreement, he ought not be burdened with the status of parent. In the case of a recanting surrogate who has married since the original Section 6 order, she will be the mother and the intended father may be the legally recognized father under the jurisdiction's ordinary paternity laws.

Subsection 9(d) should be read in connection with the parentage provision of Section 8(a). The presumption created by Section 9(d) is intended to provide a starting point for the determination of whether a child born to the surrogate was actually the product of the assisted conception performed pursuant to the agreement. For example, a surrogate may assert that the child was created by the union of her egg and her husband's sperm. She and all other persons who have notice of the birth are given 180 days to commence an action to assert that the child was not the product of the assisted conception. It is intended that the substantive and procedural law governing such actions will be governed by the otherwise relevant state statutes concerning disputed parentage of a child.

Subsection 9(e) is designed to provide an incentive to the parties to the surrogacy to make hospital personnel aware of the existence of the arrangement and to protect the health care providers in case such notification has not been made.
[END OF ALTERNATIVE A]

ALTERNATIVE B

COMMENT

A state that chooses Alternative B shall consider Sections 10, 11, 12, 13, 14, 15, and 16, renumbered 6, 7, 8, 9, 10, 11, and 12, respectively.

[SECTION 5. SURROGATE AGREEMENTS. An agreement in which a woman agrees to become a surrogate or to relinquish her rights and duties as parent of a child thereafter conceived through assisted conception is void. However, she is the mother of a resulting child, and her husband, if a party to the agreement, is the father of the child. If her husband is not a party to the agreement or the surrogate is unmarried, paternity of the child is governed by [the Uniform Parentage Act].]

COMMENT

This section should be utilized by a jurisdiction which chooses not to give any efficacy to surrogacy arrangements. It recognizes, however, that some such agreements will continue to be achieved even though they are not enforceable at law. Therefore, it makes provision for the maternity and paternity of children who are born pursuant to such agreements. Note that Alternative B's Section 5 substitutes for Alternative A's Sections 5-9.
[END OF ALTERNATIVE B]

SECTION 10. PARENT AND CHILD RELATIONSHIP; STATUS OF CHILD.
(a) A child whose status as a child is declared or negated by this [Act] is the child only of his or her parents as determined under this [Act].
(b) Unless superseded by later events forming or terminating a parent and child

relationship, the status of parent and child declared or negated by this [Act] as to a given individual and a child born alive controls for purposes of:

(1) intestate succession;

(2) probate law exemptions, allowances, or other protections for children in a parent's estate; and

(3) determining eligibility of the child or its descendants to share in a donative transfer from any person as a member of a class determined by reference to the relationship.

COMMENT

This provision is parallel to those provisions in adoption statutes which provide that once an adoption creates or negates a parent-child relationship, that relationship or negation of a relationship applies in all circumstances.

SECTION 11. UNIFORMITY OF APPLICATION AND CONSTRUCTION. This [Act] shall be applied and construed to effectuate its general purpose to make uniform the law with respect to the subject of this [Act] among states enacting it.

COMMENT

While strictly speaking this section may be redundant in light of Section 10, it is included because of the importance of the situations listed herein. The introductory clause primarily is designed to deal with situations where a parent-child relationship established under this Act is later severed through the placement of a child for adoption or, conversely, situations where a parent-child relationship is negated by the Act but is later established by an adoption.

SECTION 12. SHORT TITLE. This [Act] may be cited as the Uniform Status of Children of Assisted Conception Act.

SECTION 13. SEVERABILITY. If any provision of this [Act] or its application to any person or circumstance is held invalid, the invalidity does not affect other provisions or applications of this [Act] which can be given effect without the invalid provision or application, and to this end the provisions of this [Act] are severable.

SECTION 14. EFFECTIVE DATE. This [Act] shall take effect on _____. Its provisions are to be applied prospectively.

SECTION 15. REPEALS. Acts or parts of acts inconsistent with this [Act] are repealed to the extent of the inconsistency.

SECTION 16. APPLICATION TO EXISTING RELATIONSHIPS. This [Act] applies to surrogacy agreements entered into after its effective date.

APPENDIX IV
STATEMENTS OF POLICY ON SURROGACY

A. The American Civil Liberties Union

Introduction

Persons involved in surrogate parenting agreements have important civil liberties at stake. The U.S. Supreme Court has enumerated a fundamental right to choose 'whether to bear or beget a child.' Both women and men have the right to reproductive choice, which includes the freedom to enter into an agreement to produce a child through surrogacy. Men and women entering into surrogacy arrangements also have the right not to be discriminated against on such grounds as sexual preference, economic status, marital status, mental or physical disability or physical condition. The gestational mother as a matter of her right to privacy and bodily integrity, has the right to decide whether and when to use her body for procreation and whether to carry a pregnancy to term. Both the gestational mother and the genetic father (and the genetic mother if any) have, upon birth of the child, full parental and associational rights and responsibilities. Finally, any child born as a result of a surrogacy arrangement has the right not to be sold as a chattel.

In this policy on surrogate parenting, the civil liberties of the parties are the dominant concern. The Union believes that the fundamental civil liberties at stake override any notion that a deal is a deal.

For the purposes of this policy, the following definitions have been adopted:

Gestational mother—A woman who agrees to gestate and bear a child for another person with the intention of giving up her rights to the child after birth. For purposes of this policy, the term gestational mother refers both to arrangements: (1) where the gestational mother donates genetic material and is therefore both the genetic and gestational mother; and (2) where someone other than the gestational mother provides the genetic material. The gestational mother enjoys full parental rights at the time of the child's birth, regardless of whether she is also the genetic mother.

Genetic father—A man who enters into a surrogacy agreement with the gestational mother to bear a child with the intention to become the legal and custodial parent of the child upon birth. The genetic father always donates sperm on a non-anonymous basis and is for purposes of this policy, always the legal father regardless of the marital status of the gestational mother. Genetic fathers have parental rights upon the birth of the child.

Genetic mother—A non-anonymous woman other than the gestational mother who donates genetic material, i.e. an egg, with the intention of becoming a legal and custodial parent of a child born from a surrogacy arrangement. Genetic mothers have parental rights upon the birth of a child.

A. *Prohibition or Criminalization of Surrogacy*

The state may not prohibit or criminalize all surrogacy arrangements. The participants in a surrogacy arrangement intend to exercise their rights to procreative choice and intimate association with the future offspring, forms of protected privacy under the Constitution.

The gestational mother has the fundamental right to reproductive choice. She has a protected right to the intimate and private experience of physically caring for the growing fetus, carrying it to term, and giving birth. The U.S. Supreme Court's abortion decisions speak of a woman's private informed choice which is only for her and her physician to make.

The genetic father and his partner use the surrogacy arrangement for the purpose of having a child. In doing so, they are exercising a highly personal choice in order to procreate and to obtain the right to intimate association with the future offspring.

The gestational mother, genetic father and separate genetic mother, if any, have fundamental human and constitutional rights. These parties should have the right to undertake conduct to enable them to exercise their rights to privacy and future association. The ACLU believes that procreative decisions concerning whether, how and when to bear a child are private decisions protected by the U.S. Constitution. The state has no demonstrably compelling interest in prohibiting or criminalizing an intimate private arrangement between consenting parties seeking to produce a child. Thus, the ACLU takes the position that surrogacy arrangements may not be prohibited or criminalized.[1]

B. *Payment for Gestational Services*

The ACLU takes the position that a provision of a surrogacy agreement that conditions payments to the gestational mother on her termination of parental rights is void. The Union believes that such provisions mandate the equivalent of the sale of a child. Children have a right not to be sold as chattel.

The American Civil Liberties Union does not, however, oppose agreements to compensate the mother for providing gestational services.[2]

The mother, therefore, can be paid for conception, gestation and birth of the child. The genetic father may offer this payment in consideration for the opportunity to become a biological parent and the possibility of intimate association with the child. This possibility arises from the fact that the genetic father has the same parental rights upon the birth of a child through a surrogacy agreement as any biological father would.

The ACLU believes that, provided that contract provisions for termination of parental rights are void and the payment to the mother is not conditioned upon her giving up parental rights, the child's constitutional rights have not been violated. The child is not sold as a chattel where: the genetic father and his partner cannot purchase physical custody of the child, have no guarantee that the gestational mother will relinquish her parental rights, and have no entitlement to exclusive enjoyment of parental rights.

The Union believes that a legal prohibition or a state prohibition against payment for reproductive services, lost wages and medical costs of the gestational mother would be a *de facto* prohibition on surrogacy and thus violate the rights of the gestational mother and genetic father.

C. *Discrimination*

The state cannot discriminate against a person who seeks participation in a surrogacy arrangement on the basis of age, race, sex, sexual orientation, economic or social status, religion, marital status, or physical or mental condition. In particular, the state cannot discriminate in any of the following ways.

First, the state may not restrict the right of lesbians or gay men to participate in surrogacy arrangements. The ACLU is opposed to governmental discrimination on the basis of sexual or affectional orientation. (Policy #264) Therefore, the ACLU would oppose any law limiting access to surrogacy arrangements to heterosexuals.

Second, the state may not limit surrogacy arrangements to married couples. The civil liberties to be exercised in surrogacy arrangements are individual liberties which should be respected without regard to whether a person is married or has a partner.

Third, the state may not restrict the right to participate in the surrogacy arrangement based upon a diagnosis of infertility of the contracting father's partner. Decision about human reproduction should be a matter of voluntary choice free of government compulsion.

D. *Waiver of Rights to Privacy and Bodily Integrity*

Contract provisions that purport to waive a woman's privacy rights and right to bodily integrity and control are void and unenforceable.[3]

An agreement to waive a fundamental right in the future should be unenforceable; waiver is inappropriate until a person is in a position to know the meaning, importance, or value of a particular right.

Many surrogacy contracts, for example, contain provisions restricting the woman's right to choose, or not choose an abortion. As provided by ACLU Abortion Policy (#263), however, the decision of whether or not to continue a pregnancy should be one in the woman's personal discretion in conjunction with her doctor. Strong legal arguments exist that allowing a woman to waive her right to abortion would violate her constitutional privacy rights, along with the Thirteenth Amendment's prohibition against involuntary servitude. The ACLU has long supported the right of a woman to choose to have an abortion. Further, many legal commentators have persuasively argued that the abortion right can never be waived.

Likewise, the right to refuse or to consent to medical treatment is an essential element of the personal right to bodily integrity, a right that cannot be waived. Because a woman cannot waive her right to abortion or bodily integrity, she cannot be bound by a contract provision to give up those rights.

We should note that the potentially coercive nature of for-profit surrogacy arrangements intensifies our concerns about waiver in the case of commercial surrogacy. The fee payment serves as an inducement for women who are poor, and often uneducated, to opt for surrogacy because of financial need. There are particularly strong grounds in these cases to doubt the adequacy of the waiver.

E. *Waiver of Parental Rights*

A gestational mother's waiver of parental rights prior to the birth of the child is also unenforceable. This is true whether or not she is also the genetic mother. Waiver of parental rights is enforceable only if the waiver occurs after the rights have come into existence, i.e., after the birth.

There are two separate, but not unrelated reasons supporting this policy. One is that the woman's constitutionally protected parental rights are at stake and those rights cannot be waived enforceably prior to their existence, for the reasons discussed above.[4]

The other reason has to do with the rights of the child and the policy against the sale of babies. As provided in Section B above, the ACLU opposes payment for the sale of parental rights—which is the equivalent of the sale of a child—while not opposing payment by their father to the gestational mother for her labor in becoming pregnant, gestating, and giving birth to the child. If the contract is deemed enforceable either by specific performance or by way of damages when the mother decides not to turn over the child after its birth, or if payment to the gestational mother is conditioned on her surrender of parental rights, then the subject of the contract is the child, not the gestation. While the father has the right to pay someone to assist him in becoming a parent, his parenthood is dependent only on the birth of the child, not on obtaining sole custody nor on the termination of parental rights by the gestational mother. If there is a dispute over custody, that should be settled pursuant to the policies outlined in Section F below.

Furthermore, those surrogate contracts that incorporate provisions by which the gestational mother waives all parental rights to the child, thus purporting to give the father the legal right to force her relinquishment of the child, draw into issue the woman's fundamental rights to legal custody of her children and her right to parent. The legal standards governing involuntary termination of parental rights require a showing of parental unfitness or abandonment of the child by clear and convincing evidence before parental rights may constitutionally be terminated, and no court has ever found a surrogate contract to be *prima facie* evidence of such unfitness or abandonment.

As in the adoption context, a gestational mother's surrender of her parental rights should not be enforceable unless made after her child's birth. All states currently have laws that prevent a birth mother from terminating her parental rights or consenting to the adoption of her child until after the child's birth. Some states require an additional waiting period after the birth, before the execution of a consent to adoption. Some states' statutes also create a period after the execution of the consent during which the mother retains the right to change her mind.

When a surrogacy arrangement involves an adoption because the genetic father has a partner, these protections ought to apply. When no adoption is involved (because the genetic father has no partner and he is already a legal parent) these protections afforded in the adoption context ought to apply nonetheless, if the genetic father seeks to terminate the gestational mother's parental rights. The effect of these protections is to prevent the prebirth waiver of her parental rights.

F. *Custody*

If, upon birth of the child, a gestational mother chooses not to relinquish her parental status through adoption, she remains the legal mother of the child. The father who provided the sperm also remains a legal parent.[5]

These parents, not wed to each other, may want the other's parental rights terminated and may each want custody of the child. In such a situation, one or the other is likely to seek resolution of the dispute in court. In these circumstances, the termination of parental rights as well as questions of custody and visitation should be resolved by the principles generally applied to such disputes, insofar as those principles are consistent with the civil liberties of the parties. Parental rights may not be involuntarily terminated unless a parent is unfit or has abandoned the child. Provided that neither of these is the case, the primary issues will be custody and visitation.

Today, the universal standard for resolving custody disputes is the best interests of the child, a standard which focuses on the child's welfare rather than on the parents' rights. Yet custody questions have civil liberties implications: many experience the relational rights and responsibilities between parent and child as at least as profound and significant as other rights and responsibilities. Moreover, the broad best interests standards has been given difficult content by different jurisdictions and even different judges within jurisdictions; they often use criteria for deciding the best interest question that implicate civil rights that have been a traditional concern of the ACLU.[6]

The ACLU believes that status criteria such as age, religion, sex, sexual orientation, race, disability, economic status and marital status of a parent should not be used as proxies for an individual child's best interests. None of these factors, standing along, or in combination, can automatically be equated with the relevant substantive criterion—the best interest of the child. It is tempting in custody disputes (whether or not they arise in the surrogacy context) to resort to bright line rules for resolving these contests because such rules offer a mechanism for avoiding prolonged and harmful battles between the parents. These rules, however, evade the deeper inquiry into what is in the best interest of the particular child before the court, and, from a civil liberties perspective, permit child custody to be based on status criteria, traditionally used to discriminate against individuals, that violate ACLU anti-discrimination policy. Moreover, they decide the exercise of the fundamental right to association with one's children by presumption rather than individual determination.

Sex and economic status in particular are characteristics that could become factors in the surrogacy context. For most of our history, custody was explicitly based on sex of the parent. Originally, these rules took the form of preference for the father; later, the paternal preference was replaced in part by a preference for the mother of a child of tender years. In the surrogacy context, the obvious candidates for automatic rules are (1) that the woman who gestates the newborn receives custody (unless unfit for parenthood) because of her special role as prenatal nurturer, or (2) the man who contracted to bring the child into existence and provided his sperm should get the benefit of his bargain (unless he is unfit) at least to the extent of custody. Each of these automatic rules like the earlier, general preference for mother or father, contravenes the ACLU policy against sex discrimination and thus jeopardizes the civil liberties of one or the other parent.

An economic status test for best interest generally favors fathers, an effect which would likely be even stronger in the surrogacy context than in others because the economics of surrogacy arrangements virtually guarantees a marked disparity in the wealth of the father and gestational mother. Material advantage may not be a proper measure of the best interest of a child; moreover, use of such a test has a discriminatory effect on women.

An additional issue, unique to the surrogacy context, is what role if any the surrogacy agreement should be allowed to play in the custody determination. The ACLU takes the position that the gestational mother's entry into a surrogacy agreement should not be treated as evidence of unfitness or abandonment. If she has a right to reserve the question of whether she will relinquish rights until the child is born, and upon the birth of her child exercises her right to retain her parental status, that decision renders her previous intention irrelevant. In addition, holding her to that previous intention chills the exercise of her right to reproductive choice (the entry into a surrogacy arrangement) and penalizes the exercise of her relational right (her decision not to relinquish the child). Similarly, the fact that the father entered into the surrogacy agreement should not give him an equitable right to custody arising from his thwarted expectation that the mother would relinquish her parental rights. To do so would give partial effect to an aspect of the agreement which is, on civil liberties grounds, unenforceable, namely, the provision concerning relinquishment of the mother's parental rights.[7]

Finally, most surrogacy custody disputes involve infants, and infants pose special questions for application of the best interest standard. To the extent that past and present relationship to the infant (rather than an assessment of the quality of future relationships) provide the basis for assignment of custody, questions about what constitutes relationship become paramount. Certainly, physical contact (including gestation and birth) can be indicia of relationship; so too are acts directed towards creating a parent-child relationship, such as financial support, preparing a place at home for the baby and the father's entry into a surrogacy arrangement, to the extent any or all of these factors in the context of the particular case are in fact indices of parental caretaking and connection.[8]

Notes

1. ACLU Policy # 262 states that the whole question of human reproduction should be a matter of voluntary decision and that women and men should enjoy freedom of choice concerning reproduction. *See also* ACLU Policy # 210 opposing the criminalization of victimless crimes.

2. The ACLU sees no *per se* civil liberties bar to the state regulation or prohibition of third party intermediaries, except if such regulation or prohibition substantially interferes with the rights of individuals to pursue surrogacy as a reproductive option.

3. We use "waiver" in this policy to refer to both waiver and alienation. Waiver is "[t]he intentional or voluntary relinquishment of a known right," and involves a unilateral act with nothing in return from the party benefiting from the waiver. Black's Law Dictionary 1751–2 (4th ed. 1968); Kreimer, Allocational Sanctions: The Problem of Negative Rights in a Positive State, 132 U. Pa. L. Rev. 1293, 1383–85 (1984). Alienation of a right involves the voluntary and complete transfer of the right in exchange for a proffered benefit.

4. In contrast, we believe that a sperm or egg donor can enforceably surrender any future claims to parental rights at the time of gamete donation. The difference is that the gestational mother's waiver occurs long in advance of her final act of surrendering the child, and intervening events of gestation, birthing, and possible bonding constitute a change in circumstance so substantial as to create doubt that the prior waiver was knowing and intelligent. A gamete donor's waiver, on the other hand, occurs roughly at the same time as the final donative act, and the events normally intervening between waiver and donation do not constitute such a change in circumstance as to cast doubt on the quality of the waiver. Moreover, once donation has occurred, the donor usually knows nothing further of the use of his or her gametes. Thus, there are no further events that the donor experiences connected with the donation that would render the prior waiver less than knowing and intelligent.

5. If the child is the product of egg as well as sperm donation, he or she may have a third legal parent. An anonymous egg donor, like an anonymous sperm donor, would have no parental rights. But equal protection principles dictate that an egg donor mother who, like the sperm donor father, participates in a surrogacy arrangement, contributing genetic material for the purpose of becoming a parent, be like the father, a parent to the resulting child.

6. Because issues of custody and visitation at their core concern the relational rights of parents and children, but courts do not necessarily adopt stances consistent with civil liberties, an ACLU policy on custody and visitation would be appropriate. At such time as a custody policy is adopted, its principles will be relevant and applicable to custody disputes in the surrogacy context, particularly if sufficiently broad in scope to encompass the questions of what the best interest standard should mean in the case of infants and what the rights of parents not wed to each other should be.

7. By contrast, the surrogacy agreement may be considered relevant to the question of whether the father sought to establish a relationship to his child and acted as a father toward the child. "Acting as father" may be the criterion for determining whether a father not wed to the mother can contest custody (cf. *Lehr v. Robertson*, 463 U.S. 248 (1983)), and if so whether he has a viable custody claim.

8. Initial physical custody frequently becomes the basis for assigning long term legal custody, which means that leaving an infant with the gestational mother

initially gives her an advantage in the custody dispute. Taking the infant from the gestational mother and giving him or her to the father pending resolution of the custody question only shifts the advantage to him. A third possibility, which seems untenable, is initial placement of an infant with foster parents so mother and father will go into the custody dispute on an equal footing. The concern that neither parent be given an unwarranted "thumb on the scales" by initial physical custody, weighs in favor of a relatively short period after birth during which the gestational mother can decide whether or not she wishes to retain her parental status and, if she does, an accelerated custody trial.

B. The American College of Obstetricians and Gynecologists

Ethical Issues in Surrogate Motherhood

The American College of Obstetricians and Gynecologists recognizes that there is current interest in the reproductive alternative known as "surrogate motherhood." A surrogate mother may be defined as a woman who conceives and carries a pregnancy for another woman. In the most common example, a couple in which the husband is fertile but the wife is not contracts with a fertile woman for her to be inseminated with the husband's sperm. This woman carries the pregnancy until delivery, and then gives over the child to the contracting couple.

The obstetrician-gynecologist may be requested to participate in surrogate motherhood in a variety of ways, each of which raises ethical issues: (1) the provision of obstetric care to the pregnant surrogate, (2) participation in the process of insemination of the surrogate, (3) recruitment or screening of potential surrogate mothers, (4) counseling or referral of couples who could be candidates for such a procedure and (5) participation directly or indirectly with an organization that provides such services.

One way of examining the ethical issues involved in surrogate motherhood is to compare and contrast it with a procedure that is, in many ways, its logical counterpart: artificial insemination by donor (AID). AID has become a commonly accepted solution for problems of male infertilty, although the ethical issues surrounding it are not completely resolved. The ethical issues surrounding surrogate motherhood, however, can and must be considered while its practice is relatively limited.

Issues Shared with Artificial Insemination by Donor

The wide acceptance of AID is based in part on the assumption that couples choosing this course have the same motives and aspirations in seeking to have a child as do fertile couples. Couples who seek surrogate motherhood because of female infertility probably have similar motives, also. Nonetheless, both AID and surrogate motherhood present ethical concerns:

1. Both depersonalize reproduction to some extent. This may affect the particular couple adversely, and with widespread use may lead to a change in the way society views childbearing.
2. Both procedures may create stress in the relationship of the infertile couple. It is generally believed that this is not a serious problem in successful AID pregnancies; it may or may not be cause for concern in the surrogate mother situation.
3. Both the sperm donor and the surrogate mother risk undergoing psychological stress. Despite the wide experience with AID, this concern has not been investigated in sperm donors. Preliminary evidence suggests that a significant risk may exist for surrogate mothers.
4. Both procedures could be misused in programs for eugenic manipulation. However, both procedures may appropriately involve genetic screening for the purpose of matching surrogate phenotype with the potential parents and preventing the transmission of genetic diseases.

Originally published as "Ethical Issues in Surrogate Motherhood" (ACOG Statement of Policy 56) (Washington, D.C.: American College of Obstetricians and Gynecologists, 1983).

5. Both procedures raise concerns about adverse psychological effects on the children if their situation becomes known to them and others. There are no data that address this issue.
6. Both procedures raise questions regarding the maintenance of donor and surrogate anonymity. Legal questions such as legitimacy of the children also remain unanswered.

Concerns Not Shared with Artificial Insemination by Donor

The surrogate motherhood procedure is clearly distinguished from AID by the extent to which the surrogate herself must be personally involved. This raises several medical and ethical issues:

1. The surrogate mother undertakes two types of risks: physical and psychological. She exposes herself to potential long-term effects on her health and to all of the potential complications of pregnancy, including a remote chance of death. Psychological harm may occur when the child is separated from the surrogate. Although these kinds of risks are easily stated, they perhaps cannot be completely comprehended until experienced. Long-term psychological risks have not yet been evaluated.
2. It is not clear who should receive relevant medical information and participate in decisions affecting the welfare of the fetus and newborn. In general, the biological mother is thought to act in the best interests of the fetus, and so has the authority to make such decisions. In the instance of the surrogate mother, the motivation and the process of decision making raise complex questions. For example, may the surrogate make her own decisions about certain behaviors (such as whether to drink alcohol or smoke), or are these the decisions of the soon-to-be parents? Decisions about prenatal diagnostic and treatment procedures, and the management of the pregnancy, labor, delivery, and complications will also need to be made in concert with the physician, but it must be clarified whether they are to be made by the prospective parents or the surrogate mother.
3. The surrogate mother may change her mind and decide to have an elective abortion or to keep the child after delivery.
4. The surrogate may be confronted with a situation in which, for a variety of reasons, custody of the child returns to her by default.

Additional Concerns Raised by Financial Transactions

Most proposed agreements include financial arrangements that involve payment to the surrogate as well as to the individual or group responsible for the surrogate arrangement. These financial arrangements raise a number of ethical concerns.

1. The selling of infants is both illegal and morally objectionable. It is difficult to differentiate between payment for the service of carrying the child and payment for the child.
2. Payment to surrogates above and beyond reimbursement for expenses creates the potential for exploitation.
3. The physician who receives payment for recruiting or referring potential surrogates or parents is exploiting patients and may be in conflict of interest. The physician who invests in enterprises specializing in surrogate arrangements risks similar wrongdoing.

Special Situations

Beyond the situation of the infertile couple using the surrogate to obtain a desired child, there are other situations in which a surrogate might be employed. For example, the couple might want a child but prefers not to risk interruption of career plans, or may be unwilling to undergo the risks of pregnancy. Using a surrogate for the sake of convenience, rather than for infertility, raises a number of issues:

1. Depersonalization is increased.
2. A risk that could be borne personally is assigned to someone else.
3. The dedication of the couple to parenthood—and thereby their qualifications to rear children—is called into question.

A variety of other situations and combinations of roles in surrogate parenthood can be envisioned, each with a constellation of related problems.

Conclusions and Recommendations

The physician who participates in surrogate motherhood arrangements, provides fertility services or obstetric services for a surrogate, or provides counseling services should carefully examine all relevant issues, including legal, psychological, societal, medical, and ethical aspects. Simple, clear conclusions cannot be anticipated.

Significant ethical concerns exist even in the most uncomplicated situation involving an infertile married couple and no financial transactions. Additional concerns that result from the payment of fees and from special circumstances such as surrogate use for convenience or single parenting magnify the ethical complications.

Thus, while the decision to participate or not in the surrogate motherhood alternative is an individual one for each physician to make, the American College of Obstetricians and Gynecologists has significant reservations about this approach to parenthood and offers the following recommendations for the guidance of Fellows:

I.   Initiation of Surrogate Arrangements

   A. When approached by a patient interested in surrogate motherhood, the physician should, as in all other aspects of medical care, be certain there is a full discussion of ethical and medical risks, benefits and alternatives, many of which have been expressed in this paper.
   B. A physician may justifiably decline to participate in surrogate motherhood arrangements.
   C. If a physician decides to become involved in a surrogate motherhood arrangement, he or she should follow these guidelines:
      1. The physician should be assured that appropriate procedures are utilized to screen the contracting couple and the surrogate. Such screening may include appropriate fertility studies and genetic screening.
      2. The physician should receive only the usual compensation for obstetric and gynecologic services. Referral fees and other arrangements for financial gain beyond the usual fees for medical services are inappropriate.
      3. The physician should not participate in a surrogate program where the financial arrangements are likely to exploit any of the parties.

II.   Care of Pregnant Surrogates

   A. When a woman seeks medical care for an established pregnancy, regardless of the method of conception, she should be cared for as any other obstetric patient or referred to a qualified physician who will provide that care.

B. The surrogate mother should be considered the source of consent with respect to clinical intervention and management of the pregnancy. Confidentiality between the physician and patient should be maintained. If other parties, such as the adoptive parents, are to play a role in decision making, the parameters should be clearly delineated, with the agreement of the patient.

C. The American Medical Association

Report of the Judicial Council

Resolution 26 (A-84) asks that (1) the AMA encourage physicians and other participants in surrogate parenting programs to exercise great care and discretion, recognizing that their legal and ethical status is unclear; and (2) the AMA neither automatically endorse nor condemn surrogate parenting as an alternative for infertile couples who wish to become parents. Resolution 26 was referred to the Judicial Council.

The Judicial Council sympathizes with those individuals who wish to become parents but are unable to do so. The Judicial Council encourages those individuals to investigate various methods of becoming parents, including legal adoption. The Judicial Council also commends the progress made in the medical alleviation of infertility. Further, the Judicial Council has recognized the development of such methods of becoming parents as artificial insemination and in vitro fertilization and has provided ethical guidance as to the use of these reproductive techniques. Newer techniques such as in vivo fertilization are being developed, and it is clearly impossible to predict what further advances will occur. The Judicial Council encourages methods that are ethically and legally acceptable and that encompass the best interests of all individuals involved.

Of primary concern are the best interests of the child and of the mother. Out of concern for those interests, the Judicial Council expended over one year of study and debate and listened to testimony from various points of view on the subject of "surrogate mother" arrangements. The House of Delegates adopted Judicial Council Report C on this subject at the 1983 Interim Meeting. In that report, the Judicial Council reviewed ethical, legal, psychological, societal, and financial concerns regarding arrangements in which a women agrees to become pregnant through artificial insemination, to carry the child thus conceived to term, and to surrender the child for adoption.

Conclusion

The Judicial Council encourages people who wish to, but are unable to become parents to examine such alternatives as legal adoption and medical interventions that alleviate the causes of infertility. Where these alternatives are not possible, the Judicial Council also recognizes the potential value of those reproductive techniques that utilize the sperm or ova of donors, such as artificial insemination. However, these techniques must be utilized with the utmost concern for the welfare of all parties involved. The Judicial Council notes that the ethical questions become serious when a technique encompasses the deliberate conception of a child to be surrendered by the mother upon birth, and that those ethical questions become even more serious when the mother will be paid to relinquish her child.

No information has come to the Judicial Council's attention that would cause it to change its opinion on "Surrogate Mothers" presented to the House of Delegates at the 1983 Interim Meeting. The Judicial Council will continue to monitor surrogate parenting developments to determine whether the ethical, legal, psychological, societal, and financial concerns can be mitigated.

The Judicial Council recommends that this report be adopted in lieu of Resolution 26 (A-84).

SURROGATE MOTHERS

(Reference Committee on Amendments to Constitution and Bylaws, page 305)

HOUSE ACTION: ADOPTED

An opinion of the Judicial Council on the subject of "surrogate mother" arrangements was presented to the House of Delegates in Judicial Council Report B (I-82). The House referred Report B back to the Judicial Council. The House also requested the the Board of Trustees study the subject and report to the House.

The Judicial Council has carefully reviewed the information developed by the Board's Committee on Medicolegal Problems on the legal risks of physician involvement in surrogate parenting arrangements, as well as the article "Parenthood by Proxy," by the former AMA General Counsel, which appeared in JAMA on April 22–29, 1983. The Judicial Council has also carefully considered the excellent statement of the American College of Obstetricians and Gynecologists on ethical issues in surrogate motherhood. The Council noted the press reports in 1983 of an unfortunate incident in which a "surrogate mother" gave birth to a microcephalic child who was not the offspring of the semen donor. The Judicial Council is very much concerned about the potential legal and ethical jeopardy that physicians who participate in such arrangements face. When all considerations are brought together, these arrangements do not appear to serve societal interests.

Having received the considered views and comments of members of its panel of consultants, the Judicial Council has given additional consideration to the subject and has concluded that what have been described as "surrogate mother" arrangements do not provide a satisfactory reproductive alternative. The Judicial Council presents its opinion to the House of Delegates for information.

SURROGATE MOTHERS. "Surrogate" motherhood is an arrangement which involves the artificial insemination of a woman who agrees to give the child thus conceived for adoption by the man providing the semen and, usually, his infertile wife. The arrangement involves the services of an attorney who attends to the legal phases of the transaction, a physician who will perform or arrange for the medical services that may be required, and the person or persons seeking a child for adoption. The services of a woman who will enter into a contract for providing the services of bearing a child and delivering the child for adoption are sought. The contract customarily provides compensation for costs of the medical services and for living expenses of the surrogate mother during pregnancy, as well as for discomfort or inconvenience.

The Judicial Council is concerned about the ethical, social and legal problems that may arise in an arrangement in which a woman agrees to become pregnant through artificial insemination, to carry to term and to give the child thus conceived to other persons to serve as adoptive parents. The welfare of the child should be a foremost consideration. In ordinary adoption proceedings an appropriate agency usually investigates prospective adoptive parents to determine their fitness as parents. This precaution is not always present in surrogate motherhood arrangements.

The Judicial Council is also concerned that, if there is a subsequent birth of a defective child, a situation may arise in which prospective adoptive parents and the woman who gave birth to the child may not want to or will be unable to assume the responsibilities of parenthood.

Many other ethical, social and morally difficult situations can be envisioned. For example, the woman who has contracted to bear the child may decide to have an abortion or to refuse to give the child up for adoption. Another consideration which may be overlooked is the psychological impairment that may occur in a woman who deliberately conceives with the intention of bearing a child which she will give up.

The Judicial Council believes that surrogate motherhood presents many ethical, legal, psychological, societal and financial concerns and does not represent a satisfactory reproductive alternative for people who wish to become parents.

D. The American Fertility Society
SURROGATE MOTHERS

Background

A surrogate mother is a woman who is artificially inseminated with the sperm of a man who is not her husband; she carries the pregnancy and then turns the resulting child over to the man to rear. In almost all instances, the man has chosen to use a surrogate mother because his wife is infertile. After the birth, the wife will adopt the child.

Unlike surrogate gestational motherhood, which involves an embryo transfer after in vivo or in vitro fertilization (IVF), surrogate motherhood depends only on the technology of artificial insemination. The primary reason for the use of surrogate motherhood as a reproductive option is to produce a child with a genetic link to the husband.

The use of the term "surrogate" for the woman who is the genetic and gestational mother of the child appears a misnomer to some people, who argue that the adoptive mother is actually the "surrogate" for the biologic mother, who has given up the child. Nevertheless, a contrary position can be articulated, because the adoptive woman will be performing the major mothering role by rearing the child, with the biologic mother serving as a surrogate for her in providing the component for reproduction that she lacks. Although the term "surrogate mother" is, in any case, ambiguous and not a medical term, it has nevertheless received widespread public recognition and will be used in this report to mean a woman who conceives and gestates a child to be reared by the biologic father and his wife. The use of a surrogate mother, who provides the egg and the womb for the child, is currently much more common than the use of a surrogate gestational mother, who provides only the womb.

In comparison with the other reproductive technologies discussed in this report, surrogate motherhood has received scant attention in the medical literature. Although it has produced many more babies than have been born after cryopreservation of a preembryo or by preembryo donation after in vivo fertilization, there have been no medical articles published about the procedure, its success rate, or the mental or physical health of the children produced. There are only a few studies of the psychological ramifications of surrogate motherhood. These studies include speculation about the potential effects on the participants (Andrews, 1985b) and preliminary research on the selection of surrogate mothers and their responses to the pregnancy and subsequent relinquishment of the child (Franks, 1981; Parker, 1983).

One reason for the lack of scientific attention to the medical aspects of surrogate motherhood is that it has developed in an entrepreneurial setting, generally apart from medical institutions. Although the founders of some surrogate mother programs are physicians, the majority are lawyers, social workers, or persons with no professional training. However, most programs do use the services of a physician to perform a physical examination of the surrogate mother and to perform the artificial insemination. The extent to which these programs undertake an independent assessment of the infertility of the wife is unclear. Some couples who have

Originally published in Chapter 25, "Ethical Considerations of the New Reproductive Technologies," *Fertility and Sterility* 46 (1986): Supplement 1, 625–685. Reproduced with the permission of the publisher, The American Fertility Society, Birmingham, Alabama.

infertility problems that could be helped by drugs, surgery, IVF, or other alternatives may be employing a surrogate at a substantial fee because they do not undergo medical screening as part of the surrogate program and thus do not realize that they have other options. Existing surrogate mother programs generally perform medical screening on the surrogate, and some perform a physical on the man who will provide the sperm (Andrews, 1985).

Some women serve as surrogate mothers for an infertile friend or relative and charge no fee. In other instances, the surrogate mother is a stranger who receives compensation for her services.

The demographic studies of surrogate mothers, which deal mainly with potential paid surrogates, have found that their average age is 25. Over one-half of the women are married, one-fifth divorced, and about one-fourth single. Over one-half (57%) are Protestant and 42% are Catholic (Parker, 1983). Over one-half are high school graduates and over one-fourth have schooling beyond high school.

Polls show that the public is less favorably disposed toward surrogate motherhood as an infertility solution than it is toward IVF, artificial insemination—donor (AID), embryo donation, or adoption (Brodsky, 1983). However, surveys of the public and of child welfare professionals regarding how the law should handle surrogate motherhood indicate the most people feel that the procedure should not be banned but rather should be regulated (Child Welfare League, 1983).

Indications

When a woman is infertile, she and her husband may need the assistance of a surrogate mother to conceive and carry a child for her. Sperm from the husband of the infertile woman is used to inseminate the surrogate mother, who will carry the pregnancy and then turn the resulting child over to the couple.

The primary medical indication for use of a surrogate mother is the inability of a woman to provide either the genetic or the gestational component for childbearing, for example, a woman who has had a hysterectomy combined with removal of the ovaries. This is the only situation in which surrogate motherhood provides the sole medical solution. For other indications, other medical options are possible, although they may not be readily available.

A second indication for surrogate motherhood is the inability to provide the genetic component, for example, because of premature menopause or the desire not to risk passing on a genetic defect. Under these circumstances, the woman could alternatively have the genetic component provided through egg or embryo donation, but donors might be more difficult to find than surrogate mothers.

A third indication for the use of a surrogate mother is the inability to gestate. A woman with severe hypertension, a uterine malformation, or the absence of a uterus after hysterectomy may use the services of a surrogate mother. If that woman wanted to provide the genetic component for her child, she and her husband could create an embryo either in vitro or in vivo, then have it transferred to a surrogate gestational mother.

The use of a surrogate mother is also available as a secondary approach for women with any other type of infertility; essentially, it eliminates the need for the social mother to play any biologic role in reproduction.

Reservations About Surrogate Motherhood

The reservations about surrogate motherhood, like reservations about other reproductive technologies, focus on the potential effects on the surrogate, the couple, the potential child, and society. Because of the dearth of research on the subject, most of the potential risks are highly speculative. There is concern that it is improper to ask a surrogate to put herself through the physical hazards of a pregnancy to benefit other persons. There is also concern that the surrogate might be psychologically harmed by giving up her genetic child. There are some surrogates who go through a period of grief and mourning after giving up the child (*Psychiatric News*, 1984).

There is also a risk that, because of the uncertain legal status of the procedure, the surrogate will be required to keep (or put up for general adoption) a child for whom she did not intend to have parental responsibility. This situation might occur if a paternity test revealed that the child was not the offspring of the man who contracted with the surrogate or if the child were born with a defect so that the couple refused to take custody of the child.

In addition to the potential harm to the surrogate, there is concern that the couple might be harmed by the procedure. The woman might be harmed by not having access to medical advice to help her resolve her infertility in other ways. The couple might be at risk of harassment from the surrogate in those rare instances in which she learns the couple's identities and seeks them out after relinquishing the child. Or, if the surrogate is a friend or relative, her continued involvement with the couple may cause tension in their marital relationship. Also, the couple are financially and emotionally at risk because of the uncertain legal status of the procedure. If the surrogate keeps the child, the contracting husband might nevertheless have to pay child support because he is the biologic father. The couple who pay a surrogate might be prosecuted under criminal law in those states that prohibit payment beyond certain enumerated medical and legal expenses of a woman in connection with her giving up her child for adoption (Andrews, 1986).

The potential physical and psychological effects on the child are cause for concern as well. The child might be physically harmed if the surrogate mother passes on a genetic defect. This possibility is similar to the risk involved in using sperm donors, and it merits similar handling by appropriate screening. The surrogate mother has the responsibility not only of providing the gamete for conception but also of gestating. A surrogate mother who knows that she will not have the responsibility of rearing a child might not be sufficiently careful during the pregnancy. Moreover, the surrogate might be less likely than a woman planning to rear the child to give priority to the fetus in situations in which there is a conflict between maternal and fetal needs. For these reasons, screening of potential surrogate mothers is necessary to determine what gestational risks they present.

In addition, there are concerns about the psychological development of the child, who may feel a need for information about the surrogate mother or may want to learn her identity. If the surrogate mother is a friend or relative who maintains contact with the child, it is unclear what effect a connection with two mothers will have on the child's development or identity.

As with donation of sperm, eggs, or embryos, the use of a surrogate mother who provides an egg, as well as gestational services, raises questions about the ethics of donor involvement in procreation. There is concern that the involvement of a surrogate mother in childbearing will weaken the marital bond and undermine the integrity of the institution of the family. To some, third-party involvement in procreation is considered to be threatening to the sanctity of the marital relationship, whether or not there is provable physical or psychological harm to the participants in the process.

Some commentators have voiced the further concern that if surrogates are paid for their services, human reproduction will become commercialized, and children might come to be perceived as a "consumer item" (Hellegers, 1978).

A final reservation is that surrogate motherhood might be used for convenience when the potential rearing mother does not wish to undergo pregnancy. However, it is less likely that a woman would use a surrogate mother, rather than a surrogate gestational mother, for those purposes. With a surrogate mother, the woman gives up not only the gestational inconvenience but also the chance to be the genetic mother for the child.

Rationale for the Use of a Surrogate Mother

For some couples, of whom the wife has no uterus or ovaries, the use of a surrogate mother is the only means to have a child genetically related to one of them. In all of its applications, the use of a surrogate mother allows the infertile woman who wished to rear a child the opportunity to adopt an infant more rapidly than by waiting several years for a traditional adoption. In addition, it allows her to rear her husband's genetic child.

For the husband of an infertile woman, the use of a surrogate may be the only way in which he can conceive and rear a child with a biologic tie to himself, short of divorcing his wife and remarrying only for that reason or of having an adulterous union. Certainly, the use of a surrogate mother under the auspices of a medical practitioner seems far less destructive of the institution of the family than the latter two options.

For the child, the use of a surrogate mother gives him or her an opportunity that would not otherwise be available: the opportunity to exist. Furthermore, the child would be reared by a couple who so wanted him or her that they were willing to participate in a novel process with potential legal and other risks.

The process offers potential benefits for the surrogates as well. As in the case of organ transplantation, it offers them the chance to be altruistic. In addition, some surrogate mothers enjoy being pregnant. Moreover, one preliminary study found that about one-third of surrogate mothers may be using the process to help themselves psychologically. These are women who in the past have voluntarily aborted or given up a child through adoption and have then become surrogate mothers in order to relive the experience of pregnancy in a psychologically satisfactory way (Parker, 1983). Those women who become surrogate mothers for a fee are benefited by having another income option. For example, some divorced women with young children have chosen to be surrogates in order to support their children and to remain at home to care for them.

Although there are potential risks to surrogacy, those risks can be understood by the prospective participants. Thus informed, they can engage in competent decision making about whether or not to pursue this reproductive option. Initial data indicate that the couples and surrogates can understand in advance how they will react to the procedure. "Preliminary evidence indicates that only a few surrogates and the parental couple felt surprised by their own psychological responses after the relinquishment or by the other party's response" (Parker, 1984).

Committee Considerations

Surrogate motherhood has received extensive media attention and has raised a panoply of emotional reactions and ethical concerns. Unlike AID, which was developed in a shroud of secrecy, surrogate motherhood was thrust before the public eye, often for the pragmatic reason of needing high visibility in order to recruit potential surrogates. The use of a surrogate mother has raised a range of issues about third-party involvement in procreation, such as whether that involvement is destructive to the marital bond or psychologically harmful to the third party and whether the child has a right to learn about the history or identity of the third party. Unfortunately, there is little precedent for answering these questions; the policy of secrecy surrounding sperm donation has served to limit studies in that context that might have served as a basis for understanding the psychological implications of using third parties in reproduction generally. Nevertheless, large segments of our society view as permissible the donation of sperm to compensate for a male infertility problem. The use of a surrogate mother to compensate for a female infertility problem could similarly be viewed as permissible, unless it can be demonstrated to be significantly more risky to the participants or to society than AID or other activities that our society condones.

The Committee's main concerns about surrogate motherhood are threefold. First, there appear to be potential risks to all participants that need to be considered. There is concern that a woman who becomes a surrogate mother may be subjecting herself to too many physical and psychological risks. There is some sentiment that it is improper to ask a woman to be a surrogate mother, because she will be facing the potential physical risks of pregnancy and childbirth without receiving what seems to be a commensurate benefit. There are further concerns that a woman who is a friend or relative of the couple may be coerced into being a surrogate or that a paid surrogate may be exploited.

The perceived degree of involvement (duration, intensity, and medical risks) of the surrogate mother leads the Committee to see this third-party involvement as different from AID or egg donation. However, the Committee is mindful that society allows competent adults to take risks (for example, trying an experimental medical procedure, donating a kidney, engaging in a risky sports activity or occupation, or joining the armed services). In the medical realm, people are allowed to make risky choices as long as they have given voluntary, informed consent. With respect to surrogate motherhood, then, it is of the utmost importance to ensure that the potential surrogate mother is appropriately informed and has not been coerced into serving as a surrogate. It may be useful for the physician to interview the potential surrogate separately to ensure that she has not been coerced into participation; this may be especially important when the surrogate is a friend or relative of the couple and may have been subjected to personal pressures regarding participation.

Although the couple are not at physical risk, they may be at emotional or financial risk because the surrogate might decide to keep the child, which would require them to seek a court order to gain custody. Again, however, if voluntary, informed consent is obtained from the couple, it may be excessively paternalistic to deny them their chosen option on the speculation that it could be harmful to them.

Naturally, a prime ethical concern regarding the participants is focused on the child. A realistic assessment needs to be made of the potential physical and psychological risks to the child. Although there exists a potential for surrogates to risk harm to the child by failing to disclose a genetic defect that would disqualify them for surrogacy or by engaging in harmful behavior during pregnancy, such risk could be minimized by proper medical and psychological screening of surrogates. As is true with AID, there is little follow-up data on the health of the children born to surrogates. But the high visibility of the surrogate arrangements, as well as the fact that news about unhealthy children has been extremely rare, suggests that the potential physical risks have not frequently materialized under the current system.

As to potential psychological harm to the child, there is concern that the child's self-identity might be confused because of his or her blurred genealogy. The use of a surrogate mother does not have to have a "blurring" effect on the child's genealogy. Situations in which full disclosures are made to the child about the personal history of the surrogate (and perhaps even her identity) might provide clear knowledge of genealogy. However, it is true that any use of a third party may make the genealogy more complex and perhaps bothersome to the child. Even if there are psychological risks, most infertile couples who go through with a reproduction arrangement that involves a third party do so as a last resort. In some cases, their willingness to make sacrifices to have a child may testify to their worthiness as loving parents. A child conceived through surrogate motherhood may be born into a much healthier climate than a child whose birth was unplanned. For this reason, some of the risks caused by confused genealogy may be outweighed by possible benefits to the child of having parents who want him or her.

Concerns are also raised by payment to a surrogate. Some people may approve of voluntary surrogate motherhood but disapprove of surrogate motherhood for a fee. The ramifications of prohibiting payment are widespread, however, because there are not enough voluntary surrogates to meet the needs of infertile couples. Because a surrogate mother has a much greater involvement in reproduction than does a donor of sperm, eggs, or embryos, she usually requires remuneration. On the couple's side, spending money for childbearing does not in itself seem unethical. Even without the involvement of a surrogate, couples spend substantial sums to investigate and treat their infertility. This financial outlay does not seem to create unusually high expectations about the child that might lead to psychological problems for him or her.

Commercialization in connection with giving up a child for adoption has traditionally been banned on the grounds that it might force biologic mothers to give up children whom they do not wish to give up and that the mere willingness to pay for a child does not guarantee that the potential parent will treat the child well. Because the sperm donor is merely turning over a gamete, whereas the surrogate mother is turning over a child, the latter action may seem to fit more closely into traditional concerns about baby selling. Nevertheless, paying the surrogate a fee is readily distinguishable from paying an already pregnant women for her child. The payment to a surrogate is made in exchange for her help in creating a child, not in exchange for possession of the child. Because the decision is made before the pregnancy ensues and the arrangement is entered into with the specific intention of relinquishing the child, the woman is less likely than an already-pregnant woman to be coerced into giving up a child whom she wishes to keep. Because the child will be reared by the genetic father and his wife, it may be more likely that the rearing father will have a greater sense of responsibility for the child than if the child were turned over to a stranger. Because the surrogate's responsibilities are set out in a contract before the conception occurs, she is more likely to understand and abide by them and less likely later to harass the couple with a change of heart.

A psychiatrist who has interviewed over 500 potential surrogates and who has followed several dozen surrogates through their pregnancies and beyond has written about surrogates' financial motivation, "There is no evidence that such a motivating factor results in more adverse psychological, medical, or legal consequences" (P. J. Parker, unpublished essay, 1982).

More troublesome is the commercialization and potential for exploitation of the couples and surrogates by professionals acting as brokers. The Committee is concerned that professionals who attempt to serve both the couple and the surrogate or who receive finder's fees for surrogates may have a conflict of interest or may exploit the parties.

As a final reservation, the lack of laws protecting couples who use a surrogate leads to a reluctance on the part of practitioners to recommend it (chapter 7). This, of course, could be solved by the enactment of laws clarifying the points that the contracting couple are the legal parents and that the surrogate mother has no parental rights or responsibilities with respect to the child after birth. Such laws are already being proposed in some states. Laws that take the opposite approach and attempt to prohibit the use of surrogate mothers would likely be struck down as unconstitutional for violating the couple's right to privacy in making procreative decisions (chapter 6).

Until favorable laws are passed, the rights and duties among the parties will likely be handled by a contract that includes an agreement by the surrogate to turn the child over to the couple for adoption. Of particular importance will be the provisions for human leukocyte antigen typing of the man providing the sperm and of the child, for assurance that the surrogate did not inadvertently become pregnant by her own partner rather than through the artificial insemination procedure.

Committee Recommendations

The Committee finds that surrogate motherhood is a matter that requires intense scrutiny. The Committee does not recommend the use of a surrogate mother for a nonmedical reason, such as the convenience of the rearing mother, because nonmedical reasons seem inadequate to justify using a surrogate to undertake the risks of pregnancy and delivery. As for surrogate motherhood for medical reasons, the Committee is dismayed by the scarcity of empiric evidence about how the surrogacy process works and how it affects those involved. Nevertheless, this process offers promise as the only medical solution to infertility in a couple of whom the woman has no uterus and who does not produce eggs or does not want to risk passing on a genetic defect that she carries.

There may be individual practitioners or medical groups asked to aid a surrogate mother arrangement who find that the reservations about the procedure outweigh the benefits, i.e., that the procedure is not in the best interests of the persons integrally and adequately considered. In that circumstance, the practitioner or group could ethically decline to participate in the arrangement.

The Committee does not recommend widespread clinical application of surrogate motherhood at this time. Because of the legal risks, ethical concerns, and potential physical and psychological effects of surrogate motherhood, it would seem to be more problematic than most of the other reproductive technologies discussed in this report. The Committee believes that there are not adequate reasons to recommend legal prohibition of surrogate motherhood, but the Committee has serious ethical reservations about surrogacy that cannot be fully resolved until appropriate data are available for assessment of the risks and possible benefits of this alternative.

The Committee recommends that if surrogate motherhood is pursued, it should be pursued as a clinical experiment. Among the issues to be addressed in the research on surrogate mothers are the following:

a. the psychological effects of the procedure on the surrogates, the couples, and the resulting children
b. the effects, if any, of bonding between the surrogate and the fetus in utero
c. the appropriate screening of the surrogate and the man who provides the sperm
d. the likelihood that the surrogate will exercise appropriate care during the pregnancy
e. the effects of having the couple and the surrogate meet or not meet
f. the effects on the surrogate's own family of her participation in the process
g. the effects of disclosing or not disclosing the use of a surrogate mother or her identity to the child
h. other issues that shed light on the effects of surrogacy on the welfare of the various persons involved and on society.

In the course of the clinical experiments on surrogate motherhood, special attention should be paid to whether the surrogate and the couple have given voluntary, informed consent. Both the surrogate and the man providing the sperm should be screened for infectious diseases, and the surrogate should be screened for genetic defects (Appendices B and C).

So that potential conflicts of interest or exploitation by professionals can be avoided, the Committee recommends that professionals receive only their customary fees for services and receive no finder's fees for participation in surrogate motherhood. Although it would be preferable that surrogates not receive payment beyond compensation for expenses and their inconvenience, the Committee recognizes that in some cases payment will be necessary for surrogacy to occur.* If surrogate motherhood turns out to be useful, a change in the law would be appropriate for assurance that the couple who contract with a surrogate mother are viewed as the legal parents.†‡

---

*It has been well established that the purchasing of organs (kidney, liver, gametes, etc.) is inappropriate because of the potential for abuse. Payment for surrogacy may be viewed as rent, i.e., allied to purchase. These Committee members believe that exploitation of surrogates would be diminished if payments to surrogates were limited to compensation for expenses and inconvenience (HWJJr, C-RG).

†The subject of surrogacy receives more relative attention in this report than may be its due. The matter has attracted wide public interest, presumably because of its challenge to traditional thinking about motherhood. However, its frequency to date has been quite low and provides only minimal experience on which to base judgment. It appears likely that, barring heavy-handed commercialization, frequency will remain low. Moreover, the issue relates not so much to the morality of an innovative reproductive technology as to the possible exploitation of women—certainly an important issue in its own right (CG).

‡The issue of surrogacy is highly controversial, but this Committee member believes that the risk/benefit ratio of the surrogacy procedures does not justify their support. The probability of abuse is real, e.g., financial enticement, psychological intimidation by family members or others. When the maternal morbidity and mortality rate, albeit small, is added on, these risks outweigh the benefit to the small number of couples who will be candidates for the surrogacy procedures. Finally, given the small number of couples involved, it is unlikely that significant research will be performed (CAP).

E. The New York State Task Force on Life and the Law

.   .   .   .   .

An Assessment: The Social and Moral
Dimensions of Surrogacy

The Task Force deliberated at length about the social, moral and legal issues posed by surrogate parenting. Its members began the deliberations with a wide diversity of opinion.

Ultimately, they reached a unanimous decision that public policy should discourage surrogate parenting. Divergent and sometimes competing visions form the basis for this conclusion. Their judgments are informed by different values, concerns and beliefs. The unanimous support for the conclusion reached is no less remarkable because of the diversity of opinion that underlies it.

The Task Force members share several basic conclusions about surrogate parenting. First, when surrogate parenting involves the payment of fees and a contractual obligation to relinquish the child at birth, it places children at risk and is not in their best interests. Second, the practice has the potential to undermine the dignity of women, children and human reproduction. Many Task Force members also believe that commercial surrogate parenting arrangements will erode the integrity of the family unit and values fundamental to the bond between parents and children.

The Task Force concluded that state enforcement of the contracts and the commercial aspects of surrogate parenting pose the greatest potential for harm to individuals and to social attitudes and practices. The conclusions and concerns expressed below relate primarily to these two aspects of surrogacy.

The Interests of Children

The Sale of Babies. Many Task Force members view surrogate parenting as indistinguishable from the sale of children. They reject the practice as morally and socially unacceptable because it violates the dignity of children and the societal prohibition against the purchase and sale of human beings. That prohibition rests on basic premises about the nature and meaning of being human and the moral dictates of our shared humanity. One such premise is respect for the inherent dignity and equality of all persons. Allowing one person to purchase another contravenes this premise and should be rejected regardless of the intentions or motivations of those involved.

The fact that it is the child's father who purchases the child from the child's mother (or, at the least, purchases her right to have a relationship with her child) does not change the character of the arrangement. Euphemisms like "womb rental" or "the provision of services," developed in part as marketing techniques, disserve the public by seeking to obscure the nature of the transaction. The intended parents do not seek a pregnancy or services as the ultimate object of the arrangement; they seek the product of those "services"—the child.

The surrogacy contracts themselves make this intent unmistakably clear. For example, the contract between Mary Beth Whitehead and the Sterns specified that the Infertility Center would hold $10,000 in escrow for Mary Beth Whitehead. If Mary Beth Whitehead had suffered a miscarriage prior to the fifth month of preg-

From New York State Task Force on Life and the Law, *Surrogate Parenting: Analysis and Recommendations for Public Policy* (May 1988). Published here by permission of the Task Force.

nancy, she would not have received any money under the contract. If she had a miscarriage subsequent to the fourth month of pregnancy or if the child died or was stillborn, her compensation would have been $1,000, an amount completely unrelated to the "services" performed. Likewise, if testing indicated that the fetus had genetic or congenital anomalies and Mary Beth Whitehead had refused to have an abortion and had carried the child to term, she would have received little or no compensation. Finally, all doubt about the nature of the contract is removed by virtue of the fact that Mary Beth Whitehead was not entitled to any compensation for her "services" alone; she was only entitled to compensation if she surrendered the product of those services—the child.

The Risks Posed. The Task Force concluded that surrogate parenting presents unacceptable risks to children. First, the fact that the practice condones the sale of children has severe long-term implications for the way society thinks about and values children. This shift in attitudes will inevitably influence behavior towards children and will create the potential for serious harm.

Surrogacy also poses more immediate risks to children. Under the arrangements, children are born into situations where their genetic, gestational and social relationships to their parents are irrevocably fractured. A child may have as many as five parents, or, frequently, will have at least four—the mother and her husband and the father and his wife. Where the birth mother has no genetic link to the child, the child has two mothers.

In contemporary family life, many children are denied the benefit of an ongoing relationship with both biological parents. High divorce rates and the growing number of unwed mothers leave many children with a close connection to only one parent. When remarriage occurs, children are raised in a reconstituted family unit that does not share the bonds of genetic relationship. The same has always been true for children relinquished at birth or thereafter and raised by adoptive parents. Although some children thrive in these situations, others face greater risk of emotional harm or loss.

Unlike divorce or adoption, however, surrogate parenting is based on a deliberate decision to fracture the family relationship prior to the child's conception. Once parenthood is fragmented among persons who are strangers to one another, there is no basis to reconstruct the family unit or even to cope with alternative arrangements in the event conflict arises.

A child may be caught in the cross-fire of a fractious and lengthy court battle between his or her parents during the early years of the child's life, when stability and constant nurturing are vital. Alternatively, where the bonds of kinship are attenuated, children who are born with physical or mental anomalies are far more likely to be abandoned by both parents. Potentially, neither parent will have a bond with the child at birth; the mother because she successfully preserved her emotional distance and the father because he has not shared the pregnancy and has no relationship to the child's mother. While legislation or contractual agreements can apportion financial responsibility, they cannot compensate for the high risk of emotional and physical abandonment these children might face. Other potential dangers for children include the harm from knowing their mothers gave them away and the impact on brothers and sisters of seeing a sibling sold or surrendered.

Advocates of surrogate parenting suggest that any risks to children are outweighed by the opportunity for life itself—they point out that the children always benefit since they would not have been born without the practice. But this argument assumes the very factor under deliberation—the child's conception and birth. The assessment for public policy occurs prior to conception when the surrogate arrangements are made. The issue then is not whether a particular child should be denied life, but whether children should be conceived in circumstances that would place them at risk. The notion that children have an interest in being born prior to their conception and birth is not embraced in other public policies and should not be assumed in the debate on surrogate parenting.

The Dignity of Women and Human Reproduction

The gestation of children as a service for others in exchange for a fee is a radical departure from the way in which society understands and values pregnancy. It substitutes commercial values for the web of social, affective and moral meanings associated with human reproduction and gestation. This transformation has profound implications for childbearing, for women, and for the relationship between parents and the children they bring into the world.

The characterization of gestation as a "service" depersonalizes women and their role in human reproduction. It treats women's ability to carry children like any other service in the marketplace—available at a market rate, based on negotiation between the parties about issues such as price, prenatal care, medical testing, the decision to abort and the circumstances of delivery. All those decisions and the right to control them as well as the process of gestation itself are given a price tag— not just for women who serve as surrogates, but for all women.

The Task Force concluded that this assignment of market values should not be celebrated as an exaltation of "rights," but rejected as a derogation of the values and meanings associated with human reproduction. Those meanings are derived from the relationship between the mother and father of a child and the child's creation as an expression of their mutual love. Likewise, the meaning of gestation is inextricably bound up with the love and commitment a woman feels for the child she will bring into the world.

In a surrogate arrangement, the intended parents seek a child as a way to deepen their own relationship and to establish a loving bond with another human being. In the process, however, the birth mother uses the child as a source of income and, in turn, is used by the intended parents as a vehicle to serve their own ends. They seek the biological components of gestation from her while denying the personal, emotional and psychological dimensions of her experience and self. If she succeeds in denying her emotional responses during this profound experience, she is dehumanized in the process. If she fails, her attachment to the child produces a conflict that cannot be resolved without anguish for all involved.

Proponents of surrogate parenting urge that neither the surrogate nor the intended parents should be denied their right to choose the arrangement as an extension of their claim to reproductive freedom. Yet protection for the right to reproduce has always been grounded in society's notions of bodily integrity and privacy. Those notions are strained beyond credibility when the intimate use of a third person's body in exchange for monetary compensation is involved.

Women who wish to serve as surrogates would not be limited in their private choices to conceive and bear children—they would only be denied the opportunity to make money from their gestational capacity. Some Task Force members believe that this limitation is justified by the possibility of exploitation, especially in relation to poor women inside and outside of this country. They fear the creation of a class of women who will become breeders for those who are wealthier.

Other Task Force members concluded that the risk of exploitation could be minimized, but remained concerned about the potential loss to society. They believe that societal attitudes will shift as gestation joins other services in the commercial sphere; the contribution and role of women in the reproductive process will be devalued. Abstracted from the family relationships, obligations and caring that infuse them with meaning, gestation and human reproduction will be seen as commodities. Advances in genetic engineering and the cloning and freezing of gametes may soon offer an array of new social options and potential commercial opportunities. An arrangement that transforms human reproductive capacity into a commodity is therefore especially problematic at the present time.

The Family

The Family Unit. The family has long been one of the most basic units of our society—a repository of social and moral tradition, identity and personality. It provides the structure and continuity around which many of our most profound and important relationships are established and flourish.

Social and economic forces have challenged the traditional family unit. At the same time, high divorce rates and the incidence of unwed parents have changed the permanence of the family in the lives of many. Yet, these trends do not alter the importance of the family in our personal and communal lives.

Surrogate parenting allows the genetic, gestational and social components of parenthood to be fragmented, creating unprecedented relationships among people bound together by contractual obligation rather than by the bonds of kinship and caring. In this regard, surrogate parenting, like prenuptial agreements, has been viewed as an extension of a more general social movement from status (or kinship) to contract as a basis for ordering family relationships and the reproductive process.

Although some individuals now choose to shape aspects of their personal relationships with the principles and tools of contract law, society should not embrace this trend as a prescriptive standard. It embodies a deeply pessimistic vision of the potential for human relationships and intimacy in contemporary society. It promotes legal obligations as the touchstone for our most private relationships instead of fostering commitments forged by caring and trust. Rather than accept this contractual model as a basis for family life and other close personal relationships, society should discourage the commercialization of our private lives and create the conditions under which the human dimensions of our most intimate relationships can thrive.

The Relationship of Parent and Child. Surrogate parenting alters deep-rooted social and moral assumptions about the relationship between parents and children. Parents have a profound moral obligation to care for their offspring. Our legal and social norms affirm this obligation by requiring parents to care for their children's physical and emotional well-being.

Surrogate parenting is premised on the ability and willingness of women to abrogate this responsibility without moral compunction or regret. It makes the obligations that accompany parenthood alienable and negotiable.

Many of the Task Force members concluded that society should not promote this parental abdication or the ability of some women to overcome the impulse to nurture their children. Some Task Force members reject all third party donation to the reproductive process because it encourages adults to relinquish responsibility for biological offspring. Other Task Force members distinguish surrogacy from gamete donation because of the surrogate's direct and prolonged relationship to the child she bears.

Surrogate parenting also severs the second prong of the legal relationship that binds parents and children—parental rights. In fact, the practice involves unprecedented rules and standards for terminating both parental status and rights, including the right to a relationship with one's own child. Under existing law, parental rights cannot be denied without a showing of parental unfitness. This high standard embodies society's respect for the rights that flow from parenthood and the relationship those rights seek to protect.

Surrogate parenting rejects that standard in favor of a contract model for determining parental rights. Many Task Force members view this shift as morally and socially unacceptable. The assumption that "a deal is a deal," relied upon to justify this drastic change in public policy fails to recognize and respect the significance of the relationships and rights at stake.

The Relationship Between the Spouses. Some Task Force members reject surrogate parenting and all third party donation to the reproductive process because they violate the unity and exclusivity of the relationship and commitment between the spouses. According to this view, procreation reflects the spiritual and biological union of two people; children born of that union manifest the uniqueness of the marital relationship. The involvement of a third person as a surrogate or as gamete donor contravenes the spiritual and human values expressed in marriage and in the procreative process.

Some Task Force members also believe that an imbalance may be created in the marital relationship when only one parent is genetically related to the child. This imbalance may generate tension in the family unit rather than enrich the relationship between the spouses.

The Waiver of Fundamental Rights

Under the laws of New York and other states, parental rights and status cannot be irrevocably waived in advance of the time the rights will be exercised. By placing these rights as well as others beyond the reach of an advance agreement that is legally enforceable, society seeks to preserve those rights and the values they embody.

Many Task Force members believe that parental rights, including the right to a relationship with one's own child, deserve this special status. They do not view this as a limitation of individual freedom, but as a societal judgment about how that freedom is best protected.

The Task Force's proposal is consistent with existing adoption laws, which provide that a woman cannot consent to her child's adoption until after the child is born. Surrogate parenting should not be allowed to dislodge this long-standing public policy.

Informed Consent

Many of the Task Force members support the nonenforceability of surrogate contracts, in part because they believe that it is not possible for women to give informed consent to the surrender of a child prior to the child's conception and birth. Some commentators have argued that this conclusion diminishes women's stature as autonomous adults. The Task Force members reject that assertion.

The debate on surrogate parenting focuses on the ability of women to make informed choices—not because women differ from men in making important life decisions, but because women alone can bear children. The inability to predict and project a response to profound experiences that have not yet unfolded is shared by men and women alike. This inability often stems from the capacity for growth and an openness to experience in our relationships with others. These qualities are a positive and dynamic part of our humanness.

Denying women the opportunity to change their minds does not accord them respect; it limits their options and freedoms. Other avenues exist to inform or influence social attitudes about women. These avenues can be explored without penalizing women by demanding a degree of certainty and irrevocability we do not demand of men or women in making other vital life choices.

Many Task Force members believe that enforced removal of a child from the child's birth mother under a surrogate contract involves severe consequences for the birth mother. Studies have shown that many women who voluntarily relinquish children for adoption face a lingering and deep sense of loss. The harsh consequences of a poorly informed decision to relinquish one's child require a rigorous standard for consent before consent should be considered truly informed. This is why the adoption laws do not permit an expectant mother to surrender her child for adoption and insist that she await the child's birth before making such a decision. While some women have been able to anticipate their response in advance of the child's conception, the long gestational process and the child's birth, others have not. Our policies must recognize that many women may not be able to give informed consent in these circumstances.

Recommendations for Public Policy

At the outset of its discussion about surrogate parenting, the Task Force recognized that society could choose any one of five broad directions for public policy, subject to constitutional constraints that might apply. Essentially, society could seek to prohibit, discourage, regulate or promote the practice or could take no action.

The Task Force proposes that society should discourage the practice of surrogate parenting. This policy goal should be achieved by legislation that declares the contracts void as against public policy and prohibits the payment of fees to surrogates. Legislation should also bar surrogate brokers from operating in New York State. These measures are designed to eliminate commercial surrogacy and the growth of a business community or industry devoted to making money from human reproduction and the birth of children. They are consistent with existing family law principles on parental rights and adoption.

The Task Force proposes that surrogate parenting should not be prohibited when the arrangement is not commercial and remains undisputed. The Task Force concluded that society should not interfere with the voluntary, non-coerced choices of adults in these circumstances. Existing law permits each stage of these voluntary arrangements: a decision by a woman to be artificially inseminated or to have an embryo implanted; her decision after the child's birth to relinquish the child for adoption; and the child's adoption by the intended parents. The proposed legislation would also not bar the payment of reasonable medical and other expenses to surrogates, if the payment is made as part of an adoption and is permitted by existing law.

The Task Force evaluated and rejected the option of upholding the contracts under the regulatory models proposed in many states. This regulatory approach squarely places the state's imprimatur on the surrogate arrangement. It employs the authority of both the legislature and the courts to uphold the contracts. Through these two powerful branches of government, society would be enmeshed in a long series of dilemmas and problems posed by the practice.

The regulatory approach has been justified and supported as the only way to protect the children born of surrogate parenting. The practice is seen as a trend that cannot be inhibited given the existence of the underlying technologies and the intense desire of infertile couples to have children, a desire that now fuels a growing black market in the sale of children. According to this view, regulation does not facilitate surrogacy, but merely accepts and guides its inevitable proliferation.

The Task Force found this justification for regulating and upholding the practice unpersuasive. The difficulty of discouraging a practice does not dictate social acceptance and assistance. Society has not legalized the purchase and sale of babies to establish a better marketplace for that activity despite the fact that both the children and intended parents might be better protected. The laws against baby selling embody fundamental societal values and doubtlessly minimize the practice even if they do not eliminate it.

Public policy on surrogate parenting should also reflect basic social and moral values about the interests of children, the role of the family, women and reproduction. A commitment by society to uphold the contracts removes the single greatest barrier to those considering the practice. In contrast, voiding the contracts, banning fees, and prohibiting brokering activity will drastically reduce the number of persons who seek a commercial surrogate arrangement. Given the potential risks to the children born of surrogacy, children are best served by policies designed to discourage the practice.

The Task Force members feel deep sympathy for infertile couples, many of whom experience a profound sense of loss and trauma. Nevertheless, the Task Force concluded that society should not support surrogacy as a solution. The practice will generate other social problems and harm that reach beyond the infertile couples who seek a surrogate arrangement.

While treatment is increasingly sought by and available to infertile couples, few initiatives to prevent infertility have been taken by the public or the private sector. The Task Force recommends that measures should be undertaken to reduce the incidence of infertility through public education and public support for research about its causes. Broader awareness among health care professionals and members of the public about the causes of infertility, especially infertility related to sexually transmitted diseases, could prevent some couples from ever facing the problem. Other couples would benefit from an increased understanding of the causes of infertility and new treatments for it.

F. Institute on Women and Technology
Women and Children Used in Systems of Surrogacy: Position Statement of the
Institute on Women and Technology

Introduction

Surrogacy is a practice of sex-discrimination. It threatens the health, welfare, and
equality of women and the welfare of those children who may be born from surrogate arrangements. Surrogate brokers induce women into contractual agreements
to bear children for customers who can afford the price. In doing this, surrogacy
systematically validates a class of women who can be bought and sold as breeders.
Surrogate arrangements cast women into the role of alternative reproductive vehicles, rented wombs, human incubators, and mere receptacles for sperm. Rather
than granting a woman control over her body, these arrangements transfer control
of a woman's body to brokers and clients. They deprive women of the right to
control their bodies. To defend surrogacy as consistent with reproductive liberty,
is to equate freedom with slavery. To hire a woman's body for the breeding of a
child violates a basic underpinning of international law—that human rights must
be based on human dignity.

Exploitation of Women

Social and Political

The image of woman as reproductive object, as the image of woman as sexual
object, is rooted in most societies. It is this image of woman as reproductive object
at the disposal of men which must be changed. Surrogacy targets women in vulnerable situations: women who are both emotionally and economically vulnerable.
The harm of surrogacy includes the de-humanization, the objectification and the
commodification of women. It contributes significantly to lowering the human dignity, worth, and civil status of women, and undermines women's equal exercise
of civil rights by the constraints of the surrogate contract. By contract it subordinates
women to the wishes of the sperm donor.

Surrogate contracts set up an inequality in which the sperm donor has control.
He has both money and management power, backed up by the institution of the
broker's agency. The so-called surrogate has none of this power. She is reduced to
contributing mere egg and uterine environment. She becomes an instrument that
is purchased as raw material from which something—the child—is manufactured.
Her value is a use-value.

Indeed, the very language of "surrogate" mother privileges the male immediately.
It reinforces the sperm donor as the real, natural, biological parent before he does
anything which contributes to parenting beyond the mere contribution of sperm.
Meanwhile the real natural biological mother is rendered a mere surrogate. Her
generation of the egg, gestation of the fetus, and giving birth to the child are
rendered as substitute activities. Surrogate contracts establish the sperm-donor's
entitlement to the child on the grounds of genetic contribution alone.

Economic

Surrogacy is a market, and a very lucrative one. The merchandise involved is
women's bodies and what issues from them. The market is created by demand
which is met by supply. The demand comes from the client, who is technically, in
[   ]ng, a sperm donor. The supply is provided by women who are called

surrogates. The most commanding figure in this market, however, is the market organizer, that is the surrogate broker/business man. He is, in actuality, a procurer of women.

Surrogacy has been justified as an option for women's economic survival, portrayed as necessary women's work. It is universally true that jobs defined as women's work carry low pay, low status, and little security. The earnings gap between women and men is universal and growing, in spite of equal pay laws. Women everywhere earn less than men, so much so that we now talk about the feminization of poverty. It is only in this context of women being denied economic dignity and survival elsewhere that the selling of women's wombs appears as one of women's economic options.

Personal

Surrogacy exploits the limited roles and the personal identities given to women in a gender-defined society. It reinforces the cultural definition which leads women into motherhood at any cost to themselves. It takes advantage of the altruistic and self-giving female ideal that having a baby for another is the greatest gift that a woman can give. Many women used in systems of surrogacy may have experienced abortion as a trauma or the ambivalence of giving up a child for adoption. The surrogacy brokers manipulate women's desire to resolve these past experiences.

Systems of surrogacy exploit a woman's *relationship* with a child. Motherhood is not a biologically determined bond. It is not a woman's essence, mystical state of being, or historically unchanging. Motherhood is a relationship which occurs within a social, political, and historical context. A woman who revokes a surrogate contract and claims her child asserts that her relationship to the child privileges her claim. The sperm donor's relationship and contribution to the fetus becoming a child are not equal to the woman's. The sperm donor does not assume the risks of conception, pregnancy, and birth. Nor does he do the work of carrying the fetus for 9 months.

Physical

Surrogacy contracts routinely require prospective mothers to submit to hormone injections, amniocentesis, and an array of genetic probes and tests at the discretion of the client. The agreements often stipulate that the woman agree to abort the fetus on demand if and when the client desires to terminate the "service." These contracts also contain written provisions which make the woman liable for all the "risks." Indeed, one women involved in a surrogacy agreement died in her eighth month of pregnancy due to a congenital heart condition known to the broker. Women who sign surrogacy agreements are treated as "alternative reproductive vehicles."

Effect on Children

Another victim of surrogacy is the child. Children born of surrogate arrangements are also objects of a commercial transaction. The child is treated as a means to an end—the creation of a family for the sperm donor and his genetic fulfillment. Unlike adoption, which resolves a crisis with the best interests of the child in mind, surrogacy creates conditions in which a child may suffer crises of identity, worth, and trust. Surrogacy teaches children the limited value of women and children, given in such commercial arrangements of surrogacy. Further, what kind of a society wants its girl children born into a world where there is a breeder class of women, where they too can be so-called surrogate mothers? Are these the kind of aspirations we want girl children to have?

Conclusion: Regulation Vs. Prohibition of Surrogate Contracts

Many people have opposed surrogacy because they view it as baby-selling. Far fewer people have noted that surrogacy is primarily a system of buying and selling of women. Children are not always born of surrogate arrangements. Women are always used in systems of surrogacy. Therefore, legislation in opposition to surrogacy must not only oppose commercialized childbearing.

The condition of women and children is very tied together. Legislation is needed which opposes women being used as reproductive vehicles and commodities and which prevents children from being born under these conditions. Therefore, we support legislation that *prohibits* contractual surrogate arrangements.

We cannot be satisfied with *regulatory* legislation. Regulation will not save women from being treated as reproductive vehicles. Regulating surrogacy is like regulating slavery so it won't be so obviously oppressive, so there will be better slaves, so slavery will be less haphazard. Regulatory legislation is exactly what the surrogate industry wants. The surrogate agencies want regulation of the contract because regulation gives them more legal sanction than they ever had. It also gives them a stable marketing environment, less susceptible to being challenged. The surrogate industry cannot survive and succeed as a business without regulatory legislation.

There is no way that a surrogate contract can be made anything other than an inherently unequal relationship between broker, sperm-donor, and a woman involving the objectification, sale, and commodification of a woman's body. Therefore, we support federal legislation making surrogate contracts void and unenforceable and contrary to public policy.

H. Patricia Hynes, Director
Dr. Janice G. Raymond, Associate Director
Gena Corea, Associate Director

G. Testimony of Gena Corea
Associate Director of the Institute on Women and Technology, before California Assembly Judiciary Committee, April 5, 1988.

JUNK LIBERTY

We hear lots of high-minded talk about "rights" and "liberty" from the defenders of the human breeding industry. It's a man's right to exercise his constitutionally protected and newly invented "procreative liberty" to hire a woman to bear a child for him. It's a woman's right to sell her body if she so chooses.

We are repeatedly told that legalizing the sale of women protects the freedom our forefathers died for.

Gary Skoloff, attorney to William Stern in the Baby M surrogacy case, is one of the many new single-issue defenders of women's liberation.

"If you prevent women from becoming surrogate mothers and deny them the freedom to decide . . . ," he says, "you are saying that they do not have the ability to make their own decisions, but *you* do. It's being unfairly paternalistic, and it's an insult to the female population of this nation" (Snyder, 1987).

The U.S. Constitution, written by a number of slave-holders, safeguards "protective liberty"—a concept articulated by University of Texas law professor John Robertson.[1]

"Since hiring a surrogate gestator is an exercise of procreative liberty on the part of the couple," he writes, "there is a strong case for a constitutional right to employ a surrogate."

He argues: "Prohibition of such arrangements would interfere with the woman's and couple's right to procreate, for there is no other way for them to have offspring of their genes. Harm to the offspring or the surrogate does not appear great enough to justify limitation of the arrangement" (Robertson, 1988, pp. 189, 186).

The notion that hiring a breeder is an exercise in liberty is repeated in a host of official reports on surrogacy.

Attorney Lori Andrews, who wrote the new reproductive technologies report for a women's rights law project based at Rutgers University and also served on the ethics committee of the American Fertility Society, has been a major disseminator of the liberty line (Andrews, 1987).

This liberty line has been eagerly grabbed by the surrogacy industry. For example, in his testimony before the Pennsylvania House Judiciary Committee hearing on surrogacy in 1987, William Handel, director of the Center for Surrogate Parenting in Los Angeles, stated: " . . . The right to procreate, which encompasses the right to conceive, bear and rear children, is one of society's most highly cherished and constitutionally protected rights. . . . Surrogate parenting . . . is an alternative that should be protected as vehemently as normal reproduction. After all, the first amendment right of procreation does not protect the *act* of procreation, but rather the fundamental nature and importance of having a child" (Handel, 1987).

Various legislatures and courts, including the New Jersey lower court that ruled in the Mary Beth Whitehead case, have also embraced "protective liberty" as a rationale for male use of a female breeder caste. Judge Harvey Sorkow, citing John Robertson and quoting him at length, wrote in his Baby M decision: "It must be reasoned that if one has a right to procreate coitally, then one has the right to

In a slightly altered form, "Junk Liberty" was submitted before the California Assembly Judiciary Committee in Sacramento, California, on April 5, 1988. In its present form, "Junk Liberty" was presented on December 4, 1988 at the Colloque International: L'Ovaire Dose? (Paris, France), sponsored by the Mouvement Français pour le Planning Familial.

reproduce non-coitally. . . . This court holds that the protected [reproductive] means extends to the use of surrogates. . . . It is reasoned that the donor or surrogate aids the childless couple by contributing a factor of conception and for gestation that the couple lacks" (Sorkow, 1987, p. 941).

Legal action invalidating the surrogate contract does more than just interfere with the couple's liberty, he argued. "The surrogate who voluntarily chooses to enter such a contract is deprived of a constitutionally protected right to perform services" (Sorkow, 1987, p. 93).

In its 1986 ethics report on the new reproductive technologies, the American Fertility Service, a professional association of some 10,000 U.S. physicians and scientists who work in reproductive biology, reveals itself as another defender of "procreative liberty".[2]

"Couples" have a right to hire breeders, the American Fertility Society tells us.[3]

Building on the work of feminist author Kathleen Barry, Janice Raymond, associate director at the Institute on Women and Technology, challenges the "rights" justification for surrogacy: "It is a fundamental postulate of international law that human rights must be based on human dignity. A surrogate arrangement offers no dignity to women and therefore cannot be called a real right. It violates the core of human dignity to hire a woman's body for the breeding of a child so that someone else's genes can be perpetuated" (Raymond, 1987a).[4]

Raymond, a professor of women's studies at the University of Massachusetts, has further written in regard to the surrogacy promoters: "Give the female creature abstract rights—rights that don't really benefit women politically as a class—but don't give her dignity" (Raymond, 1987b).

Human dignity. Alejandra Muñoz, the Mexican woman brought across the border illegally to serve as a so-called surrogate, inseminated and, once pregnant, kept confined in the home of the buying couple, Mario and Nattie Haro, knows her dignity was violated. So does Mary Beth Whitehead, protagonist in the Baby M case. And Nancy Barrass, the so-called surrogate now fighting in California to see her child. And Patty Foster, fighting in Michigan for her child. And Elizabeth Kane, billed as America's first legal surrogate. And Laurie Yates, the young woman in Michigan who struggled long, hard, and in vain to keep the twins she bore after having been superovulated like a cow. That is, the surrogate company's doctor gave her fertility drugs because she apparently didn't get pregnant fast enough (whether for the doctor or the man hiring her is not clear).

There are many issues to discuss surrounding surrogacy: the opening up of the reproductive supermarket that the burgeoning surrogate industry is a part of; the use of so-called surrogates as "living laboratories" for the development of various new reproductive technologies; the eugenic implications of surrogacy—the search for "perfect" children of the right race, genetic material, and degree of physical perfection; the coming expansion in the traffic in women internationally when, with the use of embryo transfer technology, Third World women are used as cheap breeders for white, Western men (and at least one surrogate entrepreneur has concrete plans now for this international traffic[5]); the expansion of father rights that surrogacy represents, and the curtailment of mother rights; the new polygamy—two women doing for one man; the erosion of self-esteem in future female children who—if the surrogate industry is not stopped—will be born into a world where there is a class of breeder women. But now I am making one point only: Human rights must be based on human dignity, and surrogacy, which violates human dignity, is no "right."

—Mary Beth Whitehead: "I thought because the Sterns had hired me, they could tell me what to do. So even though my doctor said I didn't need amniocentesis or a Tay Sachs test, I had them because the Sterns insisted on it. Even when Betsy

Stern wanted to take blood from my arm several times, and I didn't know why, I allowed it. When we were sitting in a car and she was drawing blood from me, I felt used and exploited." (Whitehead, 1987)

—Alejandra Muñoz: "The Haros said they were willing to give me $1,500. Mario Haro said he thought that was enough money for what he called an 'uneducated, uncivilized ignorant woman.' [My cousin] Angela told him that here in the United States, surrogate mothers are paid up to $10,000. He said, 'For that price, I could have gotten someone intelligent.' " (Muñoz, 1987)

—American Bar Association committee drafting a model surrogacy law and deciding neither the court nor legislation should control the fee paid to the so-called surrogate: "Here the committee took somewhat of a commerical position that the market place should control. It was felt that the services of some surrogates would be worth more than the services of others."[6]

—Harvey Berman, former attorney to "surrogate" Alejandra Munoz, commenting on the fee that should be paid to the so-called surrogate: "I guess it depends on the woman's station in life. The $10,000 works out to a couple of bucks an hour. Well, what would that person be doing if she were not pregnant? It the woman is a famous writer who commands some money, then it's not fair. If she is a homemaker who has no economic earning capacity anyway, it's not so unfair." (Corea, 1987)

—Elizabeth Kane began to feel exploited, she told me, when the head of Surrogate Parenting Associates, Dr. Richard Levin, brought couples in from all over the world, "dripping in mink and diamonds," to view potential surrogate mothers in sessions that the women privately called "cattle night." Levin would point proudly to the impeccably dressed and made-up "surrogates" and tell his clients: "I can get you a woman just like this."

IT IS A FUNDAMENTAL POSTULATE OF INTERNATIONAL LAW THAT RIGHTS MUST BE BASED ON HUMAN DIGNITY.

—Alejandra Muñoz: "The Haros never took me anywhere—to a park or anywhere—and they didn't want me to leave the house. They told me that immigration would pick me up. I think they didn't want me to leave the house because most of Mario's family thought that it was Nattie [his wife] who was pregnant, not me. Nattie would wear a little pillow under a maternity gown when she visited Mario's mother." (Muñoz, 1987)

—Millionaire private investigator Frank Monte of Sydney, Australia, who has gone into the surrogacy business, is determined that the women used by his company will not refuse to give up their children, the magazine *New Idea* reports. Monte intends to keep the inseminated women under constant surveillance by his private detectives throughout the nine months of their pregnancies. Monte told the magazine: "If we're going to do the job 100 percent, we're going to have to keep tabs on the women."

New Idea reported: "The type of volunteers he's looking for, he says, would be quiet girls from the country, aged 25–30, probably a little down on their luck and who 'need the money and don't mind going through the experience.' " (Bicknell, 1988)

—American Bar Association committee's draft of model surrogacy law, 11 b: "If the intended parent or parents prove that the child is not as intended, that is, not genetically related to the intended providers of genetic materials, then the intended parent or parents shall not be required to assume custody of the child or to make any payments pursuant to the terms of the agreement. If, however, the child is not as intended because of physician or laboratory error, then the intended parent or parents shall be required to assume custody and shall be required to make all payments pursuant to the terms of the agreement."[6]

A "surrogate" baby born seropositive for the HIV antibody, a baby with a high likelihood of developing AIDS, was not as intended. Both the mother and the contracting couple refused custody of the child, as physicians from Howard University Hospital report (Frederick et al., 1987). If the couple had intended to have a sick child, they could have adopted one. The indignity of treating the child as property is obvious. The indignity of treating the woman like a mother machine, like a manufacturing plant for the production of a child to specifications, an "as intended" child, is not visible to many.

When "surrogate mother" Patty Nowakowski delivered twins—a girl and a boy—in 1988, one child was as intended and the other not. The Michigan man who hired Nowakowski to be inseminated with his sperm wanted a girl. So he took the girl and left the boy behind. He had ordered a pink one, not a blue one. The boy was put into a foster home until Nowakowski, pained at his fate, claimed him as her own (Belloli, 1988).

A SURROGATE ARRANGEMENT OFFERS NO DIGNITY TO WOMEN AND THEREFORE CANNOT BE CALLED A REAL RIGHT.

—Nancy Barrass, in a letter to the customer couple (I'll give them the pseudonyms "Bob" and "Judy"), commented on a baby shower given for the three of them during Barrass' pregnancy. The invitation had read "Judy and Nancy and Bob are having a baby." In her letter, Barrass wrote of the pain she had felt in being ignored at the shower. The friends toasted the customer couple and the baby without ever mentioning Barrass' name.

Barrass wrote: "Sue toasted to Judy, Bob and their baby and to its aunts and cousins in the room who'd be a part of its growing up. But she talked as if the baby were not even there. . . . The baby they were referring to was in reality within eye sight, only a few feet away, but to those people it could have been a million miles away growing in an incubator somewhere. Not one had the decency to point out that the baby was there—alive, well, and kicking up a storm. Not one person even glanced at me. All eyes were on Judy. . . .

"Judy's friends all rant and rave about how wonderful her having a baby is—how exciting it is for her—which is true. But I am the one who went through morning sickness, was given drug overdoses to conceive, lost jobs due to the pregnancy, had to deal with both a cyst and a tumor. . . .

"Why was my name even on the invitation when no one was able to acknowledge my and my baby's presence? I knew that someday I, the birth mother, would be forgotten, but never in my wildest dreams did I think I'd be forgotten in the presence of others with the baby still in me." (Barrass, 1986)

—Patty Foster, a so-called surrogate mother, describing an incident a few days after the birth of her son [I'll call him Joseph], whom she unwillingly gave to the customer: "The nurse came in one night when I was playing with Joseph and she said, 'You *look* like a good mother.' I thought: 'Oh my God, this what they think of us.' This is the thing that nobody tells you—that these people think that you are garbage. On the one hand, they're saying you are a saint, you are giving the gift of life. On the other hand, you're garbage because you're giving up your child. After you give birth, the sperm donor and his wife treat you like a piece of trash. You're no longer the saint." (Corea, 1988)

—Attorney Harvey Berman: "I think that was permeating Mr. Haro's thinking: the fact that he comes from the Mexican culture and here was a woman balking at him. I saw that underneath, he was boiling, just seething. And I felt sympathetic for the reason that he did not get what he originally bargained for. He thought he was going to pay a family member a mere pittance and get a child that was solely his. And now he was going to be perhaps forced to share." (Corea, 1987)

—Nancy Barrass: "The center's doctor prescribed Clomid, a fertility drug. After taking the drug, I developed a cyst in my ovary which lasted throughout my pregnancy. The doctor then prescribed antibiotics for the bacteria infection [I got from the father's sperm at one insemination]. With that particular infection, it is very difficult to become pregnant. However, rather than wait until the infection was cured, he prescribed a triple dose of Clomid and continued to inseminate me.

"The triple dose of the drug had serious side effects for me. I experienced dizziness, blurred vision, a severe facial rash and intense pain in my left ovary. I was unable to walk because of the pain." (Barrass, 1987)

IT VIOLATES THE CORE OF HUMAN DIGNITY TO HIRE A WOMAN'S BODY FOR THE BREEDING OF A CHILD SO THAT SOMEONE ELSE'S GENES CAN BE PERPETUATED.

—From The Bionetic Foundation's 1982 catalog of women available as so-called surrogates: "Sue. Address: San Luis Obispo, Ca. . . . Status: married. Career: clerical (spouse: computer operator). Birth date: April 11, 1953. Height: 5' 6". Weight: 150. Racial origins: caucasian (1/4th Italian). . . . Insurance: Blue Shield (full coverage for pregnancy)." (Bionetics, 1982)

—An American Bar Association committee's June 1987 draft of a model surrogacy law would require a woman to carry with her—at all times after the sixth month of pregnancy—a court paper ordering the hospital to give her baby only to the "intended" parents, that is, the people who paid for it.[6]

—Patty Foster: "I had asked the hospital staff not to let the sperm donor's wife, 'Alice,' in the delivery room. But right before the delivery, my husband Brent went into the waiting room and told her the baby would be coming in five minutes. She grabbed a gown, put it on, left Brent with her coat and purse, ran in, grabbed hold of my hand, and said, 'I'm here.' This is a woman I've seen twice before in my life and both times she acted as though it were an inconvenience for her to be there. Do you know what it was like? I had no dignity anymore. My body was—they took over everything." (Corea, 1988)

—Mary Beth Whitehead: "When I refused to give Sara up, five cops stormtrooped my house to get her while Bill and Betsy Stern waited outside in the car. I was in my nightgown breastfeeding the baby when they came. I was still bleeding from the delivery. The put me in handcuffs and threw me in the police car while the neighbors stood around and watched. Tuesday, my 11-year-old daughter, ran to the Sterns' car and said to them, 'Please don't take my mother's baby.' They said nothing." (Whitehead, 1987))

—Nancy Barrass: "Two months before my pregnancy due date I told the sperm donor and his wife of my need not to have them present in the delivery room. I felt no special closeness at this point with these people because of prior conflict with them, and had no desire to share with them something so vulnerable and intimate as my giving birth. They responded that their presence at the birth was part of what they paid for." (Barrass, 1987)

GIVE THE FEMALE CREATURE ABSTRACT RIGHTS—RIGHTS THAT DON'T REALLY BENEFIT WOMEN POLITICALLY AS A CLASS—BUT DON'T GIVE HER DIGNITY.

—Patty Foster: "The time in the hospital after the birth was supposed to be my time alone with the baby. But Alice and her husband 'Ralph' were in my room all day. I was emotionally a wreck then. I didn't sleep. I didn't eat. I cried constantly. I didn't want to give up the baby but just a little while earlier, Judge Sorkow had ruled in Mary Beth Whitehead's case that surrogate contracts were legal and binding. All the lawyers told me I had to give up my baby; I had no legal right. My own lawyer told me that too. He was the lawyer the baby broker recommended to me and he was supposedly independent. But after I signed the contract, I found out he was an associate in the baby broker's office.

"The last day I was in the hospital, the gynecologist for the surrogate company came into my room. I was sitting there crying. Alice was holding my baby. She wouldn't let me hold him. She said to the doctor, 'By the way, I'm Harry's wife.' And he said to her: 'Oh, I'd like to congratulate you.' I'm sitting there and I'm crying and he's congratulating this bitch. In front of me. Congratulating her for what? Showing up?" (Corea, 1988)

—Attorney Harvey Berman: "One of the problems you're going to have [in setting up a surrogate business] is getting surrogates of quality. I'd like to keep the genetic quality of the surrogate as high as we possibly could. But I'm sure that some people who can afford to pay less will have to take less." (Corea, 1987)

—John Stehura, president of Bionetics Foundation, who has plans to use Mexican women as particularly low-priced breeders and who explains that, because of the women's distrust of gringos, he will need to do more than just advertise to get "surrogates": "I suspect I'd really have to customize the program for Mexico. Make it very specialized. In other words, perhaps rent a house and offer a medical clinic. Have a doctor come in once a week. Do all of these U.S. charity-type things but direct it towards pregnancy and surrogacy. . . . It might look something like a Children Home Society which would be a non-profit type of adoption agency. That's my best guess for Mexico at the moment. [It would be] very much like the food programs, like the medical aid programs where U.S. medical doctors go there on weekends to help in poor neighborhoods. So I would literally be mimicking something like that. . . . That's the proper presentation of surrogate parenting for a place like Mexico. The thing needs to have the right image, basically, to function." (Corea, 1987b)

—Dr. Lee M. Silver, associate professor at Princeton University, testifying before a Congressional hearing on reproductive technology in 1988: "There is also the possibility of using chimpanzees or gorillas as gestational surrogates for human embryos. The feasibility of this approach is supported by analogous experiments in other mammals that are as similar to each other as humans are to chimpanzees. . . . I imagine that surrogate apes would only be considered if the use of surrogate women was made illegal. However, this is one technology that I hope is never used. Aside from the psychological impact on the child, an equally important consideration is the diminishing number of great apes alive in the world today. If we require them to gestate our children instead of their own, we will only hasten their extinction." (Silver, 1988)

Apes are too valuable to be used in that way. So let's use women.

—Elizabeth Kane: "I had been agitated several days earlier when Dr. Levin, told me he had arranged for Sarah and Dale [a reporter and photographer from *People* magazine] to be present at the insemination. . . . " All during the insemination, while Kane lay on a table with her legs spread, the photographer from *People* snapped photos.

Nine months later, when Kane entered the birthing room with surrogate company director Dr. Richard Levin, she found a small television camera on a tripod. Levin told her it was for pictures of the labor and delivery: "You knew I was going to have a photographer here after we canceled the NBC camera pool last week. Don't worry about him," Levin said, indicating a man Kane had never before seen. "Paul's my cousin. He'll be discreet. . . . "

Kane wrote: "I wanted to shriek in protest at the lack of privacy I would have for the birth" (Kane, 1988).

IT IS A FUNDAMENTAL POSTULATE OF INTERNATIONAL LAW THAT HUMAN RIGHTS MUST BE BASED ON HUMAN DIGNITY.

—John Stehura, president of the Bionetics Foundation, discussing his plans to use Mexican women as breeders: "You know, you could buy a house in Mexico, a wonderful new house right on the ocean for $20,000. If you go inland a bit, not quite as nice, they'll build a house for you for $5,000 or $6,000. . . . You can literally give a young lady a brand new house and say, 'If you have the child. . . . ' You could devastate them with money and things—you know, whatever they need. And they'd be delighted. It would save them 20 years of scratching. So the bargain could be extraordinarily unique for the adoptive parents and for the woman having the child in Mexico." (Corea, 1987b)

—Paul Gerber, bioethicist at Queensland State University in Australia, suggested in June 1988 that brain-dead "neo-morts," or newly dead women, could be kept on life-support systems so their bodies could be used to gestate babies. Later, their bodies could be harvested for organ transplants.

In vitro fertilization could be used to join the egg and the sperm and then the embryo could be implanted in the brain-dead woman, Gerber said at a medical ethics conference in Queensland. He added: "I can't see anything wrong with it and at least the dead would be doing some good. It's a wonderful solution to the problems posed by surrogacy and a magnificent use of a corpse" (UPI, 1988).

—Pat Mounce, mother of "surrogate" Denise Mounce who died in the eighth month of her pregnancy: "My grandchild is in a coffin. There is an adopting couple out there who have a piece of paper with Denise's name on it as their surrogate mother. They sent no flowers. They sent no sympathy card. They sent no money to pay for Denise's funeral or for the baby's. They did not ask for the baby so they could bury it. They wanted that baby when it was alive. And when it was dead, it was nothing to them." (Corea, 1988)

Surrogacy is a violation of human dignity. As Janice Raymond points out, many women themselves don't recognize this is part of the problem, not part of the solution.

Those in the surrogate industry and their many champions argue that surrogacy has a 99 percent success rate. The Mary Beth Whitehead case was an aberration, they say. The Laurie Yates case was a fluke. Alejandra Munoz was an exception.

So was Nancy Barrass.

Elizabeth Kane was too.

And Kathy Hoppe.

Denise Thrane.

Judy Stiver.

Denise Mounce. Mounce is dead now. Twenty-four years old and dead of heart failure in the eighth month of her "surrogate" pregnancy. (No one noticed.) (Gordon, 1987; Powers, 1988; Corea, 1988)

They were a few unhappy women who should never have become contract mothers in the first place. Proper screening and counseling would have weeded these women out, the human breeding industry says.

Surrogacy critics, they say, are obsessed with the bad apples and ignore the hundreds of cases where there were no problems and the mothers were perfectly happy and gave up their babies without a murmur.

The cases which are alleged to be smooth and happy are the ones I worry about the most. Those are the cases in which the woman never causes anyone any trouble, never recognizes any violation of her human dignity.

She does what the contract tells her to do. She thinks of herself as an impersonal instrument of the desires of a man who has more money, education, and status than she.

She hears herself described as a variety of inanimate objects—a receptacle, an alternative reproduction vehicle (that's what Judge Harvey Sorkow called Mary Beth

Whitehead), a surrogate uterus (psychiatrist Lee Salk's description of Whitehead), a rented womb, an incubator, a kind of hatchery, rented property, plumbing, a therapeutic modality, "the woman attached to the rented womb," a factor for reproduction, a function. She hears herself described as a chicken hatching another chicken's eggs. She protests none of this.

The surrogate industry calls her, not a mother, not even a "surrogate mother," but simply a "surrogate". It calls the sperm donor "the natural father," or sometimes "the natural and biological father." This use of language is a vital part of the process of turning women into objects. Not only does she not object to this denigration of her role in procreation and the elevation of the role of the sperm donor, she does not even notice it.

If she has a miscarriage and is depressed, she seeks counseling and pays for it herself.

She develops no relationship with the child growing within her or, if she does so, she does not burden anyone with this knowledge.

She goes to all the doctor's appointments scheduled for her, gets up on the table, lets a needle pierce her womb so that the quality control test on the fetus can be done efficiently.

If the sperm donor reads the test results and tells her to abort, she obeys. In some contracts, she will receive no money after having undergone months of insemination, the morning sickness of early pregnancy, and then the abortion. Nor is she entitled to any compensation for lost wages during this time. She raises no objections.

If the fetus passes the test, she continues the pregnancy.

If she has a splitting headache, she obtains her physician's written permission before taking an aspirin, as some contracts require. Maybe she had to drive downtown to get the aspirin permit. Not a word of protest passes her lips. She's a reproductive vehicle. She must do what she is told to safeguard the valuable contents of her valueless body.

If the doctor tells her he wants to do a cesarean section, she submits without question.

She gives the baby to the father and goes away.

She does not burden anyone by reporting any pain she may feel.

If, six weeks after the birth, she suffers ill effects from the pregnancy, she does not ask the man who hired her or the company that procured her to help her pay for the resulting medical bills. Some contracts stipulate that she is not entitled to any payment for medical expenses related to the pregnancy after that date. She scrapes the money together and pays the bills herself.

The women who fight—the Alejandra Muñozes, the Laurie Yates, the Nancy Barrasses, the Mary Beth Whiteheads, the Patty Fosters, the Elizabeth Kanes—they will be all right. They will suffer greatly. They will be heaped with ridicule. All their supposed character defects will be held up for international scorn. But they will be all right. They are alive and kicking. They could not act as if they were blocks of wood. They asserted their humanity. They couldn't do what the contract told them to do: to be THINGS.

It is the "happy surrogates," the "Stepford surrogates," I worry about. The ones who don't cause anyone any trouble. The ones who hear, "You are a thing," and who think, "I am a thing."

Selling women as breeders, setting up a class of breeder women, violates human dignity. When the mechanisms of violating human dignity are so firmly established that no one objects to them or even finds them remarkable, which is the case in the "successful" surrogacy cases, then we are living in a society in which a woman's life is held in utter contempt.

But no. We are told that we are living in a country that protects liberty—"pro-creative liberty."

It is junk liberty.[7]

We know what junk food is. It's made of junk ingredients. Nutrients have been processed out of it, leaving it with little substance, bulk. It does not nourish. Sometimes it looks and tastes good. But it can make you sick. It can leave you hungering for something real, something that can sustain your life, something that can strengthen you. Junk food has the appearance of food without the reality.

Junk liberty looks and sounds good. Even noble. But human dignity has been processed out of it. Anything of real substance, anything that can nourish and sustain a woman's Self, her soul, her life, has been processed out, leaving behind only the appearance of liberty.

Junk liberty is full of artificial preservatives, "junk rights." Women have the right to be treated as commodities. We have the right to subject our most intimate feelings and relationships to contract law. We have the right to be sold.

Junk liberty is for the people the patriarchy would like us to be: junk people, junk women. Women without dignity or substance. Women who can't feel joy or pain or love or hate or anger. Women who act like machines. Women who let themselves be used and then quietly throw themselves on the junk heap.

Junk liberty is a key concept in the marketing strategy of the surrogate industry. It is a concept used to cover up a crime against humanity.

Junk liberty. ("The triple dose of the drug had serious side effects for me [including] . . . intense pain in my left ovary. I was unable to walk because of the pain.")

Junk liberty. (A surrogate mother would be required to carry with her, at all times after the sixth month of pregnancy, a court paper ordering the hospital to give her baby only to the people who paid for it.)

Junk liberty. ("When I refused to give Sarah up, five cops stormtrooped my house to get her. . . . They put me in handcuffs and threw me in the police car. . . . ")

Junk liberty. (" . . . I told the sperm donor and his wife of my need not to have them present in the delivery room. . . . They responded that their presence at the birth was part of what they paid for.")

Junk liberty. ("You could devastate them [poor Mexican women] with money and things—you know, whatever they need.")

The real question is not whether women have the "right," the "liberty" to sell our bodies or not. The question is not whether surrogacy is forced or voluntary. The question is this: What is surrogacy? As Janice Raymond writes, it is "an inherently unequal relationship involving the objectification, sale, and commodification of a woman's body" (Raymond, 1987a).

Kathleen Barry, author of *Female Sexual Slavery*, demonstrates that prostitution is a crime against women. Following her argumentation, surrogacy—reproduction prostitution—is also a crime against women. The crime is turning a whole class of people—women—into a commodity exchange and, in so doing, violating our human dignity. The customers and the surrogacy brokers are those who commit this crime against women. The customer is buying time on a woman's body, and the broker is enabling it.

Surrogacy is not liberty. It is crime.

Women will not settle for junk liberty. We want real freedom—the substance, not just the appearance. We want real nourishment for our spirits. We want human dignity. We want it for *all* of us. We want it for women in Thailand and Bangladesh and Mexico as well as for the women who have not yet been born. We want human dignity. We will not stop fighting until we have it.

References

1. Andrea Dworkin, author of *Pornography: Men Possessing Women*, has often made the point that the U.S. Constitution was written by a number of slave-holders.

2. A bit of backgroud on the AFS ethics report on the new reproductive technologies: In November 1984, the American Fertility Society's board decided the organization needed "to take a leadership position in addressing ethical issues in reproduction" and in publicizing its views. So it appointed an ethics committee led by Dr. Howard Jones. Jones is co–lab parent of the U.S.'s first test tube baby and a leading practitioner and proponent of reproductive technology.

The eleven-member committee (ten men, one woman) consisted of two attorneys, two ethicists, and seven "technodocs," a term conceived by the head of the Yale University IVF team to describe himself and his colleagues. Among the technodocs were the chief of a California in vitro fertilization team who is experimenting in human embryo freezing, and Jones's colleague, the scientific director of the Jones Institute of Reproductive Medicine.

Surprise: After 18 months of serious deliberation, the technodocs determined that what they do is ethical.

Some quotes on "procreative liberty" from the AFS ethics report: " . . . several international declarations of human rights speak about the right of men and women of full age . . . to marry and found a family." On several occasions, it adds, the U.S. Supreme Court has indicated strong support for procreative liberty, particularly of married persons. It adds:

> Although these cases have not involved state attempts to prevent married couples from reproducing, they do suggest that the court would recognize such a couple's right if it were ever faced with a direct limitation on a married couple's desire to reproduce by sexual intercourse. The language in these cases is broad and presumably would extend to both coital and noncoital reproduction, even if the latter were not contemplated at the time.
>
> The values and interests underlying a right of coital reproduction strongly suggest a married couple's right to non-coital reproduction as well and, arguably, to have the assistance of donors and surrogates as needed. (p. 3)
>
> The married couple's right to reproduce should thus extend to noncoital means of conception, which include the wide range of choices made possible by developments in IVF. The couple would then have the right to create, store and have transferred to them extracorporeal preembryos created by their egg and sperm. They would have the right to determine whether their gametes would be used for reproduction and determine the disposition of preembryos created with their gametes, which would include a right to donate preembryos to other couples. . . . (p. 4)

In a footnote on the "right to procreate", the ethics committee observes: "Severe overpopulation might constitute the compelling interest necessary to uphold interference with reproduction by sexual intercourse, as might the situation in which a couple knowingly and avoidably conceives and brings to term a severely handicapped child, then passes to others the cost and burdens of rearing that child."

3. The AFS Ethics Committee stated: "Strictly analyzed, the logic of marital procreative liberty would require the state to enforce such contracts. . . . Refusal to enforce a reproductive contract or a ban on payments would amount to an interference with procreative liberty because it would prevent couples from acquiring the donor or surrogate assistance needed to acquire a child genetically or gestationally related to themselves" (American Fertility Society, 1986).

4. Kathleen Barry's work has been central in conceptualizing the relationship of human rights to human dignity. See Barry, Bunch, and Castley, 1983.

Janice Raymond, who has applied Barry's insights to surrogacy, has written the most trenchant articles I have read on surrogacy. Her work, listed in the bibliography, is on the cutting edge in analysis of this issue. In particular, see "The Spermatic Market: Surrogate Stock and Liquid Assets."

5. John Stehura, head of a surrogacy operation, maintained in an interview with me in 1983 that surrogacy was too expensive for the U.S. middle class. The way to bring the price down, he said, was to use poverty-stricken women in the U.S. who would accept even less than the then current (and still current) $10,000 fee. Even less could be paid women, he said, once it was possible to cross international boundaries.

Asked what countries he had he mind, he replied, "Central America would be fine" (Corea, 1985).

In a more recent interview (December 1987), Stehura, president of Bionetics Foundation in Santa Monica, California, discussed his current work.

His plans for expanding surrogacy include:

a. Bringing the cost of surrogacy down (the "engineering angle") by providing clients with the information they need to find a "surrogate" mother themselves, largely through advertising.

He is completing a listing of all the newspapers in the U.S. that will run advertisements for existing pregnancy adoptions and surrogacy. The listing will include each newspaper's circulation and cost per line for classified ads.

Then he will do listings for England, Scotland, the rest of Europe and Thailand and the Philippines ("I've had the data for some time now").

b. Seek women in the economically depressed north of England as so-called surrogates.

c. Seek women in Thailand and the Philippines.

d. Open up a surrogacy agency in Mexico that mimics a U.S. charitable organization in order to win the trust of Mexican women who have, until now, been fairly unresponsive to advertisements for breeders.

e. Locate a Filipino or Mexican physician, finance a short course for him in in vitro fertilization and embryo transfer in the United States and send him back to his country to open a clinic there. U.S. couples could then travel to that country for a variety of inexpensive procedures, including the use of these technologies on Mexican or Filipino so-called "surrogate" mothers (Corea, 1987b).

6. The Model Reproductive Services Act is the act drafted by the Executive Adoption Committee of the Family Law Section of the American Bar Association for approval by the Family Law Section Council at its 1987 annual meeting in San Francisco. In a letter dated Sept. 4, 1987, to Robert L. Gletzer, chairman of the Science and Technology Section of the ABA, Joseph Gitlin, Chair, Ad Hoc Surrogacy Committee, wrote: "I am writing to you in behalf of the Family Law Section to solicit your section's support for the Family Laws Section's Model Reproductive Services Act (Surrogacy). The Model Reproductive Services Act was approved by the Family Law Section Council in August of 1987, subject to 'refinement' by the section's Ad Hoc Surrogacy Committee."

Since Gitlin wrote, the Model Act has been refined considerably.

The draft states, on page 8, that the reproductive services agreement shall "State that the surrogate shall arrange to give birth to the child in a health facility that previously has been given a certified copy of the order provided for in Section 9 below and that the surrogate shall arrange to keep a certified copy of the order with her at all times after the sixth month of pregnancy."

According to Robert Arenstein, a member of the Ad Hoc Surrogacy Committee, that provision of the draft has now been removed.

On page 15 of the draft, Section 11 a reads: "The child and intended providers of genetic materials who are parties to the contract shall be tested for blood and tissue type within 14 days after receiving notice of the birth. . . . In order to avoid certification of parentage, within 14 days after the test results are mailed to the parties, the party or parties seeking to assert that the child is not as intended must file their petition, and mail or otherwise serve notice directly or on the agents of the other parties to the contract."

7. The idea of junk liberty sprang to life during a long conversation with José Juncá of David, Panama. Juncá volunteered to serve as a translator for Alejandra Muñoz in Washington, D.C., when she came to speak out at a press conference announcing the formation of the National Coalition Against Surrogacy on August 31, 1987. At the time of the conversation, Juncá was a college student in the U.S.

Bibliography

American Fertility Society, Ethics Committee. 1986, September. Ethical Considerations of the New Reproductive Technologies, 46 *Fertility and Sterility* 1S (Supp.)

Andrews, Lori B. 1987. Feminist Perspectives on Reproductive Technologies. In *Reproductive Laws for the 1990s*, Briefing Handbook. Women's Rights Litigation Clinic. Rutgers Law School, Newark, New Jersey 07102.

Barrass, Nancy. 1986, July 21. Letter to sperm donor and wife. Copy provided to the author.

———. 1987, October 12. Testimony submitted to the U.S. House of Representatives, Committee on Energy and Commerce, Subcommittee on Transportation, Tourism and Hazardous Materials.

Barry, Kathleen. 1979. *Female Sexual Slavery*. Prentice Hall. New York.

Barry, Kathleen, Charlottte Bunch, and Shirley Castley (eds). 1984. International Feminism: Networking Against Female Sexual Slavery. Distributed by The International Women's Tribune Centre, Inc., 777 United Nations Plaza, New York, New York 10017.

Belloli, Sheilia Gruber. 1988, April. Surrogate Twin in Legal Limbo. *Detroit News.*

Bicknell, Graham. 1988, May 21. Frank Monte: A Search for Surrogates. *New Idea* (Australia)

Bionetics Foundation. 1982. *Surrogate Mother: Spring 82 Directory*. Malibu, California.

Corea, Gena. 1985. *The Mother Machine*. Harper and Row. New York.

———. 1987a. Tape-recorded interview with Harvey Berman.

———. 1987b, December 15 and 22. Tape-recorded interviews with John Stehura.

———. 1988. Interview with Patricia Foster.

———. 1988, April 27. Showdown for the Surrogate Industry. *The Age* (Melbourne, Australia).

Frederick, Winston R., et al. 1987, Nov. 19. HIV Testing of Surrogate Mothers. *New England Journal of Medicine.* 1351–52.

George Washington University Medical Center. 1988. Host Uterus: In Vitro Fertilization Embryo Transfer Program. Brochure.

Gordon, Cathy. 1987, Nov. 11. Secret Surrogate: Coroner Sees Negligence after Heart Attack Kills Contract Mom. *Houston Chronicle.*

Handel, William. 1987, September 3. Testimony before the Pennsylvania House Judiciary Committee, chaired by the Hon. H. William DeWeese, Pittsburgh, Pennsylvania.

Hubbard, Ruth. 1984, March/April. "Fetal Rights" and the New Eugenics. *Science for the People.*

Kane, Elizabeth. 1987, October 15. Testimony before the U.S. House of Representatives, Committee on Energy and Commerce, Subcommittee on Transportation, Tourism and Hazardous Materials.

————. 1988. *Birth Mother*. Harcourt, Brace, Jovanovich. Washington, D.C.

Muñoz, Alejandra. 1987, October 15. Testimony before the U.S. House of Representatives, Committee on Energy and Commerce, Subcommittee on Transportation, Tourism and Hazardous Materials.

Powers, Rebecca. 1988, Jan. 17. Surrogate Mom's Death Raises Troubling Questions. *Detroit News*.

Raymond, Janice G. 1987a, October. Testimony on House Bill Number 4753 before the House Judiciary Committee, State of Michigan. Lansing, Michigan.

————. 1987b. Making International Connections: Surrogacy, the Traffic in Women and De-Mythologizing Motherhood. In *Sortir la Maternité du Laboratoire*. Eds. Thérèse Mailloux, Marie Rinfret, Jocelyn Olivier, Lucie Desrochers. Conseil du Statut de la Femme. Quebec, Quebec.

————. 1988. In the Matter of Baby M: Rejudged. *Reproductive and Genetic Engineering: International Feminist Analysis*. 1 (2):175–181.

————. 1988. The Spermatic Market: Surrogate Stock and Liquid Assets. *Reproductive and Genetic Engineering: International Feminist Analysis*. 1 (1):65–75.

————. 1988. Of Eggs, Embryos and Altruism. *Reproductive and Genetic Engineering: International Feminist Analysis*. 1 (3):281–285.

Robertson, John. 1986. Embryos, Families, and Procreative Liberty: The Legal Structure of the New Reproduction. *Southern California Law Review*. 59:939.

Silver, Lee M. 1988, July 14. Statement prepared for the Human Resources and Intergovernmental Relations Subcommittee of the Committee on Government Operations of the U.S. House of Representatives.

Snyder, Sarah. 1987, March 13. Baby M Trial Hears Closing Arguments. *Boston Globe*.

Sorkow, J. S. C. 1987, March 31. Opinion in the Baby M case. Superior Court of New Jersey, Chancery Division/Family Part, Bergen County. Docket No. FM-25314–86E.

UPI. 1988, June 25. Use Brain-Dead Women as Surrogate Moms, Scientist Says. *Detroit News*.

Whitehead, Mary Beth. 1987, October 15. Testimony before the U.S. House of Representatives, Committee on Energy and Commerce, Subcommittee on Transportation, Tourism and Hazardous Materials.

APPENDIX V

BIBLIOGRAPHY

In the preparation of this bibliography, several earlier bibliographies on surrogate motherhood were consulted. These were *Surrogate Mothers: Bibliography-in-Brief,* Edith Sutterlin, Congressional Research Service, March 1988; *Surrogate Motherhood: A Selective Bibliography,* Daniel J. Jacobs, The Record of the Association of the Bar of the City of New York, October 1987; "Selected Bibliography" from *Surrogate Mothering—The Legal and Policy Perspective,* Martha Field, Harvard University Press, 1988; "A Select Bibliography on Surrogacy," Laura Peritore, *Family Law Quarterly,* 22 (2, summer 1988); and *Annotated Bibliography on Surrogacy,* The Reproductive Freedom Project of the American Civil Liberties Union.

Adlam, Diana. "The Case against Capitalist Patriarchy." In *Feminism and Materialism: Women and Modes of Production,* ed. Annette Kuhn and Ann Marie Wolpe. London: Routledge and Kegan Paul, 1978.

Allen, Anita L. "Privacy, Surrogacy, and the Baby M Case." *Georgetown Law Journal,* 76:5 (June 1988), pp. 1759–92.

American Bar Association Journal. "Life, Liberty, and Children." 73 (June 1987), p. 39.

American College of Obstetricians and Gynecologists. *Ethical Issues in Surrogate Motherhood* (A.C.O.G. Statement of Public Policy 56). Washington, D.C.: A.C.O.G., 1983.

American Fertility Society. "Ethical Statement on In Vitro Fertilization." *Fertility and Sterility,* 41 (1984), p. 12.

———. "Minimal Standards for Programs on In Vitro Fertilization." *Fertility and Sterility,* 41 (1984), p. 13.

American Fertility Society, Ethics Committee. "Ethical Considerations of the New Reproductive Technologies. *Fertility and Sterility,* 4:3 (Supplement 1), 1986.

American Law Institute. *Restatement (Second) of Contracts.* St. Paul, 1981.

Andrade, Jane Carroll. "The Law and Surrogate Motherhood." *State Legislature,* 13 (July 1987), p. 24–26.

Andrews, Lori B. "The Aftermath of Baby M: Proposed State Laws on Surrogate Motherhood." *Hastings Center Report,* 17 (October–November 1987), pp. 31–40.

———. *Between Strangers: Surrogate Mothers, Expectant Fathers, and Brave New Babies.* New York: Harper and Row, 1989.

———. "Brave New Baby." *Student Lawyer* (December 1983), p. 25.

———. "Law and the Stork: New Reproductive Methods Raise New Legal Problems for Lawyers, Clients." *Los Angeles Daily Journal,* August 30, 1984, p. 4, col. 3.

———. *New Conceptions: A Consumer's Guide to the Newest Infertility Treatments, Including In Vitro Fertilization, Artificial Insemination, and Surrogate Motherhood.* New York: Ballantine, 1985, xvii, 330 p.

———. "Removing the Stigma of Surrogate Motherhood." *Family Advocate,* 4 (Fall 1981), pp. 20–27.

———. "Stork Market: The Law of the New Reproductive Technologies." *American Bar Association Journal*, 70 (August 1984), pp. 50–56.

———. "Surrogate Motherhood: Should the Adoption Model Apply?" *Children's Legal Rights Journal*, 7 (1986), pp. 13–20.

———. "When Baby's Mother is Also Grandma—and Sister." *Hastings Center Report*, 15 (October 1985), p. 29.

———. "Yours, Mine, and Theirs." *Psychology Today*, 18 (December 1984), p. 20.

Angel, Carol. "Natural Mother Stripped of Rights in Baby 'M' Case: Historic Ruling May Bolster Business of Surrogate Parenting: Others Decry Decision." *Los Angeles Daily Journal*, April 1987, p. 1, col. 6.

Annas, George J. "The Baby Broker Boom." *Hastings Center Report*, 16 (June 1986), pp. 30–31.

———. "Baby M: Babies (and Justice) for Sale." *Hastings Center Report*, 17 (June 1987), pp. 13–15.

———. "Death without Dignity for Commercial Surrogacy: The Case of Baby M." *Hastings Center Report*, 18 (April–May 1988), pp. 21–24.

———. "Law and the Life Sciences: Contracts to Bear a Child: Compassion or Commercialism?" *Hastings Center Report*, 11 (April 1981), pp. 23–24.

———. "Making Babies without Sex: The Law and the Profits." *American Journal of Public Health*, 74 (1984), pp. 1415–17.

———. "Pregnant Women as Fetal Containers." *Hastings Center Report*, 18 (December 1986), p. 13.

———. "Social Policy Considerations in Noncoital Reproduction." *Journal of the American Medical Association*, 255 (January 3, 1986), pp. 2–8.

Annas, George J., and Sherman Elias. "In Vitro Fertilization and Embryo Transfer: Medico-Legal Aspects of a New Technique to Create a Family." *Family Law Quarterly*, 17 (1983), p. 199.

Aral, S., and W. Cates. "The Increasing Concern with Infertility." *Journal of the American Medical Association*, 250 (1986), p. 2327.

Arditti, Rita. "The Surrogacy Business." *Social Policy*, 18 (Fall 1987), pp. 42–46.

———. "Surrogate Mothering Exploits Women." *Science for the People*, May–June 1987, pp. 22–23.

Areen, Judith. "Baby M Reconsidered." *Georgetown Law Journal*, 76:5 (June 1988), pp. 1741–58.

Arms, Suzanne. *To Love and Let Go*. New York: Alfred Knopf, 1986.

Armstrong, Stephen M. "Womb and Board: Medical Advances in Reproduction—At What Costs?" *Medical Trial Technology Quarterly*, 33 (1987), p. 465.

Asche, Justice. "Ethical Implications in the Use of Donor Sperm, Eggs and Embryos in the Treatment of Human Fertility." *Law Institute Journal*, 57 (1983), p. 714.

Atallah, Lillian. "Report from a Test-Tube Baby." *New York Times Magazine* (April 18, 1976), pp. 16–17, 48, 51–52.

Atwood, M. *The Handmaid's Tale*. New York: Fawcrest, Ballantine, 1986.

Australian Law Journal. "Legislation in Regard to Surrogate Motherhood." 59 (1985), pp. 306–308.

———. "Surrogate Motherhood—The Warnock and Waller Reports." 58 (1984), pp. 683–685.

Avery, P. A. "Surrogate Mothers: Center of a New Storm." *U.S. News and World Report*, 94 (June 1983), p. 76.

Barnett, Daniel L. "In Vitro Fertilization: Third Party Motherhood and the Changing Definition of Legal Parent." *Pacific Law Journal*, 17 (1985), p. 231.

Barrett, Michele, and Mary McIntosh. *The Anti-Social Family*. London: NLB, 1982.

Beck, W. W. "Two Hundred Years of Artificial Insemination." *Fertility and Sterility*, 41 (1984), p. 193.

Bettenhausen, Elizabeth. "Hager Revisited: Surrogacy, Alienation and Motherhood." *Christianity and Crisis,* 47 (May 4, 1987), pp. 157–159.

Bhimji, S. "Womb for Rent: Ethical Aspects of Surrogate Motherhood." *Canadian Medical Association Journal,* 137 (December 15, 1987), pp. 1132–35.

Bick-Rice, Judith. "The Need for Statutes Regulating Artificial Insemination by Donors." *Ohio State Law Journal,* 46 (1985), pp. 1055–76.

Billig, R. L. "High Tech Earth Mothering: Legal Aspects of Biomedical Ethics." *District Lawyer* (July/August 1985), pp. 56–63.

Billiter, Bill. "State May Set Rules on Motherhood: Could Become First to Legalize, Control Use of Surrogates." *Los Angeles Times,* June 20, 1982, p. I-3.

———. "State Studies Surrogate Mother Law: L.A. Hearing Vents Views on Growing Nationwide Practice." *Los Angeles Times,* November 22, 1982, p. I-23.

———. "Surrogate Mother Protection Bill Tabled in Senate." *Los Angeles Times,* August 4, 1982, p. I-21.

———. "Surrogate Mothers Bill Dead for Session," *Los Angeles Times,* August 5, 1982, p. II-12.

Bird, Kathleen. "Model Law Recommends Court Approval for Surrogacy Pacts." *New Jersey Law Journal,* 4 (June 4, 1987), pp. 18–19.

———. "Parental Rights at Issue: Baby M Ruling's Boldness May Invite Appellate Attack." *New Jersey Law Journal,* 4 (April 9, 1987), pp. 26–27.

———. "Ruling Sparks Legislative Debate." *New Jersey Law Journal,* 109 (April 9, 1987), p. 2, col. 1.

———. "Surrogate Motherhood: Hers? Yours? Ours?" *California Lawyer,* 2 (February 1982), pp. 20–25.

Birzon, Paul I., and Grace M. Ange. "Whose Baby Am I Anyway? The Impact of Baby M in New York." *Manhattan Lawyer,* 4 (May 11, 1987), p. 38.

Bitner, Lizabeth A. "Wombs for Rent: A Call for Pennsylvania Legislation Legalizing and Regulating Surrogate Parenting Agreements." *Dickinson Law Review,* 90 (Fall 1985), pp. 227–259.

Black, Robert C. "Legal Problems of Surrogate Motherhood." *New England Law Review,* 16:3 (1980–81), pp. 373–396.

Blair, Betty. "Surrogate Motherhood Gains Acceptance, Won't Go Away." *Los Angeles Times,* December 16, 1982, p. IV-4.

Blakely, Mary Kay. "Surrogate Mothers: For Whom Are They Working?" *Ms.* (March 1983), pp. 18–20.

Blank, Robert. *Redefining Human Life: Reproductive Technologies and Social Policy.* Boulder, Colo.: Westview, 1984.

Blodgett, Nancy. "Surrogate Parent Rights: Alternative Reproduction Laws Proposed." *American Bar Association Journal,* 72 (December 1986), pp. 33–34.

———. "Who is Mother? Genetic Donor, Not Surrogate." *American Bar Association Journal,* 72 (June 1986), p. 18.

Blumberg, Patricia. "Human Leukocyte Antigen Testing: Technology versus Policy in Cases of Disputed Parentage." *Vanderbilt Law Review,* 36 (November 1983), pp. 1578–1631.

Bolick, Nancy O'Keefe. "The New Faces of Adoption." *Boston Magazine* (October 1986), p. 152.

Bonavoglia, Angela. "The Ordeal of Pamela Rae Stewart." *Ms.* (July–August 1987), pp. 92–95, 196–204.

Boskey and McCue. "Alternative Standards for the Termination of Parental Rights." *Seton Hall Law Review,* 9 (1978), p. 1.

Boston Women's Health Book Collective. *The New Our Bodies, Ourselves.* New York: Simon and Schuster, 1985.

Bowal, Peter. "Surrogate Procreation: A Motherhood Issue in Legal Obscurity." *Queens Law Journal*, 9 (Fall 1983), pp. 5–34.

Brahams, Diana. "The Hasty British Ban on Commercial Surrogacy." *Hastings Center Report*, 17 (February 1987), pp. 16–19.

———. "Surrogacy: A Criminal Offence?" *Medico-Legal Journal*, 52 (1984), p. 248.

———. "Surrogacy, Adoption, and Custody." *Lancet*, 1 (April 4, 1987), p. 817.

Brakel, L. A. "A Modern 'Solution' to the Oedipal Problem: A Fantasy of Surrogate Motherhood." *Psychoanalytical Quarterly*, 57 (January 1988), pp. 87–91.

Brighton Science Collective. *Alice through the Microscope (The Power of Science over Women's Bodies)*. London: Virago Press, 1980.

Brody, E. B. "Reproduction Without Sex—But With the Doctor." *Law, Medicine, and Health Care*, 15 (Fall 1987), pp. 152–55.

Bronner, Ethan. "Advances Elevate Status of Fetus." *Boston Globe*, July 21, 1987, p. 1.

Brophy, Katie M. "A Surrogate Mother Contracts to Bear a Child." *Journal of Family Law*, 20 (1982), pp. 263–291.

Brown, Bridgett. "Surrogate Parenting Law: The Applicability of LA-R.S. 14–286 towards Providing a Constitutionally Reasonable and Legitimate Means by Which the State May Address Surrogate Contracts." *Southern University Law Review*, 13 (1986), p. 125.

Brown, Hutton, et al. "Legal Rights and Issues surrounding Conception, Pregnancy, and Birth." *Vanderbilt Law Review*, 39 (1986), pp. 597–850.

Buchanan, J. *Baby "M" and Surrogate Motherhood: A Resource Guide*. 1987.

Buser, Paul J. "The Cutting Edge—Most Current Topics in Family Law." *Advocate* (Idaho), 29 (1986), p. 16.

Business Week. "Adoption: It's Not Impossible" (July 8, 1985), p. 112.

Bustillo, M. "Nonsurgical Ovum Transfer as a Treatment in Infertile Women: Preliminary Experience." *Journal of the American Medical Association*, 251 (1984), p. 1171.

California Legislature Committee on Judiciary. "Surrogate Parenting Contracts: Hearing of November 19, 1982; Whittier College School of Law, Auditorium, 5353 West Third Street, Los Angeles, California." (1982), v, 230 p.

Cappuccio, Mark S. "Surrogate Motherhood in Ohio: A Dangerous Game of Baby Roulette." *Capital University Law Review*, 15 (1985), p. 93.

Capron, Alexander M. "The New Reproductive Possibilities: Seeking a Moral Basis for Concerted Action in a Pluralistic Society." *Law, Medicine, and Health Care*, 12 (October 1984), pp. 192–198.

CBS News. "Surrogate Mother." Produced by Suzanne St. Pierre. New York: CBS, Inc., 1982. 11 leaves.

Chambers, D. R. "No Primrose Path." *Medicine, Science, and Law*, 27 (1987), p. 151.

Christensen, Steven A. "Adoption Procedures of Minor Children in Colorado." *Colorado Lawyer*, 12 (1983), pp. 1057–66.

Clark, Natalie Loder. "New Wine in Old Skins: Using Paternity-Suit Settlements to Facilitate Surrogate Motherhood." *Journal of Family Law*, 25 (1986–87), pp. 483–527.

Cohen, Barbara. "Surrogate Mothers: Whose Baby Is It?" *American Journal of Law and Medicine*, 10 (Fall 1984), pp. 243–285.

Cohen, B., and T. L. Friend. "Legal and Ethical Implications of Surrogate Mother Contracts." *Clinics in Perinatology*, 14 (June 1987), pp. 281–92.

Coleman, Phyllis. "Surrogate Motherhood: Analysis of the Problems and Suggestions for Solutions." *Tennessee Law Review*, 50 (Fall 1982), pp. 71–118.

Columbia Journal of Law and Social Problems. "Surrogate Motherhood and the Baby-Selling Laws." 20 (1986), p. 1.

Condie, Karen T. "Surrogacy as a Treatment for Infertility." *Journal of the Law Society of Scotland*, 31 (1986), p. 469.

Cook, Alberta. "Lawyers Debate Impact of Baby 'M' Ruling." *National Law Journal*, 9 (April 13, 1987), p. 3, col. 1.

Corbin, Arthur L. *Contracts*. 12 vols. St. Paul: West, 1950–64.

Corea, Gena. *The Mother Machine: Reproductive Technologies from Artificial Insemination to Artificial Wombs*. New York: Harper and Row, 1986.

Cox, Gail. "California Surrogate-Mother Case Settles, Munoz v. Haro." *National Law Journal* (March 1, 1987), p. 6, col. 1.

Crow, Carol A. "The Surrogate Child: Legal Issues and Implications for the Future." *Journal of Juvenile Law*, 7 (1983), pp. 80–92.

Council for Science and Society. *Human Procreation: Ethical Aspects of the New Techniques*. 1984.

Cullen, Kevin. "Law Orders Coverage for Infertility." *Boston Globe*, October 9, 1987, p. 1.

Curie-Cohen, Martin, Lesleigh Luttrell, and Sander Shapiro. "Current Practice of AID in the United States." *New England Journal of Medicine*, 300 (1979), pp. 585–590.

Cusine, Douglas J. " 'Womb-Leasing': Some Legal Implications." *New Law Journal*, 128 (1978), pp. 824–825.

Dart, John. "Ethicist Examines Social Issues of Surrogate Motherhood: Says Traditional Ideas of Parenthood Might Change Radically." *Los Angeles Times*, January 2, 1982, p. II-4.

D'Aversa, Carmina Y. "The Right of Abortion in Surrogate Motherhood Arrangements." *Northern Illinois Law Review*, 7 (1987), pp. 1–39.

Davis, Linda. "Surrogate Parenting." *New Law Journal* (Great Britain), 134 (1984), pp. 707–708.

Denton, L. "Surrogate Parenting." *American Psychological Association* (April 1987).

Dickens, Bernard. "Artificial Reproduction and Child Custody." *Canadian Bar Review*, 66 (March 1987), p. 49.

Dickman, S. "West German Reactions over U.S. Surrogacy Company." *Nature*, 329 (October 15–21, 1987), p. 577.

Dodd, Bette J. "The Surrogate Mother Contract in Indiana." *Indiana Law Review*, 15 (1982), pp. 807–830.

Donovan, Patricia. "New Reproductive Technologies: Some Legal Dilemmas." *Family Planning Perspectives*, 18 (March-April 1986), pp. 57–60.

Dunstan, Gordon Reginald. "Moral and Social Issues arising from A.I.D.: Law and Ethics of A.I.D. and Embryo Transfer." *CIBA Foundation Symposium*, 17 (1973), pp. 52–68.

Eaton, Thomas A. "Comparative Responses to Surrogate Motherhood." *Nebraska Law Review*, 65 (1986), p. 686.

———. "The British Response to Surrogate Motherhood: An American Critique." *Law Teacher*, 19 (1985), pp. 163–192.

Eckholm, Erik. "The Baby 'M' Case; Designing an Ethical Frame for Motherhood by Contract." *Los Angeles Daily Journal* (January 13, 1987), p. 4, col. 3.

The Economist (Britain). "Is Having Babies Bad?" 294 (January 12, 1985), pp. 14–15.

———. "Surrogacy: A Very Special Birthday." 298 (March 15, 1986), p. 58.

———. "Surrogacy: Wrong Mothers, Wrong Babies." 295 (April 20, 1985), pp. 63–64.

———. "Surrogate Mothers: Happy Families." 291 (June 23, 1984), p. 54.

———. "Take the Baby and Run." 300 (September 6, 1986), p. 27.

Ehlers, V. J. "Artificial Insemination, Surrogacy, and the Law." *Nursing RSA*, 2 (November–December 1987), pp. 31, 46.

Ehrenreich, B., and D. English. *For Her Own Good*. New York: Anchor Press, Doubleday, 1979.

Eisler, Kim Isaac. "Alternative Births: Embryonic Field for Family Law but Few Lawyers Entering Practice; Case Law Is Scarce: Issues under Study." *Los Angeles Daily Journal*, March 27, 1985, p. 1, col. 6.

Ellis, Jane Truesdell. "The Law and Procedure of International Adoption: An Overview." *Suffolk Transnational Law Journal*, 7 (Fall 1983), 361–390.

Engram, Sara. "Doctors and Surrogate Moms: Physicians Face Ethical Dilemma over Technology." *Los Angeles Times*, April 9, 1982, p. V-14.

Erickson, Elizabeth A. "Contracts to Bear a Child." *California Law Review*, 66 (1978), pp. 611–622.

Erlenbusch, Phyllis. "Planned Parenthood: The Surrogate Alternative." *Reports on Family Law*, 29 (November 1982), pp. 51–73.

Family Law (Great Britain). "Family Law Developments: An Update." 14 (1984), pp. 217–219.

―――. "Re a Baby." 15 (1985), pp. 71–72.

Family Law Quarterly. "Special Issue on Surrogacy." 22:119 (1988).

Fashing, Felicia R. "Artificial Conception: A Legislative Proposal." *Cardozo Law Review*, 5 (Spring 1984), pp. 713–735.

Feinerman, James V. "A Comparative Look at Surrogacy." *Georgetown Law Journal*, 76:5 (June 1988), pp. 1837–44.

Feldman, Walter S. "Wombs for Rent: Surrogate Mothers and Semen Donors." *Legal Aspects of Medical Practice*, 10 (May 1982), p. 8.

Field, Martha. *Surrogate Motherhood*. Cambridge, Mass.: Harvard University Press, 1988, 215 p.

Finegold, Wilfred J. *Artificial Insemination*. 2d ed. Springfield, Ill.: Charles C. Thomas, 1976.

Flaherty, James T. "Enforcement of Surrogate Mother Contracts: Case Law, The Uniform Acts, and State and Federal Legislation." *Cleveland State Law Review* 36:223. 1988.

Fleming, A. T. "Our Fascination with Baby M." *New York Times Magazine* (March 29, 1987).

Fletcher, William M. *Cyclopedia of the Law of Private Corporations*. Rev. ed. Vol. 7A. Wilmette, Ill.: Callaghan, 1978.

Flickinger, Russell N. "Surrogate Motherhood: The Attorney's Legal and Ethical Dilemma." *Capital University Law Review*, 11, pp. 593–610.

Foster, Henry H., Jr. "Adoption and Child Custody: Best Interests of the Child?" *Buffalo Law Review*, 1 (Spring 1973), pp. 1–16.

Fox, Martin. "Long Island Surrogate Mother Waives Child Custody." *New York Law Journal* (March 17, 1987), p. 1, col. 1.

Frederick, W. R., R. Delapena, G. Gray, W. L. Greaves, and C. Saxinger. "HIV Testing of Surrogate Mothers" (letter). *New England Journal of Medicine*, 317 (November 19, 1987), pp. 1351–52.

Freed, D. "As Surrogate Parenting Increases, States Must Resolve Legal Issues." *National Law Journal* (December 22, 1986), p. 28, col. 1.

Freed, Doris J., and Henry H. Foster. "Family Law in the Fifty States: An Overview." *Family Law Quarterly*, 16 (Winter 1983), pp. 289–383.

―――. "Surrogate Mothers—An Unbearable Dilemma." *New York Law Journal* (March 1, 1983), p. 1, col. 1.

Freeman, M. D. A. "After Warnock—Whither the Law?" *Current Legal Problems*, 39 (1986), pp. 33–55.

Frey, Kelly L. "New Reproductive Technologies: The Legal Problems and a Solution." *Tennessee Law Review*, 49 (1982), p. 303.

Friedrich, Otto. " 'A Legal, Moral, Social Nightmare': Society Seeks to Define the Problems of the Birth Revolution." *Time* (September 10, 1984), pp. 54–56.

Frontline. "Desperately Seeking Baby." WGBH Boston (television). March 3, 1987.

Frug, Mary Joe. "The Baby M Contract." *New Jersey Law Journal*, 119 (1987), pp. 337–338.

Furrow, Barry R. "Surrogate Motherhood: A New Option for Parenting?" *Law, Medicine and Health Care*, 12 (1984), p. 106.

Galen, Michele. "Surrogate Law: The Decision in a Novel Case in New Jersey Could Have Wide-Reaching Implications for Infertile Couples and Surrogate Motherhood." *National Law Journal*, 9 (September 29, 1986), pp. 1–10.

Gallagher, J. "The Fetus and the Law—Whose Life Is It Anyway?" *Ms.* (September 1984).

Garrison, Marsha. "Why Terminate Parental Rights?" *Stanford Law Review*, 35 (February 1982), pp. 423–496.

Gelman, D. "Infertility: Babies by Contract." *Newsweek*, 10 (November 4, 1985), pp. 74–75.

George, Ellen S., and Stephen M. Snyder. "A Reconsideration of the Religious Element in Adoption." *Cornell Law Review*, 56 (May 1971), pp. 782–830.

Georgetown Law Journal, "Developing a Concept of the Modern 'Family': A Proposed Uniform Surrogate Parenthood Act," 73 (1985), p. 1283.

Gersz, Steven R. "The Contract in Surrogate Motherhood: A Review of the Issues." *Law, Medicine, and Health Care*, 12 (June 1984), pp. 107–114.

Gest, T. "Whose Baby is 'Baby M'?" *U.S. News and World Report*, 102 (January 19, 1987), p. 15.

Gitlin, H. Joseph. "Surrogate Motherhood Raises Many Questions." *Chicago Daily Law Bulletin* (September 10, 1986), p. 2, col. 1.

Gladwell, M., and R. Sharpe. "Baby M Winner." *New Republic*, 19 (February 16, 1987), pp. 15–16.

Gold, Stephen. "Surrogacy News: The Secret Diary of Derek Kirby Johnson Aged over 18." *New Law Journal*, 135 (February 1, 1985), pp. 98–99.

Goldfarb, Carolea. "Two Mothers, One Baby, No Law." *Human Rights*, 11 (Summer 1983), pp. 26–29.

Goldstein, Joseph, Anna Freud, and Albert Solnit. *Before the Best Interests of the Child.* New York: Free Press, 1979.

———. *Beyond the Best Interests of the Child.* New York: Free Press, 1973.

———. *In the Best Interests of the Child.* New York: Free Press, 1986.

Goleman, Daniel. "Motivations of Surrogate Mothers." *New York Times*, January 20, 1987, p. C1.

Gonzaga Law Review. "Baby-Sitting Consideration: Surrogate Mother's Right to 'Rent Her Womb' for a Fee." 18 (1982), p. 539.

Goodman, Ellen. "Surrogates Could Make Pregnancy a Service Industry," *Los Angeles Times*, September 2, 1986, p. III-5.

———. "Which Mother Is Mom?" *Los Angeles Times*, April 25, 1986, p. II-7.

———. "Wombs for Rent: New Era on the Reproduction Line." *Los Angeles Times*, February 8, 1983, p. II-5.

———. "The Word That's Not Mentioned in the Baby M Case." *Boston Globe*, February 17, 1987, p. 15.

Gordon, L. "Baby M: New Questions about Biology and Destiny." *Ms.* (June 1897).

———. "Reproductive Rights for Today: Some Policy Proposals." *Nation*, 245 (September 12, 1987), pp. 230–232.

Gorlin, Cathy E., and Thomas Miley. "Surrogate Parenting." *Bench and Bar of Minnesota*, 41 (January 1984), pp. 17–22.

Graham, M. Louise, "Surrogate Gestation and the Protection of Choice." *Santa Clara Law Review*, 22 (Spring 1982), pp. 291–323.

Granelli, James S. "Surrogate Mother Sued over Custody Agreement." *National Law Journal* (New York), (April 1981), pp. 4, 33.

———. "Surrogate Mother Bill Runs into a Snag in California." *National Law Journal* (August 30, 1982), p. 5.

———. "A 'Viable Option': California Eyes Surrogate Mother Bill." *National Law Journal* (July 12, 1982), (Col.1) p. 5.

Gray, M. "A Battle of Ethics, Money and Blood." *Macleans*, 100 (January 2, 1987), p. 44.

Greenberg, Lisa J., and Harold L. Hirsch. "Surrogate Motherhood and Artificial Insemination: Contractual Implications." *Medical Trial Technique Quarterly*, 29 (1983), pp. 149–166.

Greer, William R. "The Adoption Market: A Variety of Options." *New York Times*, June 2, 1986, pp. C1, C10.

Griffin, Moira K. "Wives, Hookers, and the Law." *Student Lawyer*, 10 (January 1982), pp. 18–21, 36–39.

———. "Womb for Rent." *Student Lawyer*, 9 (April 1981), pp. 29–31.

Grobstein, C., Flower, and Mendeloff. "External Human Fertilization: An Evaluation of Policy." *Science* (October 14, 1983), pp. 127–133.

———. *From Chance to Purpose: An Appraisal of External Human Fertilization.* Reading, Mass.: Addison Wesley, 1981.

Growe, S. J. "The Furore over Surrogate Motherhood." *Macleans* (Canada), 95 (July 5, 1982), p. 48.

Grubb, Andrew, and David Pearl. "Medicine, Health, the Family and the Law." *Family Lawyer*, 16 (1986), p. 227.

Gubernick, Lisa. "Noel Keane: Babies Are His Business." *American Lawyer* (June 6, 1984), pp. 119–121.

Gustaitis, Rasa. "The Time Is Now to Decide If This Should Go Further." *Los Angeles Daily Journal*, April 7, 1987, p. 4, col. 3.

Handel, William W. "Surrogate Parenting, In Vitro Insemination and Embryo Transplantation." (Whittier Health Law Symposium '84) *Whittier Law Review* (1984), p. 83.

Handel, William W., and B. A. Sherwyn. "Surrogate Parenting: Coming to Grips with the Future." *Trial*, 18 (April 1982), p. 56.

Hanley, Robert. "Baby M Case Etches a Study in Contrasts: Different Social Classes and Family Relations." *New York Times*, February 17, 1987, pp. B1–B2.

———. "Baby M's 'Best Interests' May Resolve a Puzzling Case." *New York Times*, February 2, 1987, p. B1.

———. "Baby M's Mother Examined on Her Family and Facts." *New York Times*, February 19, 1987, p. B2.

———. "Baby M Trial Lawyers: Two Goals and Two Styles." *New York Times*, February 23, 1987, p. B1.

———. "Experts Testify on Whitehead as a Parent." *New York Times*, February 24, 1987, p. B2.

———. "Father of Baby M Thought Mother Had Been Screened." *New York Times*, January 14, 1987, p. B2.

———. "Reporter's Notebook: Grief over Baby M." *New York Times*, February 12, 1987, pp. B1, B3.

———. "Reporter's Notebook: Mother Plans to Tread Softly in the Baby M Trial." *New York Times*, February 9, 1987, p. B3.

———. "Whitehead Outlines Her Life before Baby M." *New York Times*, February 10, 1987, p. B15.

Hansbrough, Nancy. "Surrogate Motherhood and Tort Liability: Will the New Reproductive Technologies Give Birth to a New Breed of Prenatal Tort?" *Cleveland State Law Review*, 34 (1986), pp. 311–348.

Hardin, H. T. "On the Vicissitudes of Early Primary Surrogate Mothering." *Journal of the American Psychoanalytical Association*, 33 (1985), pp. 609–629.

Harding, Lorraine M. "The Debate on Surrogate Motherhood: The Current Situation, Some Arguments and Issues: Questions Facing Law and Policy." *Journal of Social Welfare* (Great Britain) (1987), pp. 37–63.

Harris, Lindsey E. "Artificial Insemination and Surrogate Motherhood—A Nursery Full of Unresolved Questions." *Willamette Law Journal*, 17 (Fall 1981), pp. 913–952.

Harrison, B. G. "Surrogate Mothers: No Way to Treat a Baby." *Mademoiselle* (January 1987), p. 3.

Harrison, M. "Bias and the Baby." *Boston Phoenix*, March 31, 1987.

Harrison, Michelle. "Social Construction of Mary Beth Whitehead." *Gender and Society*, 1 (September 1987), pp. 300–311.

Harvard Law Review. "Reproductive Technology and the Procreation Rights of the Unmarried." 98 (January 1985), pp. 669–685.

———. "Rumpelstiltskin Revisited: The Inalienable Rights of Surrogate Mothers." 99 (June 1986), pp. 1936–55.

Harvard Women's Law Journal. "Constitutional Analysis of the Baby M Decision." 11 (1988), p. 9.

Healey, J. M. "Baby M and Public Policy." *Connecticut Medicine*, 51 (July 1987), p. 481.

———. "The Baby M Case: Background and Conclusions." *Connecticut Medicine*, 51 (May 1987), p. 345.

———. "The Baby M Case: Findings and Implications." *Connecticut Medicine*, 51 (June 1987), p. 407.

———. "The Welfare of Surrogates and Others" (letter). *Hastings Center Report*, 16 (June 1986), p. 43.

Higginson, Richard. *Reply to Warnock*. Bramcote: Grove Books, 1986, 24 p.

Hilts, Philip J. "Two Embryos Transplanted in Human." *Washington Post*, July 22, 1983, p. A12.

Hirsch, B. D. "Parenthood by Proxy." *Journal of the American Medical Association*, 249 (1983), p. 2251.

Hirsh, Harold L. "Surrogate Motherhood: A Womb in Livery." *Legal Medicine* (1986), pp. 165–198.

Holder, Angela R. "Surrogate Motherhood: Babies for Fun and Profit." *Law, Medicine and Health Care*, 12 (1984), pp. 115–117.

———. "Surrogate Motherhood: Babies for Fun and Profit." *Case and Commentary*, 90 (1985), pp. 3–9.

Hollinger, Joan H. "From Coitus to Commerce: Legal and Social Consequences of Noncoital Reproduction." *University of Michigan Journal of Law Reform*, 18 (Summer 1985), pp. 866–932.

Holmes, H. B., B. Hoskins, and M. Gross, eds. *Birth Control and Controlling Birth—Women Centered Perspectives*. New Jersey: Humana Press (1980).

———. "Surrogacy with IVF Carries Biological Risks" (letter). *Hastings Center Report*, 16 (August 1986), p. 49.

———. *The Custom-Made Child: Woman-Centered Perspective*. Clifton, N.J.: Humana Press, 1981.

Houston Law Review. "Medical Decision Making during a Surrogate Pregnancy." 25 (1988), p. 599.

Hubbard, R. "Caring for Baby Doe." *Ms.* (May 1984).

————. "The Fetus as Patient." *Ms.* (October 1982).

Humphreys, Sarah A. L. "Lawmaking and Science: A Practical Look at In Vitro Fertilization and Embryo Transfer." *Detroit College Law Review* (1979), p. 429–456.

Ince. "Inside the Surrogate Industry." *Test Tube Woman: What Future for Motherhood.* Ed. Arditti, Klein, and Minden (1984), p. 114.

Iowa Law Review. "Litigation, Legislation, and Limelight: Obstacles to Commercial Surrogate Mother Arrangements." 72 (1987), pp. 415–444.

Isaacs, Stephen L., and Renee J. Holt. "Redefining Procreation: Facing the Issues." *Population Bulletin,* 42 (September 1987), 37 p. (whole issue).

Jabro, John. "Surrogate Motherhood: The Outer Limits of Protected Conduct." *Detroit College Law Review,* 1981 (1981), pp. 1131–46.

Jackson, Vicki C. "Baby M and the Question of Parenthood." *Georgetown Law Journal,* 76:5 (June 1988), pp. 1811–28.

Jacobs, Daniel J. "Surrogate Motherhood: A Selective Bibliography." *Record of the Association of the Bar of the City of New York,* 42 (October 1987), pp. 839–851.

Jacobs, Kevin. "Surrogate Mother Gives Birth to Triplets for Her Daughter." *Boston Globe,* October 2, 1987, pp. 1, 3.

Jensen, Brent J. "Artificial Insemination and the Law." *Brigham Young University Law Review,* 4 (1982), pp. 935–990.

Jewett, R. T. "The Legal Consequences of Artificial Insemination in New York." *Syracuse Law Review,* 19 (1968), p. 1009.

Jost, Kenneth. "The Innocent and the Ugly." *Los Angeles Daily Journal* (April 1987), p. 2, col. 5.

Kane, Elizabeth. *Birth Mother: The Story of America's First Legal Surrogate Mother.* San Diego: Harcourt Brace Jovanovich, 1988.

Kantrowitz, Barbara. "Who Keeps Baby M?" *Newsweek* (January 19, 1987), pp. 44–49.

Kasirer, Nicholas. "The Surrogate Motherhood Agreement: A Proposed Standard Form Contract for Quebec." *Revue de Droit* (Sherbrooke University), 16 (1985), pp. 351–387.

Katz, Avi. "Surrogate Motherhood and the Baby-Selling Laws." *Columbia Journal of Law and Social Problems,* 20 (1986), pp. 1–53.

Keane, Noel P. "Legal Problems of Surrogate Motherhood." *Southern Illinois University Law Journal,* 1980 (1981), pp. 147–169.

————. "The Surrogate Parenting Contract." *Adelphi Law Journal,* 2 (1983), pp. 45–53.

Keane, Noel P., and Dennis L. Breo. *The Surrogate Mother.* New York: Everest House, 1981.

Keech, Kristina, and Bruce W. McDougal. "Surrogate Parenting Agreements in Virginia: A Proposal for Action." *Colonial Lawyer,* 16 (1987), pp. 28–39.

Knoppers, B., and E. Sloss. "Recent Developments: Legislative Reforms in Reproductive Technology." *Ottawa Law Review,* 18 (1986), pp. 663–719.

Kolko, S. Joel. "Admissibility of HLA Test Results to Determine Paternity." *Family Law Reporter,* 9 (1983), pp. 4009–18.

Kopytoff, Barbara. "Surrogate Motherhood: Questions of Law and Values." *University of Southern Florida Law Review,* 22:205 (Winter 1988).

Krause, Harry D. "Artificial Conception: Legislative Approaches." *Family Law Quarterly,* 19 (Fall 1985), pp. 185–206.

Krauthammer, Charles. "The Ethics of Human Manufacture." *New Republic* (May 4, 1987), pp. 17–19.

Kremer, J., B. W. Frijling, and J. L. M. Nass. "Psychosocial Aspects of Parenthood by Artificial Insemination by Donor." *The Lancet,* 628 (March 17, 1984).

Krier, Beth Ann. "The Psychological Effects Are Still a Question Mark." *Los Angeles Times*, March 30, 1986, p. V-1.
———. "Surrogate Motherhood: Looking at It as Business Proposition." *Los Angeles Times*, March 30, 1981, p. V-1.
Krimmel, H. T. "The Case against Surrogate Parenting." *The Hastings Center Report*, 13 (1983), p. 35.
Kruse, Richard A. "The Strange Case of Baby M." *Human Life Review*, 13 (Fall 1987), pp. 27–34.
Lacayo, Richard. "Is the Womb a Rental Space?" *Time*, 128 (September 22, 1986), p. 36.
———. "Whose Child Is This? Baby M and the Agonizing Dilemma of Surrogate Motherhood." *Time*, 129 (January 19, 1987), pp. 56–58.
Lacey, Linda J. "The Law of Artificial Insemination and Surrogate Parenthood in Oklahoma: Roadblocks to the Right to Procreate." *Tulsa Law Journal*, 22 (1987), pp. 281–324.
The Lancet. "Non-Surgical Transfer of In Vitro Fertilization Donated to Five Infertile Women: Report of Two Pregnancies" (July 23, 1983), p. 223.
Landes, Elisabeth M., and Richard A. Posner. "The Economics of the Baby Shortage." *Journal of Legal Studies*, 7 (June 1978), pp. 323–348.
Law, Sylvia. "Women, Work, Welfare and the Preservation of Patriarchy." *University of Pennsylvania Law Review*, 131 (May 1984), pp. 1249–1339.
Law Society Journal (New South Wales). "Legal Problems of Surrogate Motherhood." 22 (1984), pp. 587–588.
———. "Parenthood and Associated Dilemmas." 23 (1985), pp. 313–315.
Lawson, Carol. "Surrogate Mothers Grow in Number despite Questions." *New York Times*, October 1, 1986, p. C1.
Leach, W. Barton. "Perpetuities in the Atomic Age: The Sperm Bank and the Fertile Decedent." *American Bar Association Journal*, 48 (October 1962), pp. 942–944.
Leavy, Morton L., and Roy D. Weinberg. *Law of Adoption.* 4th ed. Dobbs Ferry, N.Y.: Oceana, 1979.
Levine, J. "Whose Baby Is It?" *The Village Voice* (November 25, 1986), p. 15.
———. "Motherhood is Powerless." *The Village Voice* (April 14, 1987), p. 15.
Lorio, Kathryn B. "Alternative Means of Reproduction: Virgin Territory for Legislation." *Lousiana Law Review*, 44 (July 1984), pp. 1642–76.
———. "In Vitro Fertilization and Embryo Transfer: Fertile Areas for Litigation." *Southwestern Law Journal*, 35 (1982), p. 973.
Los Angeles Times. "Curbs on Surrogate Motherhood Favored by Medical Ethics Panel." September 9, 1986, p. I-5.
———. "Man Who Hired 'Surrogate Mother' Isn't Child's Father." February 3, 1983, p. I-17.
———. "Ruling Made on Daughter Born to Surrogate." September 11, 1986, p. II-21.
———. "Surrogate Mothers Form Lobby Group." November 12, 1986, p. II-6.
———. "Surrogate's Baby Born with Deformity Rejected by All." January 22, 1983, p. I-17.
Lucas, Greg. "California Bills Seek to Prevent Baby M Fight Here: Defining the Contracts." *Los Angeles Daily Journal*, April 3, 1987, p. 1, col. 2.
Lyons, Richard D. "Two Women Become Pregnant with Transferred Embryos." *New York Times*, July 22, 1983, p. A1.
MacEwen, Virginia. *In Vitro Fertilization and Fetal Medicine: Legal and Ethical Aspects of New Reproduction Technologies: Bibliography-in-Brief, 1983–86.* Washington, D.C.: Congressional Research Service, 1986.

Mady, Theresa M. "Surrogate Mothers: The Legal Issues." *American Journal of Law and Medicine*, 7 (Fall 1981), pp. 323–352.

Mandler, John J. "Developing a Concept of the Modern 'Family': A Proposed Uniform Surrogate Parenthood Act." *Georgetown Law Journal*, 73 (1985), pp. 1283–1329.

Marcus, Ruth. "The Baby Maker." *National Law Journal* (New York), (August 25, 1980), pp. 1, 17, 26.

Markoutas, Eileen. "Women Who Have Babies for Other Women." *Good Housekeeping*, 192 (April 1981), p. 96.

———. "Women Who Have Babies for Other Women." *Reader's Digest*, 119 (August 1984), pp. 70–74.

Martin, David K. "Surrogate Motherhood: Contractual Issues and Remedies under Legislative Proposals." *Washburn Law Journal*, 23 (Spring 1984), 601–637.

Mason, Stephen. "Abnormal Conception." *Australian Law Journal*, 56 (July 1982), 347–357.

Mathews, Jay. "Boy's Birth Is First from Embryo Transfer." *Washington Post*, February 4, 1984, p. A14.

Maule, J. E. "Federal Tax Consequences of Surrogate Motherhood." *Taxes*, 60 (1982), pp. 656–668.

Mawdsley, Ralph D. "Surrogate Parenthood: A Need for Legislative Direction." *Illinois Bar Journal*, 71 (March 1983), pp. 412–417.

McGoldrick, K. E. "Baby M: Surrogacy and the Law." *Journal of the American Medical Women's Association*, 43 (September–October 1988), p. 131.

McMillan, Penelope. "Natural Parents' Embryo Living in Surrogate Mother." *Los Angeles Times*, November 29, 1986, p. II-1.

Medicine and Law. "Surrogate Motherhood: The Legal Climate for the Physician." 5 (1986), pp. 151–167.

Medico-Legal Journal. "The Future of Surrogacy in Great Britain" (editorial). 55 (1985), pp. 3–5.

Meezan, William, Sanford Katz, and Eva Mankoff Russo. *Adoptions without Agencies: A Study of Independent Adoptions*. Washington, D.C.: Welfare League of America, 1977.

Mehren, Elizabeth. "A Capital Site for a Surrogate Parent Center." *Los Angeles Times*, April 19, 1983, p. V-1.

Meinke, Sue. *Surrogate Motherhood: Ethical and Legal Issues*. Washington, D.C.: Kennedy Institute of Ethics, Georgetown University, 1988.

Mellown, Mary Ruth. "An Incomplete Picture: The Debate about Surrogate Motherhood." *Harvard Women's Law Journal*, 8 (Spring 1985), 231–246.

Michigan Bar Journal. "Whither Surrogate Contracts?" 67 (1988), p. 482.

Moggach, Deborah. *To Have and to Hold*. New York: E. P. Dutton. 1987.

Montgomery, J. "Constructing a Family—After a Surrogate Birth." *Modern Law Review*, 49 (1986), pp. 635–640.

———. "Surrogacy and the Best Interests of the Child." *Family Lawyer*, 16 (1986), p. 59.

Morgan, Derek. "Making Motherhood Male: Surrogacy and the Moral Economy of Women." *Journal of Law and Society*, 12 (1985), p. 219.

———. "Who to Be or Not to Be: The Surrogacy Story." *Modern Law Review*, 49 (1986), pp. 358–368.

Moss, Debra Cassens. "Surrogate Contract OK'd: Natural Mom to Appeal Ruling Taking away Baby M." *American Bar Association Journal*, 73 (May 1987), p. 32.

———. "Surrogate Parent Debate: Baby 'M' Case Lawyers Outline Views to Family Law Section." *American Bar Association Journal*, 73 (April 1987), pp. 24–25.

Murphy, Pam. "Reaction Mixed to Baby M Decision." *Pennsylvania Law Journal Report* (April 6, 1987), p. 2, col. 2.

Nakamura. "Behind the Baby 'M' Decision: Surrogacy Lawyering Reviewed." (Monograph No. 3) *Family Law Reporter*, 13 (1987), p. 3019.

National Committee on Adoption. *Adoption Factbook.* Washington, D.C., 1985.

Nature. "Tough Talk on Surrogate Birth." 320 (March 13–19, 1986), p. 95.

New Jersey. Superior Court. Chancery Division. Family Part (Bergen County). *In the Matter of Baby M (a pseudonymn for an actual person): Briefs on Trial.* New Jersey: [s.l.:s.n.]; 1986. 1 vol. (various pagings).

————. *In the Matter of Baby M (a pseudonym for an actual person): Pleadings and Related Documents.* New Jersey: [s.l.:s.n.]; 1986. 1 vol. (various pagings).

New Jersey Law Journal. "The Baby 'M' Contract: Is It Enforceable?" (February 26, 1987), pp. 24–34.

New Jersey Law Journal. "Baby 'M' Contract Enforced in Child's 'Best Interests'." (April 1, 1987), pp. 29–41.

New York State Law Journal. "The Public Policy Response to Surrogate Motherhood Agreements: Why They Are Illegal and Unenforceable." 60:21 (1988).

New York State Legislature. Senate Committee on Judiciary. *Surrogate Parenting in New York: A Proposal for Legislative Reform,* prepared by the staff of the New York State Senate Judiciary Committee. Albany, N.Y., 1986, 59 leaves.

New York State Task Force on Life and the Law. *Surrogate Parenting: Analysis and Recommendations for Public Policy,* May 1988.

New York Times. "Group to Guard Rights of Surrogate Mothers." November 13, 1986, p. C11.

————. *The Vatican on Birth Science* (includes "Instruction on Respect for Human Life in Its Origin and on the Dignity of Procreation: Replies to Certain Questions of the Day"). March 11, 1987, pp. A1, A14–15, A17.

Newsweek, "After the Baby M Case." (April 13, 1987), pp. 22–23.

————. "Surrogate Mothers: A Newsweek Poll." (January 19, 1987), p. 48.

————. "Whose Baby Is It Anyway?" (April 6, 1984), p. 83.

O'Brien, Shari. "Commercial Conceptions: A Breeding Ground for Surrogacy." *North Carolina Law Review,* 65 (November 1986), pp. 127–153.

————. "The Itinerant Embryo and the Neo-Nativity Scene: Bifurcating Biological Maternity." *Utah Law Review,* 1987, (No. 1, 1987), pp. 1–33.

Palca, J. "U.S. Courts and Legislatures Face Implications of Surrogacy." *Nature,* 325 (January 15–21, 1987), p. 184.

Parker, Diana. "Surrogate Mothering: An Overview." *Family Law,* 14 (1984), pp. 140–144.

Parker, Phillip J. "Motivation of Surrogate Mothers: Initial Findings." *American Journal of Psychiatry,* 140 (1983), p. 117.

————. "Surrogate Motherhood, Psychiatric Screening and Informed Consent, Baby-Selling, and Public Policy." *American Academy of Psychiatry and Law Bulletin,* 12 (1984), p. 21.

————. "Surrogate Motherhood: The Interaction of Litigation, Legislation and Psychiatry." (Eighth International Congress of Law and Psychiatry—June 18–22, 1982) *International Journal of Law and Psychiatry,* 5 (1983), p. 341.

Patterson, Suzanne M. "Parenthood by Proxy: Legal Implications of Surrogate Birth." *Iowa Law Review,* 67 (January 1982), pp. 385–399.

Perloe, Mark, and Linda G. Christie. *Miracle Babies and Other Happy Endings for Couples with Fertility Problems.* New York: Rawson Associates, 1986.

Perry, Clifton. "Surrogate Contracts: Contractual and Constitutional Conundrums in the Baby "M" Case." *Journal of Legal Medicine,* 9:105 (March 1988).

Petchesky, R. *Abortion and Women's Choice.* New York: Longman, 1984.

Peterson, Iver. "Baby M Case: Surrogate Mothers Vent Feelings." *New York Times,*
    March 2, 1987, pp. B1, B4.
────. "Baby M Trial Splits Ranks of Feminists: Surrogate Motherhood Stirs Ex-
    ploitation Issue." *New York Times,* February 24, 1987, pp. B1, B2.
────. "Lawyers Await Ruling in Baby M Case Today." *New York Times,* March
    31, 1987, p. 15, col. 1.
────. "States Assess Surrogate Motherhood." *New York Times,* December 13, 1987,
    p. I-42.
Phillips, John W., and Susan D. Phillips. "In Defense of Surrogate Parenting: A
    Critical Analysis of the Recent Kentucky Experience." *Kentucky Law Journal,*
    69 (1980–81), pp. 877–931.
Pierce, William L. "Baby 'M' Decision Creates Flurry of Legislative Activity." *Family
    Law Reporter,* 13 (1987), pp. 1295–96.
────. "Surrogate Parenthood: A Legislative Update." *Family Law Reporter,* 13
    (1987), pp. 1442–44.
────. "Survey of State Activity regarding Surrogate Motherhood." *Family Law
    Reporter* (Monograph No. 1), 11 (January 1985), pp. 3001–04.
Pilel, Harriet F. "New Methods of Conception and Their Legal Status." *New York
    Law School Human Rights Annual,* 3 (1985), pp. 13–33.
Pollitt, Katha. "Contracts and Apple Pie: The Strange Case of Baby 'M.' " *The Nation,*
    244 (May 23, 1987), pp. 667, 682–686, 688.
Pollock, Donald I. "Surrogate Parenthood Arrangements." *Florida Bar Journal,* 56
    (1987). pp. 51–54.
Postell, Claudia J. "Establishing Guidelines for Artificial Conception." *Trial,* 22
    (1986), p. 93.
Radin, Margaret Jane. "Property and Personhood." *Stanford Law Review,* 34 (May
    1982), pp. 957–1015.
────. "Market-Inalienability." *Harvard Law Review,* 100 (June 1987), pp. 1849–
    1937.
Rakusen, J., and M. Davidson. *Out of Our Hands—What Technology Does to Pregnancy.*
    London: Pan Books, 1982.
Ranii, David. "Future Shock for Family Law: Can One Child Have Two Mothers?"
    National Law Journal (March 26, 1984), p. 1, col. 1.
Reagan, Leslie. "Surrogacy Is a Bad Bargain." *Against the Current,* 2 (September–
    October 1987), pp. 56–58.
Reaves, Lynn. "Surrogate Parenthood." *American Bar Association Journal,* 70 (Feb-
    ruary 1984), p. 28.
────. "To Be Born, to Die: Individual Rights in the 80's." *American Bar Association
    Journal,* 70 (February 1984), p. 27.
Rees, N., C. Thaler, and K. Hamod. *Adoption, Surrogate Mothers, and Other Legal
    and Medical Remedies for Infertility,* 1986.
Reidinger, Paul. "Lawyers Reject Surrogate Mothers' Claims: Lawpoll." *American
    Bar Association Journal,* 73 (June 1987), p. 55.
Reimer, Rita Ann. *Analysis of Legal and Constitutional Issues Involved in Surrogate
    Motherhood.* Washington, D.C.: Congressional Research Service, 1988.
Richardson, H., ed. *On the Problem of Surrogate Parenthood: Analyzing the Baby "M"
    Case,* 1987.
Roberts, Charley. "Surrogate Parents, Court Bills Endorsed by Assembly Unit." *Los
    Angeles Daily Journal,* May 29, 1985, p. 2, col. 4.
Robertson, John A. "Embryos, Families, and Procreative Liberty: The Legal Struc-
    ture of the New Reproduction." *Southern California Law Review,* 59 (July 1986),
    pp. 939–1041.

———. "Extracorporeal Embryos and the Abortion Debate." *Journal of Contemporary Health Law and Policy*, 2 (1985), pp. 53–70.

———. "Procreative Liberty and the Control of Conception, Pregnancy, and Childbirth." *Virginia Law Review*, 69 (April 1983), pp. 405–464.

———. "Surrogate Mothers: Not So Novel after All." *Hastings Center Report* (October 1985), p 28.

Robbins, Sara. *Surrogate Parenting: An Annotated Review of the Literature*. Brooklyn, N.Y.: CompuBibs, 1984, 40 p.

Rosenblatt, R. "The Baby in the Factory." *Time*, 121 (February 14, 1983), p. 90.

Rosner, F., E. J. Cassell, M. L. Friedland, A. B. Landolt, L. Loeb, P. J. Numann, F. V. Ora, H. M. Risemberg, and P. P. Sordillo. "Ethical Considerations of Reproductive Technologies." *New York State Journal of Medicine*, 87 (July 1987), pp. 398–401.

Ross, Andrew. "Raising a 'Surrogate' Issue." *Pennsylvania Law Journal Report* (April 6, 1987), p. 2, col. 2.

Rothman, Barbara Katz. *The Products of Conception: The Genetic Tie*. New York: Viking Press (1985).

———. "Surrogacy: A Question of Values." *Conscience* (May–June 1987).

———. *The Tentative Pregnancy*. New York: Viking, 1986.

———. *The Tentative Pregnancy, Prenatal Diagnosis and the Future of Motherhood*. New York: Everest House, 1981.

Rovner, Sandy. "Ethical Choices in Reproductive Technology." *Washington Post Weekly of Medicine, Health and Fitness* (September 9, 1986), p. 15.

Rushevsky, Cynthia A. "Legal Recognition of Surrogate Gestation." *Women's Rights Law Reporter*, 7 (Winter 1982), pp. 107–142.

Rust, Mark. "Whose Baby Is It? Surrogate Motherhood after Baby M." *American Bar Association Journal*, 73 (June 1987), pp. 52–56.

St. Louis University Law Journal. "What Money Cannot Buy: Commercial Surrogacy and the Doctrine of Illegal Contracts." 32 (1988): 1171.

Saltarelli, Joseph J. "Genesis Retold: Legal Issues Raised by the Cryopreservation of Preimplantation Human Embryos." *Syracuse Law Review*, 36 (1985), pp. 1021–53.

Saltus, Richard. "Embryo Research Provokes Debate on Ethical and Legal Issues." *Boston Globe*, July 22, 1987, p. 1.

———. "Guidelines Urged for Fetal Tissue Transplants." *Boston Globe*, July 22, 1987, p. 9.

Samuels, Alec. "Warnock Committee: Human Fertilization and Embryology." *Medico-Legal Journal* (Great Britain), 51 (1983), p. 174.

Sappideen, Carolyn. "The Surrogate Mother: A Growing Problem." *University of New South Wales Law Journal*, 6 (1983), pp. 79–102.

Schmeck, Harold M. " 'Pre-Natal Adoption' Is the Objective of New Technique." *New York Times*, June 14, 1983, p. C1.

Schuck, Peter, "Some Reflections on the Baby M Case." *Georgetown Law Review*, 76:5 (June 1988), pp. 1793–1810.

Scott, Janny. "Pair Duped Her on Surrogate Mother Pact, Woman Tells Court." *Los Angeles Times*, February 20, 1987, p. I-22.

Seidman, L. M. "Baby M and the Problem of Unstable Preferences." *Georgetown Law Review*, 76:5 (June 1988), pp. 1829–36.

Shannon, Thomas. *Surrogate Motherhood: The Ethics of Using Human Beings*. New York: Crossroads, 1988, 191 p.

Shapiro, Daniel. "No Other Hope for Having a Child." *Newsweek*, January 19, 1987, pp. 50–51.

Sherman, Rorie. "Guardian *ad litem* Role Unclear." *New Jersey Law Journal* (March 5, 1987), p. 1, col. 5.

Sherwyn, Bernard A. "Attorney Duties in the Area of New Reproductive Technologies." *Whittier Law Review*, 6 (1984), pp. 799–810.

Shipp, E. R. "Death Draws Public's Eye to Adoption." *New York Times*, November 29, 1987, p. B1.

Simpson, Laurence Packer. *Handbook of the Law of Contracts*. 2d ed. St. Paul: West, 1965.

Singer, Peter, and Helga Kuhse. "The Ethics of Embryo Research." *Law, Medicine and Health Care*, 14 (September 1986), pp. 133–137.

Singer, Peter, and Deane Wells. *Making Babies: The New Science and Ethics of Conception*. New York: Scribner, 1985.

Sloman, Susan. "Surrogacy Arrangements Act 1985." *New Law Journal* (Great Britain), 135 (October 1985), pp. 978–980.

Slovenko, Ralph. "Obstetric Science and the Developing Role of the Psychiatrist in Surrogate Motherhood." *Journal of Psychiatry and Law*, 13 (1985), pp. 487–518.

Sly, Karen Marie. "Baby-Sitting Consideration: Surrogate Mother's Right to 'Rent Her Womb' for a Fee." *Gonzaga Law Review*, 18 (November 1983), pp. 539–565.

Small, M. "Baby Sellers or Sisters of Mercy? Surrogate Mothers Give Birth to a Legal Debate." *People Weekly*, 19 (June 13, 1983), p. 47.

Smith, David. "Wombs for Rent, Selves for Sale?" *Journal of Contemporary Health Law and Policy*, 4:23 (Spring 1988).

Smith, George P. II. "Australia's Frozen 'Orphan' Embryos: A Medical, Legal, and Ethical Dilemma." *Journal of Family Law*, 24 (1985–86), pp. 27–41.

———. "The Razor's Edge of Human Bonding: Artificial Fathers and Surrogate Mothers." *Western New England Law Review*, 5 (Spring 1983), pp. 639–666.

Smith, George P. II, and Roberto Iraola. "Sexuality, Privacy and the New Biology." *Marquette Law Review*, 67 (1984), pp. 263–291.

Smith, Ruth Bayard. "Choosing Sides." *Boston Globe Magazine*, January 3, 1988, p. 30.

———. "The Baby Broker." *Boston Globe Magazine*, January 3, 1988, pp. 20–28, 31.

Snyder, Sarah. "Baby Case Spurs Debate of Surrogate Mothers—Despite Custody Fight, Couples Seek Service." *Boston Globe*, February 22, 1987, pp. 1, 10.

Sokoloff, B. Z. "Alternative Methods of Reproduction: Effects on the Child." *Clinical Pediatrics*, 2 (January 1987), pp. 11–17.

Sorkow, Harvey R. *In the Matter of Baby M (a pseudonym for an actual person)*. Opinion . . . [Bergen County, N.J.]. Superior Court of New Jersey. Chancery Division. Family Part. 1987, 121 p.

Spann, G. A. "Baby M and the Cassandra Problem." *Georgetown Law Review*, 76:5 (June 1988), pp. 1719–40.

Steadman, J. H., and G. T. McCloskey. "The Prospects of Surrogate Mothering: Clinical Concerns." *Canadian Journal of Psychiatry*, 32 (October 1987), pp. 545–550.

Steiber, S. "Public Opinion Divided on Surrogate Parenting." *Hospitals*, 61 (August 5, 1987), p. 114.

Stetson, Susan. "Whose Children Are They? The Moral and Legal Dilemmas of Surrogate Parenting." *Empire State Report*, 13 (May 1987), pp. 56–58.

Stevens, Kristy. *Surrogate Mother: One Woman's Story*. London: Century, 1985, 181 p.

Stoxen, John M. "The Best of Both 'Open' and 'Closed' Adoption Worlds: A Call for Reform of State Statutes." *Journal of Legislation*, 13 (Spring 1986), pp. 292–309.

Stumpf, Andrea E. "Redefining Mother: A Legal Matrix for New Reproductive Technologies." *Yale Law Journal*, 9 (1986), pp. 187–208.

Suender, John M. "Surrogate Motherhood Agreements and the Law in Pennsylvania." *Dickinson Law Review*, 91 (1987), pp. 1085–1111.

Sutterlin, Edith. *Surrogate Mothers: Bibliography-in-Brief*. 1981–87. Washington, D.C.: Congressional Research Service, 1987, 6 p.

Swerdlow, Marian. "Class Politics and Baby M." *Against the Current*, 2 (September-October 1987), p. 53.

Taub, S. "Surrogate Motherhood and the Law." *Connecticut Medicine*, 49 (October 1985), pp. 671–674.

Taylor, Shereen. "Conceiving for Cash: Is It Legal? A Survey of the Laws Applicable to Surrogate Motherhood." *Human Rights Annual*, 4 (1987), pp. 413–444.

Timnick, Lois. "Surrogate Mother Wants to Keep Her Unborn Baby." *Los Angeles Times*, March 21, 1981, p. I–1.

Townsend, Margaret D. "Surrogate Mother Agreements: Contemporary Legal Aspects of a Biblical Notion." *University of Richmond Law Review*, 16 (Winter 1982), 467–483.

Turk, A. Marco. "If Baby 'M' Were a Californian . . . Our Courts Have Not Ruled on Surrogate Contracts, but the Issue Is Gestating." *California Lawyer*, 7 (1987), pp. 78, 80, 82.

Turner, Paula Diane. "Love's Labor Lost: Legal and Ethical Implications in Artificial Human Procreation." *Journal of Urban Law*, 58 (1981), p. 459.

Tweeton, Leslie. "They Get a Baby, She Gets $10,000." *Boston Magazine*, 77 (June 1985), pp. 137–138, 189–195.

USA Today. "Surrogate Motherhood." 11 (November 1987), pp. 66–71.

United States Congress. Senate. *Adoption and Foster Care, 1975: Hearings before the Subcommittee on Children and Youth of the Senate Committee on Labor and Public Welfare*, 94th Cong., 1st sess., 1976, p. 6.

University of Iowa College of Law, New Biology Seminar. *Model Human Reproductive Technologies and Surrogacy Act*. 1987.

U.S. News and World Report. "After Baby M, Motherhood is Not for Sale: Surrogate Births." 104 (February 15, 1988), pp. 11–12.

Van Hoften, Ellen L. "Surrogate Motherhood in California: Legislative Proposals." *San Diego Law Review*, 18 (1985), pp. 341–385.

Vermont Law Review. "The Rights of the Biological Father: From Adoption and Custody to Surrogate Motherhood." 12 (1987), p. 87.

Vieth, Perry J. "Surrogate Mothering: Medical Reality in a Legal Vacuum." *Journal of Legislation*, 8 (1981), pp. 140–159.

Wadlington, Walter. "Artificial Conception: The Challenge for Family Law." *Virginia Law Review*, 69 (1983), pp. 465–514.

Walker, Louis. "Borne for Another" (transcript of Eighth Oscar Mendelsolm lecture, delivered at Monash University on March 1, 1981). *Monash University Law Review* (Australia), 10 (1984), pp. 113–130.

Wallis, Claudia. "A Surrogate's Story." *Time* (September 10, 1984), p. 53.

Walsh, Elizabeth. "Warnock and After." *Family Law* (Great Britain), 15 (1985), pp. 138–139.

Walters, L. "Ethical Aspects of Surrogate Embryo Transfer." *Journal of the American Medical Association*, 250 (1983), p. 2183.

Warnock, Dame Mary. *A Question of Life: The Warnock Report of the Committee of Inquiry into Human Fertilization and Embryology*. London: United Kingdom Department on Health and Social Security, July 1984. (Cited as the Warnock Report.)

Warren, David G. "The Law of Human Reproduction: An Overview." *Journal of Legal Medicine*, 3 (March 1982), pp. 1–57.

White, A. G. *The Law, Public Administration and Artificially-Procreated Humans: A Selected Bibliography*. 1983.

Whitehead, M. B. "A Surrogate Mother Describes Her Change of Heart—And Her Fight to Keep the Baby Two Families Love." *People Weekly*, 26 (October 20, 1986), pp. 46–48.

William Mitchell Law Review. "Surrogate Parenthood: An Analysis of the Problems and a Solution: Representation for the Child," 12 (1986), pp. 143–182.

Williams, Helen E. "Legislative Guidelines to Govern In Vitro Fertilization and Embryo Transfer." *Santa Clara Law Review*, 26 (1986), pp. 495–518.

Williams, Jack F. "Differential Treatment of Men and Women by Artificial Reproduction Statutes." *Tulsa Law Journal*, 21 (Spring 1986), pp. 463–484.

Wilson, Andrew B. "Adoption, It's Not Impossible." *Business Week* (July 8, 1985), pp. 112–113.

Winkler, Robin, and Margaret van Keppel. *Relinquishing Mothers in Adoption*. Melbourne, Australia: Institute of Family Studies, 1984.

Wolf, Susan. "Enforcing Surrogate Motherhood Agreements: The Trouble with Specific Performance." *Human Rights Annual* 4:375 (Spring 1987)

Wong, Doris Sue. "Mass. Couple asks for Va. Ruling in Surrogate Case." *Boston Globe*, January 14, 1987, p. II-23.

Woodruff, Elizabeth. "Irrevocability of Consent to Surrender of a Child for Adoption (C.C.I. v. The Natural Parents)." *Mississippi College Law Review* (Spring 1982), pp. 423–445.

Wright, Moira. "Surrogacy and Adoption: Problems and Possibilities." *Family Law Review*, 16 (April 1986), pp. 109–116.

Wrigley, Julia. "Whose Baby Is It Anyway?" *Against the Current*, 2 (September–October 1987), pp. 53–55.

Yale Law Journal. "Lawyering for the Child: Principles of Representation in Custody and Visitation Disputes arising from Divorce." 87 (1978), pp. 1126–90.

———. "Redefining Mother: A Legal Matrix for New Reproductive Technologies." 96 (1986), p. 187.

Younger, Judith T. "Medicine and the Law: Making Excellent Time but Lost." *Bench and Bar of Minnesota*, 44 (1987), p. 14.

Yovich, J. "Surrogacy" (letter). *Lancet*, 1 (June 13, 1987).

Zegel, Vikki, and Irene Smith-Coleman. *Biomedical Ethics and Congress: History and Current Legislative Activity; Issue Brief*. Washington, D.C.: Congressional Research Service. Updated regularly. 10 p.

Zeilmaker, G. H., et al. "Two Pregnancies following Transfer of Intact, Frozen-Thawed Embryos." *Fertility and Sterility*, 42 (1984), p. 293.

Zinkula, Thomas. "Termination of Parental Rights: Should Nonpayment of Child Support Be Enough?" *Iowa Law Review* (1982).

Zuckerman, A. *Surrogate Parenting*. 1988.

CONTRIBUTORS

LORI B. ANDREWS, J.D., author of *Between Strangers: Surrogate Mothers, Expectant Fathers, and Brave New Babies,* is a research fellow at the American Bar Foundation, Chicago, Illinois, and a senior scholar at the Center for Clinical Medical Ethics, University of Chicago School of Medicine.

GEORGE J. ANNAS, J.D., M.P.H., is Utley Professor of Law and Medicine at the Boston University School of Medicine, chief of the Health Law Section of the Boston University School of Public Health, and book review editor of *Law, Medicine & Health Care.*

RANDALL P. BEZANSON, JR., is dean of Washington and Lee University School of Law in Lexington, Virginia.

LISA SOWLE CAHILL, Ph.D., is professor in the Department of Theology at Boston College, Massachusetts.

A. M. CAPRON, LL.B., FCLM, holds the Norman Topping Chair in Law, Medicine and Public Policy at the Law Center and the School of Medicine, University of Southern California, Los Angeles, and recently served as president of the American Society of Law & Medicine.

R. ALTA CHARO, J.D., is assistant professor of law and medicine at the University of Wisconsin Schools of Law and Medicine.

GENA COREA is associate director of the Institute on Women and Technology and editor of *Reproductive and Genetic Engineering: Journal of International Feminist Analysis* (Pergamon Press).

LARRY GOSTIN is executive director of the American Society of Law & Medicine and editor-in-chief of *Law, Medicine & Health Care,* as well as adjunct associate professor in health law at the Harvard School of Public Health, Boston, Massachusetts. He is on the National Board of Directors of the American Civil Liberties Union and is chair of the ACLU Special Committee on Surrogate Parenting.

ANGELA R. HOLDER, LL.M., is professor of pediatrics (law) at Yale University, counsel for medicolegal affairs at Yale–New Haven Hospital, and a past president of the American Society of Law & Medicine.

RUTH MACKLIN, Ph.D., is professor of bioethics at Albert Einstein College of Medicine, Bronx, New York.

JOAN MAHONEY, J.D., is professor at the University of Missouri–Kansas City School of Law.

M. J. RADIN, M.F.A., J.D., is Carolyn Craig Franklin Professor of Law at the Law Center, University of Southern California, Los Angeles, California.

JOHN A. ROBERTSON, J.D., is the Baker and Botts Professor of Law at the University of Texas School of Law, Austin.

KAREN H. ROTHENBERG, J.D., M.P.A., is associate professor of law and director of the Law and Health Care Program at the University of Maryland School of Law, Baltimore.

GEORGE P. SMITH, II, J.D., is professor at the Catholic University Law School, Washington, D.C.

NADINE TAUB, LL.B., is professor of law and director of the Women's Rights Litigation Clinic at Rutgers University School of Law, Newark, New Jersey. For the past three years, she has directed the Project on Reproductive Laws for the 1990s.

INDEX